Revisiting Ibn Sina's (Avicenna) Heritage

Kadircan H. Keskinbora (ed.)

# Revisiting Ibn Sina's (Avicenna) Heritage

PETER LANG

**Bibliographic Information published by the Deutsche Nationalbibliothek**

The Deutsche Nationalbibliothek lists this publication in the Deutsche Nationalbibliografie; detailed bibliographic data is available online at http://dnb.d-nb.de.

**Library of Congress Cataloging-in-Publication Data**

A CIP catalog record for this book has been applied for at the Library of Congress.



ISBN 978-3-631-83056-7 (Print)
E-ISBN 978-3-631-85547-8 (E-PDF)
E-ISBN 978-3-631-85548-5 (EPUB)
DOI 10.3726/b18457



Peter Lang – Berlin · Bern · Bruxelles · New York · Istanbul · Oxford · Warszawa · Wien



This publication has been peer reviewed.

www.peterlang.com

In the memory of the beloved Ibn Sina (Avicenna), the Giant of Medicine and Philosophy, whom all writers accept as their teacher.

# PREFACE

Ibn Sina – or Avicenna as he is known in the Latin West - is perhaps the most representative figure of medicine and philosophy in the world. His influence was not limited to the East, extending profoundly also to the West.

Even well after his lifetime, Ibn Sina was renowned, not just in medicine or philosophy, but in other areas, especially in the Islamic world. In brief, he was an authority in the Islamic East, or an "*auctoritas*". However, in the west, his work was massively influential in not only the medical education curricula, but also in the important, innovative doctrines in philosophy. The most fundamental sections of his major encyclopedia, *al-Shifâ* being translated into Latin as early as the 12th and 13th centuries and spreading throughout universities dispersed this impact rapidly. The second factor was lbn Sina's efforts to blend Greek and Islamic thought. This led Christianity to begin formulating its own fusion with Greek philosophy.

Large sections of his major encyclopedia, al-Shifâ, were translated into Latin. To translate accurately was - and still is - a difficult task. There are many versions of translations of Ibn Sina's work into Latin. Therefore, it is likely that the Latin translators first produced a literal translation, then revised it to create a more 'readable' text. During these translations, the scholastic scholars became familiar with Ibn Sina's thought, through which they learned about ancient philosophers.

More important was the direct impact of Ibn Sina's innovative ideas. Historians of philosophy have noted the extent of Ibn Sina's influence on important scholars like Albert the Great and Thomas Aquinas. Gundissalinus, Albert the Great and Roger Bacon are among the western thinkers whose works incorporate elements of lbn Sina's thought especially in relation to the character of the human will. No doubt, these effects highlighted the impact of Ibn Sina's thought among the Latin philosophy circles. Ibn Sina's legacy is so rich and complicated that many aspects remain as yet undiscovered and others await further critical investigation.

lbn Sina's thought had a clear and strong impact on the science, literature and philosophy of both the east and west. The many commentaries produced relating to his works and ideas, whether they embraced or rejected his thought, show the influence of his philosophical thought. Even criticism of his ideas did not keep his critics from utilizing many of his ideas. Only two examples among many are Gazali's 1) logic and 2) philosophy terminology, which are largely taken from lbn Sina.

It should also be recalled that lbn Sina did not only write his major encyclopedia, al-Shifâ, as the manifesto of the systematized version of rationalism called the "Peripatetic Islamic Philosophy (*al-Falsafa al-Mashsha'iya*)" in Islam, he also compiled explanations and defenses for mysticism and knowledge in the last sections of his work "Remarks and Admonitions (*al-Isharat wa'l Tenbihât*)", wrote commentaries on the Qur'an, visited the tombs of the righteous, wrote treatises on the hereafter, and was the first to write a series of biographies in the history of Islamic thought.

Ibn Sina placed great importance on insight and some people's talent for unification without actively utilizing intelligence or persuasion, and applied "holy intellect", "holy faculty [or power]" and "the power [or faculty] of [a] holy soul" to a high degree of divination. As Ibn Sina wrote, if a person "burns" with insight to the extent that he effortlessly obtains immense scientific knowledge from active intelligence, he likes intellectual prophecy, "the highest of divination powers".

As Gutas determined, Avicenna masterfully brought together the dominant understandings of the tradition of Islamic philosophy before him, the basic texts of Plotinus and Proclus, the Neoplatonism of the Kindi circle, and the Fârâbî school in a philosophically dynamic and theoretically convincing system. He included all the intellectual interests of the Islamic society, such as the nature of prophecy, life after death, and the phenomenon of religion, in his philosophical system, and dealt with these issues in the concepts he developed. In his works, he used a writing style that is fully compatible with the needs of the intellectual discourse in society and is open to experimenting with different styles.

In experimental fashion, Ibn Sina incorporated some sections of his system with short allegorical stories. One of these is *Hayy Ibn Yaqzan*, meaning "Son of the Awake One Lives"; "Living" is active intelligence and it is a son of the first reason, which is always awake as a kind of emanation. Active intelligence is personified in the allegory as a wise old man instructing the narrator, who represents the rational human spirit about the nature of the universe.

Known as "the prince of physicians", Ibn Sina is the writer of the Canon of Medicine (*al-Qānūn fi-al-Tibb*), which became a medical standard in the Christian west as well as the Islamic world. Ibn Sina also wrote a series of scientific investigations into general medicine as well as specific diseases in addition to his masterpiece. He also wrote a book in which the principles of medicine were written in verse for medical students to learn more easily. While respecting the Hippocratic and Galenic traditions, he made the following revisions:

1. He blended the basic principles of Greek and Roman medicine and interpreted these within an Islamic framework.
2. He ensured that the theoretical and practical aspects of medicine represented parts of an integrated whole.
3. He documented the effects of medicines on the body. He commented on the necessity of, and applied, a methodology in the research of pharmacological problems.
4. He introduced a series of medicines and treatments unknown to the Greek.

Ibn Sina believed that the science of medicine was divided into two, i.e., practical and theoretical. Illnesses arose due to external or internal causes. It was an imbalance in the nature of the human body that led to disease. These causes could also be the result of psychological elements. Ibn Sina recommended various treatments and medicines for issues as wide ranging as psychotherapy and diet to exercise.

This book offers the reader 17 different topics concerning the philosophical as well as the medical works of Ibn Sina, written by experts who viewed the information in the light of modern knowledge.

I extend my gratitude to the outstanding authors of this collection for their invaluable contributions.

As one may expect, despite all efforts, books can feature minor typing errors. I thank the reader in advance for their understanding. I look forward to comments and contributions and hope that our book will benefit science and scientists.

Sincerely,
Prof. Dr. Kadircan H. Keskinbora
kadircan.keskinbora@gmail.com
REVISITING IBN SINA'S HERITAGE

# Contents

# List of Contributors

**Hamed Arezaei, Ph.D.**
University of Medical Sciences, School of Traditional Medicine, Dept. History of Medical Sciences Tehran-Iran

**Prof. Dr. Dana Baran, M.D., Ph.D.**
"Grigore T. Popa" University of Medicine and Pharmacy, Iasi - Romania

**Prof. Dr. Mehmet Bayrakdar**
Yeditepe University, Faculty of Arts and Sciences, Department of Anthropology Istanbul-Turkey

**Glen M. Cooper, Ph.D.**
Brigham Young University Department of Philosophy, U.S.A.

**Engin Erdem, Assoc. Prof.**
Ankara University, Faculty of Divinity, Ankara, Turkey

**Ömer Faruk Erdoğan, Assoc. Prof.**
Dumlupinar University, Faculty of Divinity, Department of Islamic Philosophy, Kütahya - Turkey

**Prof. Dr. Esin Kâhya**
Emeritus Professor, Ankara University Faculty of Languages, History and Geography, Dept. History of Science Ankara-Turkey

**Prof. Dr. Kadircan H. Keskinbora, M.D., Ph.D.**
Bahcesehir University School of Medicine, Istanbul-Turkey

**Prof. Dr. Salahaddin Khalilov**
Chairman of the Presidium of the Azerbaijan Association of Philosophy and Socio-Political Sciences (AFSEA). Honorary Chairman of International Philosophical Research Centre (UFAD) in Istanbul - Turkey

**Ferdi Koç, Assoc. Prof.**
Sakarya University, State Conservatory, Turkish Music Department, Adapazari-Turkey

**Prof. Dr. Roida Rzayeva Oktay**
Azerbaijan National Academy of Sciences Baku-Azerbaijan

**Peter Starr, Ph.D.**
Istanbul Technical University Faculty of Human Science Istanbul-Turkey

**Prof. Dr. Michael Such, O.M.D, C.M (I.A.TCM)**
Lecturer at the "East West" College Tel Aviv - Israel

**Prof. Dr. Ahmet Hakkı Turabi**
Marmara University Faculty of Divinity, Turkish Religious Music Department Istanbul-Turkey

**Prof. Dr. Yavuz UNAT**
Kastamonu University, Department of Philosophy Kastamonu-Turkey

Prof. Dr. Kadircan H. Keskinbora, M.D., Ph.D.*

# Medicine in the Medieval Era and Early Renaissance: A Most Influential Teacher, Ibn Sīnā (Avicenna)

This section will discuss important topics in medical education, which sprouted in the Middle Ages and early Renaissance period. The history of the medical school curriculum, the approach to medical education, and influential scholars who still stood out, most importantly Ibn Sīnā, will be investigated in terms of his influence on medical education.

In the eighth and ninth centuries, after the conquests, the Islamic world witnessed substantial commercial and economic growth as well as the development of flourishing cities that prompted the intellectual milieus to assimilate the Greek philosophy and science into the Islamic intellectual context. The Greek materials were integrated with their own observations that drew on botanical pharmacology of oriental or Iberian origin, resulting in a synthesis that produced large encyclopedic works that investigated pathology and therapies. Most Muslim medical writings were large encyclopedic works that surveyed all aspects of the subject.[1] Despite the fact that the Greek and Hellenistic antiquity passed down their materials to both Western Europe and the Muslim world, the two societies differed greatly in terms of the use of inherited medical knowledge.

The association between medicine and philosophy that pervaded the ancients, notably in the Galenic corpus and the Aristotelian works, persisted strongly among Muslim writers like Ibn Sīnā (Avicenna) and Ibn Rushd (Averroes), whose philosophical views affected their medical works.

---

* ORCID ID: 0000-0003-1940-1026; Google Scholar: https://scholar.google.com/scholar?hl=tr&lr=lang_tr&as_sdt=0%2C5&q=%22Kadircan+Keskinbora%22&btnG=

1 Fuat Sezgin, *Geschichte des arabischen Schrifttums* 3 (Leiden, 1970): 21–171, provides details regarding translations of medical books from Greek into Syriac and Arabic and dissemination in the Muslim world, and on the development of Islamic medicine.

Ibn Sīnā's tendency to connect different religious, cultural and intellectual concepts caused him to identify the instances where views on important physiology topics converged and to reconcile Aristotle and Galen's perspectives. This presented a contrast to, for example, Ibn Rushd (Averroes), who often took on Aristotelian views in his medical *Colliget*. Regardless of their philosophical leanings, the writers of the Arabic medical texts were concerned with medicine. Their views, and their descriptions of illnesses, symptoms and systematic explanations were invaluable for Islamic and later Western Medicine and the *Materia Medica* collections.[2]

## Medicine and the "Twelfth-century Renaissance"

The study and practice of medicine was influenced by the rapid development in Western Europe that took place between 1050 and 1225, often referred to as "twelfth-century Renaissance". The population growth, urbanization and the development of more sophisticated forms of secular and ecclesiastical government led to the broadening of philosophical, scientific and all around deepened interest in medicine that demanded sophisticated medical literature.[3]

The need for a more comprehensive and sophisticated medical literature caused the establishment of a medical practice center in the mid-900s in Salerno, Italy. At the end of the 10th century, Salerno became well known in northern France. Among the Salernitan practitioners in the tenth and eleventh centuries were many clergymen as well as famous "Salerno women".[4] Modern resources about the Salernitan male and female practitioners contain anecdotes highlighting not only their learning but their healing skills. However, throughout the 12th century, Salerno's medicine became more theoretical, more official and academic in terms of the medicine training.[5]

The growth of centers of medical study was in turn intimately connected with the multiplication of medical books and their accumulation, in an age in which the circulation of books was still limited, in particular places. The available Latin medical literature began to expand at the beginning of the late eleventh century through the translations of Arabic texts and subsequently Greek

---

2 Siraisi, Nancy G (1990). *Medieval and Early Renaissance Medicine: An Introduction to Knowledge and Practice*. Chicago: Chicago University Press, p.11,12.

3 Siraisi, ibid, p.16.

4 Green, Monica H. 1989. "Women's Medical Practice and Medical Care in Medieval Europe." *Sign* 14:434–73.

5 Kristeller, Paul O. Studi *sulla scuola medica salernitana* (Naples, 1986), 19–49.

texts, to include substantial parts of the corpus of Greek medical writing, especially of works attributed to Hippocrates and Galen as well as the major recent Arabic contributions. There were many very important translators and centers of translation. Near Salerno, a Monte Cassino monk named Constantinus Africanus (d. 1087) translated Pantegni and many other texts from Arabic. In the 12th century, Gerard of Cremona and his students in Spain translated the works of Galen, Rāzī (Rhazes), Abu al-Qasim al-Zahrawi (Albucasis) and Ibn Sīnā (Avicenna) from Arabic. Burgundio of Pisa, who traveled between Italy and Istanbul, translated Galen's work from Greek. At around the same time, an enlarged and alphabetized version of the Latin Dioscorides became available. In these developments, of course, medicine paralleled other fields, notably logic, natural philosophy, astronomy, and geometry.[6]

Medicine was integrated into the efforts to ensure access to the entire Greco-Arab philosophy and science, which characterized western education between the end of the 11th century and the beginning of the 13th century. As in the other fields mentioned, in medicine as well, it could be assumed that the interest of scientists in acquiring new materials was both a reason and a result of new translations. Medical books did not just offer practical benefits but also contributed to the clergy intellectualism and general scientific culture in the 12th century.[7]

The strong tradition of literate, learned Jewish medicine drew on both Jewish and non-Jewish sources. Under Muslim rule in Spain and elsewhere, Jewish physicians had come into close contact with learned Arabic medical culture and had access to the written heritage of Arabic medicine in the original language. Through this means, they too came to incorporate much of the heritage of Greek medicine into their own teaching and practice. Thus, for example, the medical writings of Maimonides (1135–1204), who spent his youth in Cordoba and other parts of Spain, then under Muslim rule, and most of his adult life in Egypt, were written in Arabic and show extensive knowledge of Arabic versions of works of Hippocrates and Galen.[8]

In the Iberian Peninsula, following the Reconquista, Jewish physicians lost direct access to the Arabic medical texts. Therefore, important Arabic texts were

---

6 D'Alverny, Marie-Therese. 1982. "Translators and Translations". In *Renaissance and* Renewal *in the Twelfth Century*, ed. by Robert L. Benson and Giles Constable. Cambridge, Mass, 421–462.

7 Amundsen, Darrel W. 1978. "Medieval Canon Law on Medical and Surgical Practice by the Clergy." *Bulletin of the History of* Medicine 52:39–56.

8 Maimonides, *Medical Writings*, trans. Fred Rosner (Haifa, 1984), introduction, 1–4.

translated into Hebrew. Many translations from Hebrew into Spanish or Italian are contained in over 100 handwritings of Ibn Sīnā's encyclopedic *Canon*. At the end of the 13th century, the *Canon* had two different Hebrew translations, one of which was revised around the year 1400. At the end of the 13th century, Jewish and Christian medical circles exchanged information and texts. For example, in, Montpellier around 1300, Jewish practitioners who were excluded from the university medical schools were in contact with faculty members, as a result of which some Latin medicine and astronomy books were translated into Hebrew. Despite great diversity among Jewish practitioners in terms of learnedness, it is clear that their medical ideas and techniques penetrated the Greco-Arab medical culture as did Christians'.[9]

The diversity, scope and increased depth of medical writing in local languages can be demonstrated through sources in English. Although old English from the Anglo-Saxon period contains some important medieval medical texts, Middle English contains some recipes from the 12th and 13th centuries. The Anglo-Norman (French) medical writings of the time comprise, for the most part, recipes and other short texts.[10] However, by the end of the 15th century, the medical course books translated or adapted from Latin into English contained a series of long, complicated and sophisticated works. Until then, English seems to have been as important a language as Latin in the medical book production in England. Furthermore, these works owed a lot to ancient medicine and medieval Islam and included many theoretical and explanatory materials. Translating medical and surgical books was challenging because the Latin terminology did not often have local equivalents. Just as Greek and Arabic translations into Latin had helped expand the Latin technical vocabulary before, translators came up with creative solutions and broadened the medical lexicon. By the 15th century, practitioners who owned English medicine and surgery books ranged from master physicians who could read Latin to the barber-surgeons in London.[11]

A similar story could be told of the expansion of technical writing on medicine in other vernacular languages over the same period. In the German lands, where the late foundation and small size of university faculties of medicine

9 Manfred Ullmann, *Die Medizin im Islam* (Leiden, 1970), 28–33.

10 Tony Hunt, "Recettes medicales en vers français d'apres le manuscrit 0.8.27 de Trinity College Cambridge:' *Romania* 106 (1985): 57–83.

11 Voigts, Linda E. "Editing Middle English Medical Texts: Needs and Issues" in *Editing Texts in the History of Science and* Medicine, ed. Trevor H. Levere (New York and London, 1982), 39–66.

meant that university-trained physicians were a rarity before the fifteenth century, the dissemination of medical books in the vernacular took on a special importance. For example, perhaps as early as 1280, Ortolf von Baierland (Bavaria), a practitioner in Würzburg, put together in German a comprehensive handbook of medicine in 167 chapters. It transmitted some account of physiological theory as well as information about diseases and remedies and drew on standard Latin or translated Greek and Arabic authors, Hippocrates (*the Aphorisms*), and Ibn Sīnā (*the Canon*). In the course of the fourteenth and fifteenth centuries, Ortolf's work became one of the most widely disseminated medical textbooks in Germany and central Europe; it was translated, wholly or in part, into a variety of languages, Latin among them, and in one form or another it survives in numerous manuscripts and early editions.[12]

## The Medical Curriculum and Teaching Methods

Abundant Latin medical texts of Greek and Arabic origin ranging over various genres (Commentaries, Compendia and Glossaries) could be selected as study and teaching materials. It should be noted that teachers and students could only apprehend the medical and physiological concepts through the study of longer treaties of ancient authors; however, until the fifteenth century, only a limited number of ideas from ancient medicine and Greco-Islamic materials were translated into Latin and incorporated into university curricula. Lists of books officially assigned for medical lectures at Montpellier in 1309 and 1340 and at Bologna in 1405 show a curriculum of courses on works in the *articella* collection, which continued to supply the pedagogical need for brief statements of fundamental concepts; on up to a dozen or more longer works of Galen; and on selections from Arabic writers, notably Ibn Sīnā.[13]

Lectures did not appear to be organized in order of ascending difficulty, but certain books such as the brief Galenic compendium known as *Ars parva*, Hippocratic *Aphorisms* and parts of Avicenna's encyclopedic *Canon* were deemed to be basic texts. Sections of Avicenna's *Canon* were integrated into textbooks for university lectures that contained a synopsis of physiology (Book

12 Gundolf Keil, "Das Arzneibuch Ortolfs von Baierland: Sein Umfang und sein Einfluss auf die 'Cirurgia magistri Petri de Ulma';' SA 43 (1959): 20–60. Attention is drawn to the importance of vernacular technical medical writings in *Medizin im mittelalterlichen Abendland,* ed. Gerhard Baader and Gundolf Keil (Darmstadt, 1982), 23–44.

13 Siraisi, N. 1981. *Taddeo Alderotti and His Pupils: Two Generations of Italian Medical Learning.* Princeton: Princeton University Press. *96–106.*

1, Part 1), a treatise on fevers (Book 4, Part 1), principles of disease and treatment (Book 1, Part 4) and diseases from head to toe (Book 3). The writings of Rhazes on diseases also frequently served as the basis of lectures. The exposition of the *Ars,* the *Aphorisms,* and the *Canon* was hence a major task of late medieval medical masters, as surviving commentaries on these works suggest the significant and valuable role they had in education. Professors' commentaries on assigned texts (based on their lectures) show that there was considerable room for variation and personal opinion in the way the standard works were interpreted.[14]

Without doubt, the position of university-trained professors of medicine was confined to consultative posts, assigning physical interventions and examination to their delegated assistants. Tommaso del Garbo's demeanor toward his medical duty illustrates the varied attitudes among practicing professors. According to Tommaso del Garbo's biographer, he deemed the demands of the medical practice as a distraction from study. It is recorded of Gentile da Foligno, an exceptionally prolific medical author who commented on almost the whole of Ibn Sīnā's *Canon* (which is about one million words long), that he died in 1348 during the great plague epidemic "from too constant attendance on the sick".[15]

The views on and uses of the sections from the *Canon* as medical course books in at the beginning of the 13th and 14th centuries in both Paris and Montpellier meant that the training in Montpellier was practically similar to that in Paris. This was probably true for most of the centers of medical education.[16]

The differences were real enough, being those between the physiological doctrines of Aristotle, the master of the philosophers, and those of Galen and his followers. Both Avicenna and Averroes had discussed these differences and thus helped to focus the attention of Latin authors upon them.[17]

---

14 Siraisi, *Medieval and Early*, 71–72.

15 Campbell, Anna M. *The Black Death and Man of Learning* (New York, 1966; facsimile of original, 1931 edition), 9–13, 14–17. Much of the available information about Tommaso del Garbo is summarized, and bibliography cited, in the same work.

16 Siraisi, *Taddeo Alderotti and His Pupils*, 99.

17 Keil, Gundolf. "Das Arzneibuch Ortolfs von Baierland: Sein Umfang und sein Einfluss auf die 'Cirurgia magistri Petri de Ulma'" SA 43 (1959): 20–60. Attention is drawn to the importance of vernacular technical medical writings in *Medizin im mittelalterlichen Abendland,* ed. Gerhard Baader and Gundolf Keil (Darmstadt, 1982), 23–44.

Medical writers first defined themselves as carrying the legacy of Galenic physiology. Adherence to an acquired tradition expressed throughout medical writings guaranteed a distinct identity for rational inquiry into the human body by the physician, differing from natural philosophy and as an authentic intellectual attempt.

Siraisi offers a summary of the medical teaching before 1350 in Padua when only about a dozen professors of medicine can be securely identified compared to the size and productivity of the fifteenth-century medical faculty.[18]

## Sources and Methodology – The Contributions of Ibn Sīnā

The medical approach to the study of function and structure has been strongly influenced by the physiological and anatomical presentations in basic textbooks-notably the *Isagoge* of Johannitius and sections of the *Canon* of Ibn Sīnā.[19]

The first chapter of Ibn Sina's *Canon* provides a summary of physiology and anatomy that appears to be adjoining his philosophical generalization that assumes the nature of medical knowledge is divided into theoretical and practical aspects. The physiological subject opens with a brief account of the four elements (earth, water, air and fire), components of the human body as of all other material substances, but the treatments of element theory discuss pervasive and even unrelated topics ranging from the fate of elements to that of comets and tides. This incited medieval and Renaissance Latin commentators to expound upon topics remote from medicine in general, and physiology in particular. The anatomical section deals with "Simple" members, a term applied to bones, muscles, nerves, veins, and arteries; whose anatomical significance in practice has been reduced by Latin commentators by omitting the section from consideration. The anatomy of other organs classified as "composite" parts (for example, ear, eye, liver, spleen), are discussed in Book 3, which deals, in a head-to-toe arrangement, with diseases peculiar to different parts of the body and with their treatment. Each section opens with a brief chapter on the anatomy of the organ under discussion.[20]

---

18 Siraisi, Nancy G. 1973. Arts and sciences at Padua: the studium of Padua before 1350. Toronto, Pontifical Institute of Mediaeval Studies. Chap.5.

19 Danielle Jacquart, On the *lsagoge,* "A l'aube de la Renaissance medicale des Xl-XII siecles: L'"lsagoge Johannitii' et son traducteur;' *Bibliotheque de* l'Ecole *des Charles 144* (1986): 209–40.

20 French, Roger K. 1985. Andrew Wear, Roger K. French, and Iain M. Lonie (eds.), *Berengario da Carpi and the Use of Commentary in Anatomical Teaching, The*

Thus, Ibn Sīnā's book organization merges physiology and philosophy. It does not provide a unified treatment of anatomy, either as a subject in itself or in relation to physiological function. Furthermore, though the 1st part of the book and the 3rd volume were used as university course books, they addressed different parts of the medical curriculum. Latin commentators on the *Canon*, not realizing this nuance, ignored the sections on the bones, muscles, nerves, veins and arteries in the 1st volume and reduced the importance of anatomical content with their usual practices. They intentionally covered the physiological summary in volume 1 about disease and treatment in an abstract and generalized way, whereas the summary in the *Canon* formulates the underlying theory in a clearly organized set of fundamental principles or rules.[21]

An arrangement that gave much greater prominence and unity to anatomy than did the *Canon* was, however, to be found in a number of other well-known and influential general works. The *Pantegni* adopted the division of bodily parts into simple and composite but treated them in two consecutive sections near the beginning of the work. The treatise on pathology, diagnosis, and therapy by Rhazes, known as the ninth book of the *Almansor,* begins with a section of systematic anatomical description; so (after a preface) does the *Colliget,* Averroes' survey of medicine.

Among the works originating in the West, similar introductory chapters on anatomy are found in some general books on surgery, notably the books of two leading surgical authors of the fourteenth century, Henri de Mondeville (d.ca. 1320) and Guy de Chauliac (d. 1368).[22] Henri de Mondeville clearly states that the anatomical chapters at the beginning of his surgical book (originally another set of anatomy lessons in Montpellier) are derived from the anatomical material in the code of Ibn Sīnā, but are reformulated and shortened.[23]

---

*Medical Renaissance,* ed. Wear, French, Lonie, pp. 42–74. He discusses on the use of Book 3 of the *Canon,* and commentaries on it, in anatomical teaching.

21 *De complexionibus,* trans. Burgundio of Pisa (ed. Durling), pts. 1 and 2 (p. 64, for the example cited); Avicenna, *Canon,* Book 1, fen 1, doctrina 3, fols. $2^r$-$4^v$.

22 Mondeville, Henri. 1967. Die *Chirurgie des Heinrich von Mondeville (Hermondaville)* ed. Julius Leopold Pagel (Berlin, 1892), introduction to tractatus 1, p. 16. Markwart Michler, "Guy de Chauliac als Anatom" in *Frühe Anatomie,* ed. Robert Herrlinger and Fridolf Kudlien (Stuttgart, 1967), 15–32.

23 MacKinney, Loren C. 1962. "The Beginnings of Western Scientific Anatomy: New Evidence and A Revision in Interpretation of Mondeville's Role" *Medical History* 6:233–39.

Awareness of the value of having an understanding of anatomy when studying medical issues may have been inherent in surgeons, but it was not limited to them. Gentile da Foligno complained of the practice of removing anatomical parts from lectures in the first volume of the *Canon*, and acknowledged that knowledge of anatomy was as fundamental as studying the alphabet in medicine.[24]

## The Actual Practice of Dissection and Prohibition

Along with the production of accompanying brief anatomical manuals, the first practice of dissection since antiquity took place in 12th century Salerno using pigs as dissection specimens (chosen for the allegedly close resemblance of its interior organs to those of human beings, especially in the female).[25]

In the Kingdom of Naples, a well-known decree by Frederick II dated around 1241 presumably assumed that this requirement would be fulfilled through the dissection of animals and the study of texts. But it appears that human dissection began at the end of the 13th century. It seems that in Bologna and elsewhere human dissection began for legal purposes with autopsies and was followed by the incorporation of human dissection into medical and surgical training. The term "anatomy" acquired its meaning as an exercise consisting of the dissection of an individual human body according to pre-determined rules.

The *Anatomy* of Mondino de Liuzzi, written in 1316, was designed by its author, a professor of practical medicine at Bologna, as a handbook to accompany such a dissection. Annual anatomies (that is, dissections) became part of the formal academic curriculum at both Bologna and Padua. The practice is referred to as already established in a set of university statutes from Bologna dated 1405; a year earlier, the first public anatomy in Vienna was conducted by a professor from Padua. Statutes of the arts and medicine branch of the University of Padua, dating from 1465, refer to the annual anatomy as a well-established practice. The earliest anatomies for university students took place

---

24 French, Roger. 1985. Gentile da Foligno, commentary on *Canon,* Book 1 (Pavia, 1510), fol. 51v. On Gentile's ideas about the proper training of physicians, see Roger French, "Gentile da Foligno and the *via medicorum,*" in The *Light of Nature Essays in the* History *and Philosophy of Science Presented to* A. C. *Crombie,* ed. J. D. North and J. J. Roche (Dordrecht, Boston, Lancaster, 1985), 21–34.

25 Comer, George W. 1927. *Anatomical* Texts *of the Earlier Middle Ages* (Washington, 1927), text and translations, 48–66, discussion 19–30. *Anatomia magistri Nicolai,* in Comer, *Anatomical Texts,* 67.

privately in the houses of professors or students; by the late fifteenth century, a temporary theater was being constructed for each annual anatomy at Padua.[26]

Social, technical and intellectual constraints, nevertheless did limit the impact of anatomy and dissection, yet barriers were not elucidated completely in many popular accounts: medieval lecturers on anatomy invariably delegated the actual work of dissection to assistants. There seem to have been no blanket Church prohibitions against dissection in medical schools as such, yet discouragement of dissection practices might have been due to ecclesiastical prohibitions against boiling or dismembering bodies, especially in France.[27]

In the context of instruction rather than investigation, dissection seldom functioned as a means of verifying or correcting the written word and certainly not as an independent research tool. The fact that dissections were carried out in the light of a textual tradition does not necessarily imply that the working anatomist expected habitually to be able to match details in a precise, written description with appearances in the cadaver.

Even in the most comprehensive and authoritative texts, in many cases the actual descriptions of individual organs were brief, superficial and intertwined with non-definitive descriptions. For example, Ibn Sīnā's *Canon* offered an entire chapter on the anatomy of the kidneys, which was much more informative than Pio's early 12$^{th}$ century Salernitan anatomy book, which said that urine was rubbed into the kidneys with four humors. Most of the extra information provided in the *Canon* is completely anatomical. It contains a series of details on the shape, structure, state and consistency of the kidneys but the explanatory material was given as a diffuse and secondary component in a second chapter whose main purpose was to describe the purpose and functioning of the kidneys. In this, Avicenna may have aimed to explain the wide deviations between textual descriptions and physical appearances.[28]

Connections are also often suggested between the development of Italian Renaissance art and Renaissance anatomy, although here the evidence is ambiguous. Changes in artistic style and values unquestionably made the study

---

26 Ongaro, Guiseppe. 1981. These developments are summarized, with documentation, in Giuseppe Ongaro, "La medicina nello Studio di Padova e nel Veneto; *Storia della cultura veneta*, ed. G. Arnaldi and M. Pastore, vol. 3, pt. 3 (Vicenza, 1981), 92–95.

27 Brown, Elizabeth A. R. 1981. "Death and the Human Body in the Later Middle Ages: The Legislation of Boniface VIII on the Division of the Corpse," *Viator: Medieval and Renaissance Studies* 12:250–51.

28 Ibn Sina, *Canon*, Book 3, fen 18, tractatus 1, chap. 1, fol. 336$^{r-v}$. Comer, 1927. *Anatomical Texts*, 52.

of anatomy a subject of interest to artists. The belief that artists should know anatomy had already been expressed between the 1430s and 1450s in the influential writings of Leon Battista Alberti and Lorenzo Ghiberti. Their views were a natural concomitant of the concept, especially stressed by Alberti, that the depiction of the idealized human body in its proper proportions was a major task of sculpture and painting. Ghiberti seems to have had in mind the study of anatomy as taught in the schools, since he referred to anatomy as part of the study of medicine, wrote of the desirability of "seeing" an anatomy and drew on Ibn Sīnā.[29]

By the time the topic of changes in complexion due to aging and their outcome in natural death was taken up by thirteenth-century authors, a whole cluster of elaborations and interweaving of the Galenic and Aristotelian ideas was also available from various intermediate writers, notably Ibn Sīnā.[30]

## The Humors

The humoral theory, as explained in the Hippocratic Corpus, developed because the consistency and balance of the bodily fluids helped explain physiological changes. In addition, it had a crucial role for the physician's diagnosis and therapy of the patient and occasionally advocating bloodletting.

A systematic review with elaboration of the humors theory was provided by Ibn Sīnā, categorizing the four humors into good and bad or unnatural (bad blood, phlegm, and biles being "superfluities" that should be eliminated) and adding various secondary humors.[31]

Galen and his medieval successors stressed that phlegm comes in a number of varieties with different characteristics: sweet, salty, watery, and mucilaginous, to name only a few of those listed by Ibn Sīnā. The brain was the special organ most frequently associated with phlegm (presumably the association was

---

29 Schlosser, von Julius.1912. *Lorenzo Ghibertis Denkwürdigkeiten* (I *Commentarii*), ed. Julius von Schlosser (Berlin, 1912), 1:4, 7, 222.

30 McVaugh, Michael R. 1974. The 'humidum radicale' in Thirteenth Century Medicine. *Traditio* 30:259–83. Discuss Aristotle, *On Length and Shortness of Life* 5.466a17-466b31; Galen, De *complexionibus* 1.3.

31 Avicenna, *Canon*, Book 1, fen 1, doctrina 4, fols. $4^v$-$6^v$. On *the Nature of Man*, chap. 4, in *Hippocrates*, LCL, 4:2–40. Examples (many more could be cited) of emphasis on humors, fluids, excreta in the Hippocratic corpus: On the *Sacred Disease* 7–14, explains epilepsy as a result of a bad kind of phlegm; the assumption that the physician monitors excreta is present throughout the *Epidemics*, in *Hippocrates*.

originally made because of the color and consistency of brain tissue or cerebrospinal fluid, or both); but "natural" phlegm was also described as merely a stage in the creation of blood. Red or yellow bile was identified as the fluid found in the gallbladder and said to be manufactured in the liver, along with black bile and blood; black bile, however, was provided with an imagined "receptable" in the spleen. Blood occupied a special place among the humors. The actual fluid found in the veins was considered to be a sanguineous mass consisting of a mixture of the pure humor of blood with a lesser proportion of the other three humors; changes in color and partial separation in drawn blood left standing in a container were advanced as evidence of the presence of the biles and phlegm. The other humors were generated as part of the process of the manufacture of blood; and an important function of yellow and black bile-in their "good" form was, respectively, to purify and fortify the blood. The humors filled two important functions in the body's economy. Ibn Sīnā's explanation is clear: the digested food converted into chyle in the stomach is then carried to the liver, where it is mixed (literally "cooked") into blood, two biles and sputum (four humors). The various stages of the mixture purify the blood from the excreted excess and eventually some of the blood is refined into semen. However, most of the blood is used to nourish all parts of the body. Therefore, body parts were said to be made up of the humors. Secondly, the humors also gave the skin its color. Like all body parts, the humors were representative of appearance.

The maintenance and alteration in the individual's overall complexion was thought to be the result of humoral disproportion. Hence, humoral theory provided a materialist explanation of the mental and emotional state. In late antiquity and the Middle Ages, critics looked to Galen's works for explanations for psychological dispositions. Believing the nature of the soul and moral qualities' implied in the theory of temperament or complexion were determined by material causes they objected on philosophical or religious grounds.[32]

Whatever the limitations of actual knowledge, medical theory consistently appealed to sensible models of explanation. The Galenists taught that the three main members - the heart, brain, and liver - each govern or provide for the origin or governing principle (principium) of a separate organ and function group. Testicles (a term also used for the ovaries, understood as analogous organs in females) were sometimes added to the list of main members. Rival concepts were essentially linked to different Platonic and Aristotelian views of the soul

32 Owsei Temkin, Owsei. 1973. *Galenism: Rise and Decline of a Medical Philosophy* (Ithaca, N.Y., 1973), 87–92.

and were the subject of well-known scholastic debates. However, although the ultimate main principle in the body was thought to be one or more, certain internal organs and fluids were grouped into three different systems. Virtues, operations, and faculties were also attributed to these systems. Virtues were the general action or sensory forces of each system. Operations were functions of certain organs; for example, the stomach's was digestion. Faculties were special abilities specific to various parts of the body. For example, there was an eradicator or propulsion power in both a uterus carrying a nine-month-old and intestines.

## Principal Members and Associated Systems

These schemes were simultaneously anatomical and physiological, although anatomy was usually the handmaiden of physiological theory. The influential accounts in Galen's *On the Natural Faculties* and the chapters on the virtues in the *Canon*[33] focused more on physiological function than on bodily parts. Thus, when Ibn Sīnā wrote about vital, animal, and natural virtues, he connected each of these power sets with a specific physiological system(s) and a specific group of organs. Each set of virtues, systems, or organs was administered by or originated from a "leader". Ibn Sīnā explained in such a way that he reconciled the essentially incompatible views of Aristotle and Galen, and allowed the heart to somewhat dominate the whole body, while also allowing other major ones.

Medical writers devoted considerable attention to the eye and vision. A work that was especially influential in the medieval west was *The Treatises on the Eye* by Hunain b. Ishaq (d. 873), or Johannitius, which was translated into Latin before the end of the eleventh century. Following Galen, Hunain discussed the anatomy, physiology, and diseases of the eye and the nature of sight, stressing the role of spirits within the eye and adopting Galen's (and Plato's) view that vision occurred by means of extramission of rays from the eye. The composition of these treatises was stimulated by ancient and still more by Islamic contributions to the subjects of psychological and cognitive aspects of vision and of mathematical optics, notably by the work of the mathematician Ibn al - Haitham (d. 1041), whom the Latins knew as Alhazen. An important issue in the medieval literature on optics was whether vision occurred by extramission of rays from the eye, as Plato and subsequently Galen had believed, or by

33 Avicenna, *Canon*, Book 1, fen 1, doctrina 6, fols. 23$^{r}$-25$^{r}$.

intromission, as Aristotle and subsequently Ibn Sina, and in a more complex version Alhazen had held.[34]

It should be noted that Ibn Sina was the first physician to introduce the concept of eye muscle tendon repair. He describes the visibility of objects as follows: "*. . ..it is not a beam of light that exits through the eye and hits an object, rather, it is the beams of light that are emitted by an object and pass through the transparent part of the eye, i.e. the lens; thus, making vision possible*".[35] Ibn Sīnā not only described the anatomy of the eye, but also elaborately defined the six extraocular muscles and the trigeminal nerve. His work on the eye made important contributions to the anatomical knowledge and health of this organ.[36]

## The History of Human Life

Most influential textbooks divided life into four ages, analogous between stages of human life and various sets of four: the seasons, the elements, the primary qualities. The various other six-age, five-age, and three-age schemes developed by patristic authors and subsequent Biblical exegetes, theologians, preachers, and moralists seem not to have affected medical ideas on this issue.[37]

Between the $12^{th}$ and $15^{th}$ centuries, Western European physicians and surgeons did not have a great deal of physiological and anatomical knowledge. They learnt the texts, but they lacked a methodology that might increase the available knowledge or make changes in the theory. Humanists during the Renaissance and modern experts of medical history had little regard for these texts but it remains that they were originally quite useful. Through them, Aristotelianism was integrated into the medical discourse, based on the Islamic fusions of ancient medical teaching, thereby linking medicine with natural philosophy. The physicians who used these tools to study physiology attained the following very important achievements in their time: The comprehension of some ancient science; the recognition of the differences between the physiological doctrines of the ancient authorities, following the pioneering role of Ibn Sīnā and Averroes; the introduction of the dissection of human cadavers into

34 Siraisi, *Medieval & Early,* 108.

35 Al-Qattan, Mohammad M. 2006. History of anatomy of the hand and upper limb. *Journal Hand Surgery American*, 31: 502.

36 Price, Massoume. 2001. "*History of ancient medicine in Mesopotamia and Iran*" from http://www.iranchamber.com/history/articles/ancient_medicine_mesopotamia_iran.php. accessed 03.08.2020

37 Sears, Elizabeth. 1986. *The Age of Man* (Princeton, 1986), 12–20, 25–31, 38–53.

medical education; and, most importantly, the affirmation of the study of the human body as an intellectually respected, useful and dignified activity.

## Embryology

Human genesis received much medical attention, even though the approach was inconclusive with much repetitive verbal debate. On the former topic, Aristotle had held that the male alone contributed sperm containing an active principle to conception, the female providing only the matter of the fetus; by contrast, the Galenist view was that both male and female contributed sperm, so that the offspring could have characteristics from both parents. Astrological and metaphysical consideration were also taken into consideration in embryology since the development of the fetus involves the emergence of a new, separate being endowed with virtue, morality and complexion. The Medici were less preoccupied with the theological aspects of embryogenesis. But the astrological ideas spreading by the early fourteenth century through some circles in the medical community often included the belief that heat, light, and occult influences emanating from heavenly bodies assisted in the generation of life on earth.[38]

## Disease and Treatment

In the late thirteenth or early fourteenth century, abstracts of the Latin version of Galen's long medical treatises were used as academic textbooks, along with his commentaries (e.g. the chapter on fire in Ibn Sīnā's Canon, Book 4), general theses on practical medicine, reviews by famous physicians (councils) on specific cases, medical terminology guides, guidelines on phlebotomy techniques, ingredient lists for drugs, medical recipe collections, colored charts to aid diagnosis by examining urine, calendars and tables for use in astrological medicine and manuals on specific topics such as poisons or poisons. This last was a compound of the flesh of adders and other components, supposedly a universal antidote to venom and a remedy for diseases caused by excessive melancholy and phlegm. The principles of antidote medical action, dosage determination and practical guide to its usage had been subjects of discussion at Montpellier in the late thirteenth century. This keen interest in antidotes was stimulated by descriptions of Theriac by Ibn Sīnā and Averroes.[39]

38 Siraisi, *Medieval and Early*, 110–111.

39 Michael R. McVaugh.1972. "*Theriac at Montpellier, 1285-1325*"; SA 56:113–4; Arnald of Villanova. 1985. *Epistola de dosi tyriacalium medicinarum*, ed. Michael

Although essentially similar medical ideas are found throughout, some parts of this body of writing about disease and treatment are obviously much nearer to the world of actual practice than the rest. Only a few of the most learned or pretentious physicians would be likely to consult Galen's *On the Technique of Healing* or an academic commentary on Ibn Sīnā in the course of treating patients, whereas many practitioners might find constant use for a short handbook, a pictorial diagram, or a collection of recipes for medicinal remedies. Medical theory asserted that the human body exists in health, sickness, or a neutral state between the two. Deviations from health were classified into congenital malformations (in Medieval Latin, *mala compositio* of the body), complexional imbalance *(mala complexio),* and trauma *(solutio continuitatis,* or break in the body's continuity). The triple classification of ill-health was used in Ibn Sīnā's *Canon,* Book 1, fen 2. This classification placed almost all internal illness in the domain of complexional imbalance. Relatively little attention was paid to the first of these three categories, and when surgery emerged from medicine as a separate occupation and discipline in the west during the twelfth and thirteenth centuries, the management of trauma became the characteristic task of the surgeon. Indeed, food and medicine merged. Ibn Sīnā declared, in a passage frequently cited and discussed by Latin medical writers, that the formal distinction between them was that food was assimilated by the body, whereas medicine assimilated the body to itself. But both food and medicine were complexionate and affected the complexion of the person who ingested them; in practice, not only spices but also various vegetables counted now as one and now as the other.[40] Lettuce, for example, frequently crops up as an ingredient of cold complexion in medicinal recipes; Petrus Hispanus recommended a concoction of lettuce leaves for toothaches and lettuce seed to cool an excessively active libido.[41]

In the Islamic world and then in the West, it was thought that celestial influences were responsible for changes in the health or illness of the body, either directly or for changes in the air. As Rhazes points out: "Wise men among paramedics agree that time, air, water and skin color, light, heat, and everything

---

R. McVaugh, in Arnald's *Opera medica,* vol. 3 (Barcelona, 1985), 55–91, with historical overview in the editor's introduction, 57–73.

40 Avicenna, *Canon* Book 1, fen 2, doctrina 2, summa 1, chap. 15, fols. $33^v$-$34^v$.

41 Hispanus, Petrus. 1973. *Thesaurus pauperum* in his *Obras medicas,* ed. Maria Helena da Rocha Pereira (Coimbra, 1973), XI·35, p. 145.

related to their individual characteristics and illnesses are changed by the movement of the planets."[42]

## Diagnosis

The importance of observing the clusters of symptoms and changes through the course of illness was emphasized by ancient medicine practice. This observational tradition, as seen in the Hippocratic *Epidemics,* survived into medieval times and in the Muslim world. Within the framework of this tradition, they elaborated on diseases and differentiated different illness by observing the symptoms. A famous medieval example is Rhazes' description of smallpox, which distinguished its symptoms from those of other epidemic diseases causing skin eruptions such as measles (this description was first translated into Latin by fifteenth-century humanists). Rhazes' brief treatise was translated into Byzantine Greek, and then twice into Latin. Early editions of the Latin humanist versions bore the title *De pestilentia.* The first direct translation to Latin was made in 1747, and given the title by which the work is usually known in the West, namely *De variolis et morbillis.*[43] Shortly after its production, the eighteenth-century Latin translation was in turn translated into English, and published by Richard Mead.[44] Eighteenth-century western interest in Rhazes' writings on smallpox was due to the prevalence of the disease in Europe at that time.

In the Latin West, some *consilia* of thirteenth to fifteenth-century physicians contain descriptions of clusters of symptoms in individual cases witnessed by the author. However, many other *consilia* either omit descriptions of symptoms and explanations of the diagnostic process entirely in favor of merely naming the disease and prescribing remedies, or they are based on second-hand reports about the patient's condition.

42 Rhazes, *Aphorismorum libri* 2, in his *Opera* (Basel, 1544; facsimile repr., Brussels, 1973), 524.

43 Sezgin, Fuat: *Geschichte des arabischen Schrifttums,* Cilt 1–9, Leiden 1967–1984. *Gesamtindices zu Bd. I-IX,* Frankfurt a.M.: Institut für Geschichte der Arabisch-Islamischen Wissenschaften 1995. Vol. 10–12, Frankfurt 2000.

44 Richard Mead, Richard. 1755 A *Discourse on the Small Pox and* Measles (2d ed., London, 1755).

## Music in Therapy

Most of pulse stress theory mainly involved coding the identification of qualitative impressions. However, while describing the rhythms of the pulse, the terminology of musical proportion and metric string was also applied. The heart rate monitor had to change with age. According to Pietro d'Abano, it created an emphasis on the heart rate in infants and a sense of rhythm in adults. Various influential authors, including Ibn Sīnā, claimed that there are certain musical proportions in the pulse, and that the practitioner can identify them by touch. In the West, the idea of musical proportion in the heart is sometimes referred to as "human music" (*musica humana*, an undefined category other than audible vocal or instrumental music) and "world music" (*musica mundana*, spheres) Boethius' (d. 524 or 525) *On Music*. Undoubtedly, experience in reality gave some practitioners significant sensitivity to minute changes in heart rate and the ability to relate them to the patient's general condition. Pietro also highlighted a prosaic practical advantage of relying on the pulse on the wrist as a diagnostic tool: it eliminated the need to ask the patient (especially the female patient) to undress. This description of the pulse is largely based on Pietro d'Abano.[45]

A rich vocabulary of names for disease conditions was available. But both the relation of symptom to disease and the distinction of symptom from disease remained problematic even for the few careful observers in the world of medieval Islamic and western medicine, as it had been in antiquity. To be sure, Galen had stressed the importance of carefully distinguishing between disease and symptom, but it is hard to see how he imagined this could be achieved in practice. One of Galen's medieval interpreters, Arnald of Villanova, reworked the exhortation to suggest that it is only important to distinguish disease from symptom in situations in which it can be shown that such a distinction is relevant tuberculosis treatment. Criticism of the adequacy of Galen's definitions of disease, symptom, sign, and related terms and concepts began in the sixteenth century, but even then there was still no real possibility of replacing them.[46] But whether or not the spectrum of diseases described or predicted in the medical literature was a useful guide to historical epidemiology, it was a rich source of

45 Siraisi, Nancy G. 1975. "*The Music of pulse in the Writings of Italian Academic Physicians (Fourteenth and Fifteenth Centuries)*", *Speculum* 50:689–710.

46 Siraisi, Nancy G. 1990b. *Giovanni Argenterio and Sixteenth-Century Medical Innovation between Princely Patronage and Academic Controversy*. Osiris 2nd series, 91:161–180.

information about how disease and health was understood and recognized, and the types of problems, practitioners were ready to treat. Theoretical authors analyzed the diseases according to their complex characteristics. Pietro d'Abano, taking into account conditions that affect only the whole body rather than those specific to various body parts, classified fevers as hot; paralysis and epilepsy as cold; apoplexy, wasting, cancer as dry; and moist. Again, these terms need not be exactly equal to the conditions currently known by the same names.

Among conditions regarded as diseases of the whole body, fever, the paradigmatic example of a hot "disease", occupied a special place. The subject of fever came to constitute almost a separate branch of pathology; among much-used textbooks and works of reference, a major section of Ibn Sīnā's *Canon* (Book 4, Fen 1) and the whole of Book 10 of Rhazes' general treatise on medicine, known in the west as *Almansor,* were devoted to fevers. In these works fevers were elaborately subdivided into different varieties (quartan, tertian, hectic, ephemeral, and others), and much attention was paid to the concept of periodic rhythms in fevers. Another kind of classification of diseases that was followed in many practically oriented manuals, presumably because it was useful, emphasized the concept that different diseases were peculiar to different parts of the body by adopting a head-to-toe arrangement. Although they were accepted as part of rational, learned medicine, such manuals were essentially empirical in their approach, since they simply listed symptoms and remedies in standard diagnostic categories. These books varied significantly in sophistication and complexity. The ninth book of *Almansor* was frequently used as a university textbook of practical medicine until the sixteenth century. Indeed, Vesalius, the most famous of Renaissance anatomists, found the work of sufficient interest to edit or paraphrase the twelfth-century translation. Each of the book's 115 chapters is devoted to a different condition, ranging from headaches to pain in the feet. The materialist psychology associated with the concept of complexion and humoral qualities ensured that, in the *Almansor* and similarly arranged treatises, mental complaints (frenzy, melancholy) were interspersed among other afflictions of the head. Thus, too, physicians included passionate love *(amor hereos)* among the physical diseases and enumerated the languishing lover's physical symptoms.[47]

47 Arnald of Villanova. 1986. *Tractatus de amore heroico,* ed. Michael R. McVaugh, in Arnald's *Opera medica,* vol. 3 (Barcelona, 1986), 43–54.

## Instrumental Therapy

Practitioners working within these constraints treated mental and physical illnesses with three main types of therapy traditionally classified as three "medical tools": diet, medication, and surgery. Diet was an important component in maintaining health as well as treating disease; but as the principles of nutrition were basically the same in disease and health, no further discussion was required for surgery. Although the division of labor was far from complete in terms of treatment with incision, cautery or physical manipulation, it was normally handed to surgeons, barber surgeons and barbers in the thirteenth century. However, two minor surgical procedures often recommended by physicians as part of the management of complex diseases were cautery and phlebotomy. The use of cautery for complex disorders (i.e., internal complaints such as headaches) was based on the idea of real cautery with a heated metal instrument or applying "potential" cautery with a heated metal instrument, unlike the use of surgery for wounds. To direct the good or bad humors to different parts of the body, cupping or scarification agents could be used on the skin. Cauterization was an ancient technique that probably became more prevalent in the Medieval West after Albucasis' influential surgical manual was used in Latin throughout the 12$^{th}$ century. For example, cannulas for various uses are not what has been described, but the need to also drain blood from a chest wound is discussed in Albucasis's surgical textbook.[48]

Knowledge of phlebotomy was part of medical skill, not only because some medical practitioners performed bloodletting themselves but also because an important part of any physician's task was to judge when and how phlebotomy should be performed. Phlebotomy was unquestionably one of the most frequently used forms of general therapy; presumably its less painful character made it more tolerable to patients than cautery. The principle behind this ancient and long-lived therapeutic procedure was that bloodletting drew off corrupt matter from the body.

The simple phlebotomy applications circulated in Western Europe in the early Middle Ages; however, when the works of Haly Abbas, Ibn Sīnā, and Albucasis on this subject were made available in Latin, they provided much more comprehensive explanations of Galenic theories on phlebotomy and much more detailed practical instructions. Arabic-Latin encyclopedic knowledge formed the basis of later Latin and local treatises on phlebotomy. In the

---

48 Albucasis. 1973. *On Surgery and Instruments.* Trans. M. S. Spink and G. L. Lewis. London.

opinion of Pietro d'Abano, who reviewed the technical literature on phlebotomy found in Latin at least in the 1300s, the Arab medical authors who passed on the Greek phlebotomy doctrine were a bit more conservative than Greek sources in terms of the recommendation to open veins. The author of a phlebotomy manual, probably written in Montpellier between 1150 and 1225, categorically rejected the idea that an amount of blood so large as to make the patient faint should be requested from the patient, giving the reason that ordinary people outside of medicine would fear this prospect. In about 1400, the translator of the Middle English version of the same text added a series of dire warnings about the damage that unskilled phlebotomy can do (the result of infection with a knife or scalpel), especially by accidentally cutting an artery or causing the arm to swell to death.[49]

The foundation of medieval European pharmacy – as of traditional herbal medicine in other societies – was the attribution of medicinal powers to commonly available substances, usually plants and often those that might also be used in cooking. But in Western Europe, even in the early Middle Ages, this simple "kitchen-garden" medicine was never purely empirical, local, folkloric, and handed down by oral tradition, although these characteristics must surely have been present to some extent, but seems always also to have contained elements derived from ancient medicine by way of written sources. From the early Middle Ages to the high Renaissance, medicinal recipes were the commonest form of medical writing.[50] Two volumes, the second and fifth of Ibn Sīnā's *Canon* are also on medicinal recipes.

The new medical literature that began to become available from the late eleventh century included much technical pharmacology. Principal items included an alphabetized and enlarged version of an older Latin translation of the collection of *Materia Medica* by Dioscorides, a lengthy treatise by Galen on medicinal simples (that is, individual medicinal substances), and long sections on simple and compound medicines in the Arabic encyclopedic works.[51]

Any potential practical usefulness in medicine was, however, offset by the increased possibilities of confusion in substance identification and

49 Lina E. Voigts and Michael R. McVaugh, A Latin Technical Phlebotomy And its little middle English Translation, *Transactions of the American Philosophical Study* 74(1984):1–69.

50 John M. Riddle, 1987. "Folk Tradition and Folk Medicine: Recognition of Drugs in Classical Antiquity," in *Folklore and Folk Medicina*, ed. John Scarborough (Madison, Wisconsin, 1987), 33–61.

51 John M. Riddle, "Dioscorides": CTC 4 (1980):6–8.

nomenclature provided by the multiplication of translated or transliterated plant names.[52]

Plant naming was of course not systematic in all languages involved. European practitioners were faced with numerous plant names of Latin, Greek, Arabic, and local origin. The translation of names from Greek and Arabic into Latin was carried out in some cases by translation, sometimes by different authors choosing different ways of giving the same name, and in others by transliteration. As a result, the same plant may be known by several different names, or a completely different plant may be identified with one mentioned by an ancient or Islamic author. Visual images also did not provide a consistent means of checking terminology.

Manuscripts and similar works on herbal medicines were not always illustrated with pictures. Although there were several important examples of natural plant descriptions before the 15th century, there was no well-established tradition of naturalistic illustration to aid plant identification. Medical practitioners were well aware of these difficulties, as demonstrated in the compilation of medical dictionaries and Gentile da Foligno's complaints about the incomprehensibility of some translated Arabic terms in the collection of medical recipes that made up Book 5 of the Laws of Ibn Sīnā.[53] Ibn Sīnā, in the *Canon,* was influential in enlarging the idea suggested by Galen that some medicines, simple or compound, had particular, individual effects due not to the primary qualities but to a purely idiosyncratic "specific form". The paradigmatic example of action by specific form -which was regarded as an occult property in the sense of natural but not susceptible of rational explanation- was the action of a magnet.

Frequently used remedies included wine, employed since antiquity for cleansing wounds, and various laxatives and emetics, prized because they removed superfluities or bad humors. Most ingredients came from plants, a fair number from animals, and a few from minerals. Emphasis on the medicinal use of excreta make some of the recipes using animal ingredients unappealing to a modem reader-another of the remedies collected by Petrus Hispanus suggested that the application of pig dung would stop a nose bleed but in general it seems likely that the great majority of remedies were entirely harmless. A medication

52 Beaujouan, Guy. 1968. *"Fautes et obscurites dans les traductions medicales du Moyen Age". Revue de Synthése,* 3d ser., 89:145–52.

53 MacKinney, Loren C. 1938. "Medieval Medical Dictionaries and Glossaries:' in *Medieval and Historiographical Essays in Honor of James Westfall Thompson,* ed. J. L. Cate and E. N. Anderson (Chicago, 1938), 240–68.

new to Europe in the thirteenth century was alcohol, in the form of aqua vitae. To Taddeo Alderotti, aqua vitae seemed an exceptionally powerful and effective remedy; he wrote with enthusiasm about its usefulness for external application to cleanse wounds, as a pain reliever on an aching tooth, and as a medium for cordials, and he noted approvingly its cheering psychological effect.[54]

In fact, although among the substances likely to be in common use there were few that could be trusted to produce fairly consistent, perceptible results, practitioners' ability to produce predictable effects with drugs was limited. The only way to control the amount or concentrations at which drugs were administered was crude and largely intuitive or empirical. Physicians discussed the dosage to some extent in the summary, but although some medical prescriptions state amounts, the vast majority did not. Preparation tools, when described or mentioned, often reminded one of the kitchen rather than the laboratory. Moreover, although in some cases common sense, experimental, and naturalistic folk medicine undoubtedly lay behind the repeated prescription of some common herbs for many different types of conditions, in other cases the original basis for preferring certain herbs was magical rather than naturalistic. Therefore, a modern scientist suggests that verbena (Verbena officinalis), a common herb with a magical reputation but with no real therapeutic properties, to treat a rabid dog bite, to relieve pain, induce menstruation, reduce fever, as a diuretic, to restore breast milk, stop bleeding and avoid the plague.[55] The idea that some herbs have a magical effect was one of the few ways magical beliefs and practices play a role in therapy. However, it should be emphasized that the vast majority of remedies and therapeutic applications were completely natural. Moreover, although belief in the existence of demons and evil magic was widespread, they were rarely blamed for poor health, except in the case of impotence. The belief that witchcraft and demonic possession pose significant and ever present dangers to health was a feature of the witch panic affecting parts of Europe in the sixteenth and seventeenth centuries, not earlier.

By contrast, therapeutic magic involved direct attempts to control or manipulate celestial or occult forces and was regarded with suspicion by both Jewish and Christian religious authorities. One form of learned therapeutic magic was to engrave astral images on precious stones that the patient would then wear as

54 Hispanus, 1973

55 Stannard, Jerry. 2013. Medieval Herbalism and Post-Medieval Folk Medicine. *Pharmacy in History* 55:47–54.

a talisman, a practice tried by Jewish and Christian physicians at Montpellier in the early fourteenth century.[56]

Interest in the beneficent manipulation of astral and occult forces for therapeutic purposes intensified in the fifteenth century. It was widespread at the University of Padua, then a major center for the teaching of practical medicine, and one of the most famous and influential Renaissance accounts of astral magic occurs in a work largely devoted to astrological medicine, the *Three Books on* Life (1489) by the platonic philosopher and learned physician Marsilio Ficino.[57]

## Surgeons and Surgery

According to Pietro d'Abano, some people claimed that the only part of medicine that provides certainty is surgery because only surgery could yield obvious physical results. Surgery enthusiasts who came across Pietro's views in professional and intellectual circles in Paris or Padua in the 1300s were probably trained and ambitious surgeons. The demand for surgical information and the production of specialized technical writing on surgery was a prominent feature of literate medicine in Montpellier since the late 12$^{th}$ century in Italy and the mid-13$^{th}$ century; a similar emphasis was emerging among some literate practitioners in Paris at the time Pietro wrote. Surgery was a branch of knowledge conveyed through technical writing, a profession, and a form of physical manipulation of the human body. The practice of "surgery" was considered to be more of a treatment than medicine, as well as a variety of procedures including manipulation, surgical incision or repair. A realistic assessment by surgeons of what was possible limited the scope of the actual surgical intervention to more or less the list below; This list essentially remained unchanged between antiquity and long after: Crisis intervention for external injuries; treatment of chronic complications resulting from such injuries, particularly ulcers or fistulas resulting from infected wounds, often with externally administered drugs; treatment with cuts, excisions, cautery or medication of swelling and spots on the skin; and dropping the lens for cataracts. In addition, bloodletting, cauterization and cupping were used as a treatment for internal disorders,

56 Shatzmiller, Joseph. 1982–1983."In Search of the 'Book of Figures': Medicine and Astrology in Montpellier at the Turn of the Fourteenth Century," AJS Review 7–8 (1982–1983): 383–407.

57 Marsilio Ficino, Marsilio. 1989. *Three Books on* Life, ed. and trans. Carol V. Kaske and John R. Clark (Binghamton, N.Y., 1989).

as mentioned earlier. Outside of these categories, surgical intervention could probably only be tried for a handful of sudden life-threatening or acute painful conditions, including urinary obstruction, bladder stones, and decayed teeth.[58]

According to Guy de Chauliac, the essential equipment of the surgeon consisted of knives, razors, and lancets for making incisions, cautery irons, grasping tools, probes, needles, cannulas, and a tool for trepanation (the last may seldom have been put to use).[59]

In this way, surgeons sought to protect themselves as well as to avoid inflicting pointless additional pain and raising false hopes. Textbooks taught the recognition of some malignant tumors, notably breast cancer, and contained lists of organs to which wounds were likely to be mortal; the object was to warn against attempting treatment. Some books emphasized that tooth extraction should be undertaken only as a procedure of last resort. Examples of lists of wounds that are usually fatal include: Hippocrates, *Aphorisms*; Ibn Sīnā, *Canon*, Book 4, fen 4; Bruno Longoburgo, *Cyrurgia magna*, Book 1, chapter 6, printed with Guy de Chauliac, *Cyrurgia;* Teodorico Borgognoni, *Cyrurgia*, Book 1, chapter 21. Examples of the description of malignant tumors: Guy de Chauliac, *Cyrurgia*, chapter on cancerous apostemata, and Bruno Longoburgo, *Cyrurgia magna*, Book 1, chapter. 16.

On the need for caution in tooth extraction, we should see Albucasis, *On Surgery and Instruments*, Book.[60] Also in his book, Albucasis, following ancient authors on the matter of bladder stones, called for the surgeon to insert his finger into the patient's rectum in order to work the bladder stone down toward the neck of the bladder and then to make a perineal incision through which the stone could be extracted. Evidently such an operation demanded a high level of dexterity and a good working knowledge of complex regional anatomy.

As with the rest of medicine, the stimulus for the development of literate surgery came from social and economic growth that fostered new crafts and techniques and from the reception of written material that gave a fuller account of ancient Greek and Islamic achievements. In the case of surgery, books by Arabic authors were the most important vehicles of new information. However, the Arabic translation of Paul of Aegina made in the ninth century proved of

---

58 Wangensteen, Owen H. and Wangensteen, Sarah D. *Rise of Surgery: from Empiric Craft to Scientific Discipline*. Minneapolis, 1978, 3–15.

59 Guy de Chauliac, Cyrurgie, ed. Ogden, 4–5; *Cyrurgia* (Venice, 1498), fol. 2$^r$.

60 Albucasis, On Surgery *and Instruments*, Book. 2, chap. 30, ed. and trans. M. S. Spink and G. L. Lewis (London, 1973), 276–78.

great interest to sophisticated Muslim medical scholars. Book 6, which has been described as "*the most detailed account of ancient surgical practice to have come down to us*" was extensively utilized by all the major Arabic medical encyclopaedists: Rhazes, Haly Abbas, Albucasis, and Ibn Sīnā.[61] However, the actual information about ancient and Muslim surgery contained in the translated works was by no means easy to use. There were numerous obstacles to the understanding, let alone the practical application, of much of the surgical doctrine reported by the Arabic authors. Obscurities of terminology, confusions, and repetitions abounded. The long lists of conditions and procedures were more or less faithfully reproduced from the ancient sources and did not necessarily reflect the relative prevalence of particular problems in the actual experience of the Islamic compilers, let alone in the medieval west. Although the reader was only sometimes warned off by direct injunctions, some of the more elaborate procedures repeated from ancient sources were probably never intended by the Arabic writers to be performed.

Albucasis' *Surgery* (actually part of his medical encyclopedia, although it circulated in the West as a separate work) was especially influential after its translation into Latin in twelfth-century Spain. At Montpellier, Guillaume de Congenis, who was active in about the middle of the thirteenth century, based his teaching on the *Surgery* of Roger Frugard, although Guillaume's own book shows that he also knew Rhazes' treatment of surgery; Guillaume's book was in turn the subject of a pupil's explanatory notes.[62] The authors also freely altered the emphasis accorded to particular conditions and procedures. Thus, although cautery continued to be valued to stop bleeding and wound infection and for its supposed effect on internal conditions, the general textbooks of surgery produced in the West did not devote nearly as much attention to it as had Albucasis.

Ugo and Teodorico Borgognoni and, following them, Henri de Mondeville preferred an alternative course, that of simply cleansing wounds with wine (in itself an ancient practice). After cleansing, they advocated immediate closure in cases where the wound was fresh and there was no significant loss of

---

61 Ullmann, Manfred. 1970. *Die Medizin im Islam,* 1970, Leiden, 86–87, 141–42, 150.

62 *Keil, "Mittelalterliche Chirurgie," in Medizin im mittelalterlichen Abendland,* ed. Gerhard Baader and Gundolf Keil, Darmstadt, 1982, 23–44. *49–51. The Works of Guillaume de Congenis and his student are edited* ibid., 311–384, with introductory material at 297–310.

flesh or skin. They claimed that in this way they could achieve healing by primary intention-from the surface to the depth of the wound without formation of pus.[63]

In the fourteenth to sixteenth centuries, surgery developed and flourished chiefly in the milieu of towns and guilds, where a distinct hierarchy of surgical practitioners grew up. In some instances, sharp institutional and economic rivalry characterized the relations between surgeons and academically educated physicians.

However, conceptually and technically, the separation of medicine and surgery was always partial and incomplete in important aspects. Because medicine and surgery share a common tradition of knowledge derived mainly from the same sources, they also shared a common conceptual framework. As mentioned earlier, authoritative general studies of medicine, such as the works of Haly Abbas and Ibn Sīnā included long chapters on surgery. Both the authors of scientific studies on surgery and other medical authors continued to share the belief that surgery was one of the three therapeutic sources of medicine and repeated the usual doctrine. Each method in tumor treatment had to be tried before resorting to the next one. Therefore, surgery was seen as a last resort after diet and then medication. Classification of diseases as malformations, complex disorders and breakdown maintenance included conditions treated with surgery: conditions such as bladder stones would likely fall into the first category, and wounds, fractures, and all other types of trauma would fall into the third category. In terms of professional qualifications and common activities, the relations of *Medici* and literate surgeons differed widely in different parts of Europe during the later thirteenth, the fourteenth, and the fifteenth centuries. In principle, the separation of medicine and surgery seems to have been least marked in Italy. In the second decade of the thirteenth century, the earliest time at which Bologna appears as a center of medical study and activity, the surgical practice and private teaching of Ugo of Lucca was already an important part of the medical scene there. Moreover, when the university faculty of medicine finally took shape at Bologna, probably around the 1260s, it did so in the context of a flourishing northern Italian regional tradition of literate surgery. Furthermore, university students and their teachers in Italy, unlike university communities in northern Europe, always included a substantial proportion of laymen who were unaffected by the provision of the Fourth Lateran Council

63 Mondeville, Henri. 1967. Die *Chirurgie des Heinrich von Mondeville (Hermondaville), 32.*

forbidding priests, deacons, and subdeacons from practicing "that part of surgery involving burning and cutting." (Clerics could secure dispensations from these prohibitions; Teodorico Borgognoni received papal permission to practice his art and keep the fees when he was already a Dominican friar and probably a bishop.)[64]

Perhaps as a result, at Bologna and other Italian universities, surgery secured a place, albeit a minor one with few degrees granted, in the curriculum. The curriculum in surgery prescribed in the statutes of the University of Arts and Medicine at Bologna, issued in 1405 and probably unchanged since the thirteenth century, consisted of Bruno Longoburgo's textbook and selections from Galen, Rhazes, and Ibn Sīnā. Although university students of surgery also studied other branches of medicine, their reading in their specialty was thus very similar to that of their literate colleagues outside the schools. No doubt the university students were required to add scholastic and philosophical competence to their technical learning. These qualifications enabled them to become a professor of medicine at the universities of Bologna, Padua, and Siena. At Siena "both the theory and practice of surgery magisterially" was taught as part of the regular program of the medical faculty. In a proem to his commentary on the surgical parts of the *Canon*, Dino asserted that the teaching (again, as distinct from the practice) of surgery could be considered a form of *scientia* involving theory as well as practice.[65]

The professional separation between medicine and surgery became sharp and strongly enforced in northern Europe, where craft surgical traditions and the academic study of medicine appear to have developed much more independently of one another than was the case in Italy. In Paris, the chief center of medical education in northern Europe, the establishment of a university faculty of medicine in the course of the thirteenth century took place before the emergence of a class of self-consciously literate and Latinate surgeons in the early fourteenth century. Relations between physicians and the upper echelon of surgeons were particularly poor in fourteenth-century Paris.

It is a fact that war is the best surgical school. During the twelfth and thirteenth centuries, factional conflicts in Italian cities, the Crusades, and the

64 Goddu, Andre. 1985. "The Effect of Canonical Prohibitions on the Faculty of Medicine at the University of Paris in the Middle Ages," MJ 20 (1985): 342–62. The decree is translated, with commentary, in Amundsen, "Medieval Canon Law on Medical and Surgical Practice by the Clergy,".

65 Siraisi, *Taddeo*, 109–10.

general conditions of feudal society certainly provided surgeons many opportunities to gain experience. To understand that the treatment of injuries in combat is always an important part of the surgical procedure, if not the whole, it is sufficient to look at Guglielmo da Saliceto's long list of recommended treatments for sword and arrow wounds in different parts of the body. In the next two centuries, some rulers in northern Europe assembled armies for great expeditions by the standards of the time and had some pitched battles. For example, the 1,185 pits dug for the body remains of soldiers at the Battle of Visby in 1361 unquestionably produced a significant number of dead and wounded.[66]

## Conclusion

In the early Middle Ages, insufficient knowledge in the west contrasted with the much wider acceptance and understanding achieved in the Muslim world. The advanced scientific level in Islamic geography and the European reception of books and information by such giants as Ibn Sina provided a broad chronological framework for the development of medicine in the Middle Ages and Renaissance Western Europe. New translations of Arabic medical works, which first began to emerge from Constantinus Africanus in southern Italy in the late 11th century and later from the work offices of Gerard of Cremon in Spain in the 12th century, were later accompanied by translations of antiquity Greek works.

These studies formed the basis of a new Latin medical education that was developed and refined in the university environment from the thirteenth to the fifteenth centuries. In yet another stage of transmission and reception, Latin medicine provided the conceptual and often textual basis of the growing local European medical literature produced from the late fourteenth to the sixteenth century. Finally, the efforts of a handful of medical humanists in the late fifteenth and sixteenth centuries produced a complete insight into the remaining texts of Ibn Sina's translations into Latin.

Salerno, a center of medical practice since the late tenth century, became a center of medical education in the second half of the twelfth century. In Salerno, the medical textbook curriculum began to form, and the links between medicine and philosophy took on new importance. When the medical faculties were institutionalized at the universities of Bologna, Montpellier, and Paris during the thirteenth century, key components of late medieval and Renaissance

66 Contamine, Philippe. 1984. *War in the Middle Ages*, trans. Michael Jones (Oxford and New York. 1984). 258.

advanced medical education leading to university degrees in medicine began to form.

An important contribution to the curriculum was the anatomy taught on human cadavers, a practice that may have started around 1300. From about 1300 onwards, university education was generally considered the highest form of medical education. Texts and theories developed in the Latin academic medical world formed the basis of much of the medical knowledge and literature used by other practitioners. Literate surgeons in Italy moved to Montpellier in the thirteenth century and to Paris in the early fourteenth century. Much of the content of this surgical teaching was absorbed by the numerous literate surgeons that flourished in northern Europe in the late fourteenth and fifteenth centuries but who rarely had social or institutional connections with academic circles.

Latin medical writings of the fourteenth and fifteenth centuries continued to be printed and read during the sixteenth century. As a result, learned medical humanists launched a series of scathing attacks on the reliance on medieval translations and medieval Islamic authorities in medical teaching. For example, in a work first published in 1521, Giovanni Manardo, a professor at Ferrara, characterized the *Canon* of Ibn Sīnā in its twelfth-century Latin translation as filled with "a dense cloud and infinite chaos of obscurities".[67]

Until about the mid-sixteenth century, some of the most knowledgeable and innovative minds in medicine, such as John Caius (1510–73; second founder of Gonville and Caius College and reformer of the London College of Physicians) concentrated their efforts. They explored ancient Greek medical knowledge by researching and editing Arabic and Greek medical texts, making translations into Latin, or revising them. In short, they wanted more comprehensive and more authentic information about the ancient authorities used by their medieval and Islamic predecessors. They aimed to introduce clinical training in the hospital; and to update the way old textbooks such as *Canon* were taught, or to reproduce them. In terms of knowledge, anatomy and botany were undoubtedly the most successful of these efforts. In particular, the University of Padua became an important anatomical training center in the second half of the sixteenth century; as is well known, the Paduan anatomy environment provided William Harvey's early education. Essentially, the institutions where the medieval curriculum continued to be taught were also the main centers of

67 Giovanni Manardo, Giovanni. 1540. In Galeni doctrina et *Arabum censura celeberrimi* et *optime meriti epistolarum medicinalium libri* xx (Basel, 1540).

Renaissance innovation in anatomy, physiology, and medical education. The old curriculum was changed to some extent. In Padua, more time was given to anatomy and practical medicine and less time to medical theory. In some institutions, reformers with a humanist leaning succeeded in removing the *Canon* from the curriculum, as was the case in many German institutions in the 1550s. In some Italian universities, the *Canon* was maintained as an official textbook until the eighteenth century. In the 1520s, innovative teachers used the *Canon* and other traditional texts in their classes to criticize the author or introduce new knowledge. Leading anatomists and botanists freely pointed out to what extent they collected information that was unknown to or contradicted by their predecessors. However, these Renaissance themes in medicine reflected the real change and real advances in knowledge, but the changes involved changing, not rejecting, a long-existing information system.[68]

Ibn Sīnā not only had the opportunity to discover the wide range of topics covered in Arabic writings, he also exploited the synthesis of the ancient knowledge originating from different sources in these Arabic writings. The first examples of such encyclopedic attempts include the previous work of el-Rāzi's (Rhazes) *Kitâb al-Hâvî (Continens)* and Ali Ibn Abbas's (Haly Abbas) *Kitâb al-Melikî (Liber Regius, Regalis Dispositio)*. But that of Ibn Sīnā was the most popular one and clearly outperformed its antecedents. With regard to content, the *Canon* contained the vast majority of the medical knowledge up to the eighteenth century. The writings of Ibn Sīnā were translated into other languages including Latin and were incorporated into the curriculum of certain European universities.[69]

## Ibn Sīnā as a Teacher

Nancy G. Siraisi collected her extensive studies on the content of the curriculum in European Medical Schools, particularly after year 1500, into the book, *Avicenna in Renaissance Italy: The Canon and Medical Teaching in Italian Universities After 1500*.[70] The information presented in the book indicates that approximately 80 to 90 lectures were held annually. For instance, Matteo Corti

68 Siraisi, *Medieval and Early*, 190–192.

69 Keskinbora, Kadircan H. and Keskinbora, Kader. 2016. A systematic review of Ibn Sina's (Avicenna) studies: reflections on anatomy. *European Journal of Anatomy* 20:99–105.

70 Siraisi, Nancy G. 1987. *Avicenna In Renaissance Italy: The Canon and medical teaching in Italian universities after 1500*. Princeton University Press, New Jersey.

acquired information from Section 1, Volume 1 of the *Canon* for a total of 63 lectures, while 77 lectures given by Girolamo Capodivacca were based on the information from Section 1, Volume 4 of the *Canon*. Similarly, a 277-page volume was prepared by Bernardino Paterno using the information provided in Section 4, Volume 1 of the *Canon*. As stated by Siraisi, lectures on therapeutic procedures were also included. Siraisi also states that 80 % of the printed lectures of Giambatista da Monte and long scholastic lectures of Gentile da Foligna were taken from the *Canon*.

These examples indicate that during the 16$^{th}$ century, Ibn Sina's teachings had a prominent part in the curricular content of medical schools at Padua, Bologna and Pavia, and Ibn Sīnā's *Canon* was considered a major textbook. This curricular content in Padua suggests that in 4 of the 9 main professorship chairs concerned with medical theory, *Canon*'s Section 1, Volume 1 was a major source of information.

The grandfather of Andreas, Peter Vesalius, wrote his thesis on certain works of Ibn Sīnā.[71] Peter's son John Vesalius was the private physician of the Mary of Burgundy, wife of Maximillian I, and later he taught medicine at Louvain University. After then, the children of the Vesalius family were sent to Paris University for medical education. Andreas studied Ibn Sina's writings on tumors in his first year in Padua. An eager student, Andreas's incomplete university notes reflect a comparison between Ibn Sina's work with the classical Works of Hippocrates, Galen, Paul of Aegina, and Aetius, including some corrections of his own.[72]

In addition, many teachers at Montpellier were formerly acquainted with the Islamic medicine at Salerno. For example, Roger of Salerno, the great Salernitan surgeon, first gained his widespread reputation in Salerno around 1170, and then became the Chancellor of the medical school at Montpellier. He wrote "*Practica Chirurgia*" in 1180.[73]

Here we covered the curriculum and medical education in Salerno and Padua Medical schools, which started in the Early Renaissance period in Italy and which formed the nuclei of today's modern university education. Important

71 Holomanova, Anna; Ivanova, Angelina; Brucknerova, Ingrid; Benuska Josef. 2001. Andreas Vesalius--the reformer of anatomy. *Bratislavske lekarske listy* 102:48–54.

72 Ball, James M. 2013. (Originally published in 1910) *Andreas Vesalius, the reformer of anatomy*. Forgotten Books, London.

73 Stelmaschuk A. 2001. *The School at Salerno: Origin of the European Medical university*. The Proceedings of the 10th Annual History Of Medicine Days, The University of Calgary.

topics and important names in medical education, the true origins of which date back to the Middle Ages and early Renaissance period, were investigated. It is understood that Ibn Sīnā is one of the most influential medical teachers, perhaps the most important medical teacher, with his famous book the *Canon of Medicine* and his articles.

## Bibliography

Albucasis. 1973. *On Surgery and Instruments.* Trans. M. S. Spink and G. L. Lewis. London.

Al-Qattan, M. M. (2006). History of anatomy of the hand and upper limb. Journal of Hand Surgery, 31(3), 502.

Amundsen, D. W. (1978). Medieval canon law on medical and surgical practice by the clergy. Bulletin of the History of Medicine, 52(1), 22–44.

Arnald of Villanova. 1986. *Tractatus de amore heroico*, ed. Michael R. McVaugh, in Arnald's *Opera medica*, vol. 3 (Barcelona, 1986), 43–54.

Ball, James M. (1910). Andreas Vesalius: the reformer of anatomy. Medical Science Press.

Ball, James M. 2013. (Originally published in 1910) *Andreas Vesalius, the reformer of anatomy.* Forgotten Books, London.

Beaujouan, G. (1968). Fautes et obscurités dans les traductions médicales du Moyen Âge. Revue de synthèse, 89, 145–152.

Brown, E. A. (1981). Death and the human body in the later Middle Ages: the legislation of Boniface VIII on the division of the corpse. Viator, 12, 221–270.

Campbell, A. M. (1931). The Black Death and men of learning. Columbia University Press.

Comer, G. W. (1927). Anatomical Texts of the Earlier Middle Ages: A Study in the Trans-mission of Culture. Washington, DC: Carnegie Institution of Washington, 84.

Contamine, Philippe. 1984. *War in the Middle Ages*, trans. Michael Jones (Oxford and New York. 1984). 258.

D'Alverny, Marie-Therese. 1982. Translations and translators. In: Renaissance and renewal inthe twelfth century, ed. Robert Louis Benson, Giles Constable, and Carol Dana Lanham,421-60. Cambridge, MA: Harvard University Press.

De Mondeville, H., & Pagel, J. (1892). Die Chirurgie des Heinrich von Mondeville (Hermondaville) nach Berliner, Erfurter und Pariser Codices zum ersten Male. Hirschwald.

Ficino, M. (1989). Three Books on Life, eds and trans Carol V. Kaske and John R. Clark. Binghamton: Medieval and Renaissance Texts and Studies in conjunction with the Renaissance Society of America.

French, R. (1985). Berengario da Carpi and the use of commentary in anatomical teaching. In The Medical Renaissance of the sixteenth century, 42–74.

French, R. K. (2001). Canonical medicine: Gentile da Foligno and scholasticism. Brill.

Goddu, A. (1985). The Effect of Canonical Prohibitions on the Faculty of Medicine at the University of Paris in the Middle Ages. Medizinhistorisches Journal, (H. 4), 342–362.

Green, M. (1989). Women's medical practice and health care in Medieval Europe. Signs: Journal of Women in Culture and Society, 14(2), 434–473.

Hispanus, Petrus. 1973. Thesaurus *pauperum* in his *Obras medicas*, ed. Maria Helena da Rocha Pereira (Coimbra, 1973), XI·35, p. 145

Holomanova, A., Ivanova, A., Brucknerova, I., & Benuska, J. (2001). Andreas Vesalius-the reformer of anatomy. Bratislavske lekarske listy, 102(1), 48–54.

Hunt, T. (1985). Recettes médicales en vers français d'après le manuscrit 0. 8. 27 de Trinity College, Cambridge. Romania, 106(421 (1), 57–83.

Jacquart, D. (1986). À L'aube De La Renaıssance Médicale Des XIe-XIIe E Siècles: L'«Isagoge Johannith» Et Son Traducteur. Bibliothèque de l'École des chartes, 209–240.

Keil, G. (1959). Das Arzneibuch Ortolfs von Baierland: Sein Umfang und sein Einfluß auf die, Cirurgia magistri Petri de Ulma. Sudhoffs Archiv für Geschichte der Medizin und der Naturwissenschaften, (H. 1), 20–60.

Keil, G. (1959). Das Arzneibuch Ortolfs von Baierland: Sein Umfang und sein Einfluß auf die, Cirurgia magistri Petri de Ulma. Sudhoffs Archiv für Geschichte der Medizin und der Naturwissenschaften, (H. 1), 20–60.

Keil, G. (1983). Mittelalterliche Chirurgie, in: Acta medicae historiae. Patavina, Padova,30 (1983/84), S. 45–64.

Keskinbora, K.H., and Keskinbora, K. (2016). A systematic review of Ibn Sina's (Avicenna) studies: reflections on anatomy. Eur J Anat, 20(1), 99–105.

Khalaf ibn ʿAbbās, A. A. Q., Lewis, G. L., & Spink, M. S. (1973). Albucasis on surgery and instruments (Vol. 12). Univ of California Press.

Kristeller, P. O. (1986). Studi sulla Scuola medica salernitana. Nella sede dell'Istituto.

MacKinney, Loren C. 1938. "Medieval Medical Dictionaries and Glossaries:ʿ in *Medieval and Historiographical Essays in Honor of James Westfall Thompson*, ed. J. L. Cate and E. N. Anderson (Chicago, 1938), 240–68.

MacKinney, L. C. (1962). The beginnings of western scientific anatomy: new evidence and a revision in interpretation of Mondeville's role. Medical history, 6(3), 233–239.

MacKinney, L. C. (1966). Medieval Medical Dictionaries and Glossaries. Kennikat Press.

McVaugh, M. (1974). The 'humidum radicale' in thirteenth-century medicine. Traditio, 30, 259–283.

McVaugh, M. R. (Ed.). (1985). Arnaldi de Villanova Opera medica omnia: Tractatus de amore heroico; Epistola de dosi tyriacalium medicinarum. Edicions Universitat Barcelona.

Mead, R. (1748). A discourse on the small pox and measles. J. Brindley.

Mondeville, Henri. 1967. Die *Chirurgie des Heinrich von Mondeville (Hermondaville), 32.*

Newmyer, S. (1989). Maimonides' Medical Writings. Vol. 2. Maimonides' Commentary on the Aphorisms of Hippocrates by Maimonides, Fred Rosner (Book Review). Bulletin of the History of Medicine, 63(1), 148–9.

Ongaro, G. (1981). La medicina nello Studio di Padova e nel Veneto. Arnaldi G, Pastore Stocchi M, eds. Storia della cultura Veneta. Dal primo Quattrocento al Concilio di Trento, 3, 75–134.

Price, M. (2001). History of ancient medicine in Mesopotamia and Iran. Iranchamber. com, October.

Riddle, J. M. (1986). Dioscorides on pharmacy and medicine (Vol. 3). University of Texas Press.

Riddle, J. M. (2013). Folk tradition and folk medicine: recognition of drugs in classical antiquity. Pharmacy in history, 55(2/3), 64–87.

Sears, E. (2019). The ages of man: Medieval interpretations of the life cycle (Vol. 5449). Princeton University Press.

Sezgin, F. (1967). Geschichte des arabischen Schrifttums: Mathematische Geographie und Kartographie im Islam und ihr Fortleben im Abendland: historische Darstellung. Teil 1. Inst. für Geschichte der Arabisch-Islamischen Wiss.

Sezgin, F. (1970). Geschichte des arabischen Schrifttums: Medizin, Pharmazie, Zoologie, Tierheilkunde bis ca. 430 H (Vol. 3). EJ Brill.

Shatzmiller, J. (1982). In Search of the "Book of Figures": Medicine and Astrology in Montpellier at the Turn of the Fourteenth Century. AJS Review, 383–407.

Siraisi, N. G. (1973). Arts and sciences at Padua: the Studium of Padua before 1350 (pp. 379–404). Toronto: Pontifical Institute of mediaeval studies.

Siraisi, N. G. (1975). The music of pulse in the writings of Italian academic physicians (fourteenth and fifteenth centuries). Speculum, 50(4), 689–710.

Siraisi, N. G. (1990). Giovanni Argenterio and sixteenth-century medical innovation: between princely patronage and academic controversy. Osiris, 6, 161–180.

Siraisi, N. G. (2009). Medieval and early Renaissance medicine: an introduction to knowledge and practice. University of Chicago Press.

Siraisi, N. G. (2014). Avicenna in Renaissance Italy: the Canon and medical teaching in Italian universities after 1500. Princeton University Press.

Siraisi, N. G. (2019). Taddeo Alderotti and his pupils: Two generations of Italian medical learning. Princeton University Press.

Stannard, J. (2013). Medieval Herbalism and Post-Medieval Folk Medicine. Pharmacy in history, 55(2/3), 47–54.

Stelmaschuk, A. (2001). The School at Salerno: Origin of the European Medical university. Hıstory Of Medicine Days, 65.

Temkin, O. (1973). Galenism Rise and Decline of a Medical Philosophy.

Ullmann, M. (1970). Die Medizin im Islam (Handbuch der Orientalistik, 1. Abt., Ergänzungsband VI/1). Leiden/Köln, 54.

Ullmann, M. (1972). Die Natur- und Geheimwissenschaften im Islam. Leiden, EJ Brill.

Voigts, L. E. (1982). Editing Middle English medical texts: Needs and issues. Editing texts in the history of science and medicine, 39–68.

Voigts, L. E., and McVaugh, M. R. (1984). A Latin technical phlebotomy and its Middle English translation (Vol. 72). American Philosophical Society.

Von Schlosser, J. (1912). Lorenzo Ghibertis denkwurdigkeiten (I commentarii): zum ersten male nach der handschrift der Biblioteca Nazionale in Florenz vollstandig. Bard.

Wangensteen, O. H., and Wangensteen, S. D. (1978). The rise of surgery: from empiric craft to scientific discipline. Minneapolis, MN: University of Minnesota Press.

## Short Biography of Kadircan H. Keskinbora

He has studied medicine at Hacettepe University, Faculty of Medicine (Ankara/ Turkey). He became an Ophthalmologist in 1987, an associate professor in 1999 and a professor in 2007. He concluded his second Ph.D. in "Deontology, History of Medicine and Medical Ethics" in 2006. He still is a professor at Istanbul Bahcesehir University, School of Medicine, Head of Dept. History of Medicine and Ethics. He is a member of various national and international scientific or non-governmental organizations. His Published Books:

**Ophthalmology:** Oftalmolojide Sorularla Eğitim (Education in Ophthalmology with Questions), Oftalmolojide Sınava Doğru (Towards Exam in Ophthalmology), Oftalmoloji İle Kesişen Bilim Dalları (Scientific Areas that Intersect with Ophthalmology)

**History of Medicine:** Göz Nurunun Anahtarı ve Sevinç Hazineleri (Key to Eye Light and Treasures of Joy), Esat Işık: Bilimde, Siyasette, Milli Mücadelede Bir Işık (Esat Isik: A Light in Science, in Politics, in National Struggle), Kanûn-u Sagir of Ibn Sina (The Little Canon of Avicenna), The Little Qanun of Ibn Sina (Peter Lang Publish.).

**Literature:** Düşünen Beyinlerin İnsanlığa Mirası: Özdeyişler (Inheritance of Thinking Minds to Humanity: Aphorisms), Yaban Gülü (Brier Rose - poem book), Mardin Düşünceleri (Thoughts on Mardin - poem book), Ben Suyum (I am water - poem book), İddia (Claim - poem book).

Because of his studies on Avicenna (Ibn Sina), he was awarded the **"International Avicenne Prize"** in Paris/France in 2016.

e-mail: kadircan.keskinbora@gmail.com
hidirkadircan.keskinbora@med.bau.edu.tr

Prof. Dr. Mehmet Bayrakdar

# Half Understanding of Ibn Sīnā's Two Concepts: al-Wâjib al-Wujûd and Wâjib al-Wujûd

The most important philosophical and metaphysical terms of the famous Turkish philosopher Ibn Sīnā (Avicenna, 980 Afshana-Ozbekistan-1037 Hamadan-Iran) for our investigation are two foremost concepts of him as al-wâjibu'l-wujûd and wâjibu'l-wujûd. But unfortunatly these two concepts have been understood until today as if they were the same and one concept for nearly 1000 years by all the editors of Ibn Sīnā's works, his translators, and the all the experts on his philosophy, whether they are easterners or westerners, whether they are medieval scholars or modern scholars. This is well pointed out by the famous French scholar and Avicennist Amélie-Marie Goichon (1894-1977) in the following saying: "Wâjib is here preceded by the article; elsewhere it is not, but the meaning is the same."[1], when translating into French this statement of Ibn Sīnā:

"أن الواجب الوجود هو الموجود الذي متى فرض غير موجود عرض منه محال... . ." [2]

(*Certes l'Etre nécessaire est l'être qui, lorsqu'il est supposé inexistant, donne lieu à une contradiction* = Certainly the Necessary Being is the being which, when it is supposed to be nonexistent, gives rise to a contradiction). Similarly George F. Hourani (1913–1984) informed us that wâjib al-wujûd is variously translated into English as necessary of existence, necessary being, necessarily existent, that whose existence is necessary.[3] As we see, for Goichon, like for all others, al-wâjib al-wujûd and wâjib al-wujûd are the one and same concept, and both concepts mean the Necessary Being or Existence, which is eventually God.

Almost twenty years ago while rereading the Ilâhiyât (metaphysics) section of Ibn Sīnā's book al-Shifâ', these two concepts attracted my attention. And

---

1 Goichon (A.-M.) : "Wâjib est ici précédé de l'article; ailleurs il ne l'est pas, mais le sens est le même", Lexique de la Langue Philosophique d'Ibn Sînâ (Avicenne), Paris, 1938, p. 417.

2 Ibn Sīnā: An-Najât, Cairo, 1913, p. 366.

3 Hourani (G.F.) : "Ibn Sînâ on Necessary and Possible Existence", the Philosophical Forum, New Series, vol. 4, No: 1, 1972, p. 75.

rethinking a lot about theme, I got the idea that these two concepts, although they are very very similar to each other from every aspect, must be to some extent different in meaning. For nearly twenty years from that day to this day, I have looked for whether there are some scholars, who had already seen some difference in meaning between two concepts. And I could not find any person. And then I have decided to write this little work, in which I wanted share my idea with the academic public. I am concentrated only on the accurate and adequate understanding of the concepts. In following my intention is not to expose what they are in the metaphysics of Ibn Sīnā; and therefore I shall not discuss here the functions of the concepts in his metaphysics and other related problems. So, my primary concern is to show that al-wâjib al-wujûd and wâjib al-wujûd are not the same concept, but two different concepts.

To begin with, we want to know firstly whether Ibn Sīnā is the creator of these concepts. Some people like Mr. Zarkasyi have claimed that wâjib al-wujûd is a term coined by Ibn Sīnā.[4] But according to Ibn Sīnā himself this is wrong; because he says: "*. . ...The first Cause named in the philosophers to be Necessary Existence (wâjib al-wujûd). ..*"[5] Ibn Sīnā did not mention the philosophers by name; but modern scholars, like Goichon for example, say that one of them is Aristotle.[6] The other philosophers are al-Fârâbî (872–950) and al-Amirî (913–992) ; they used the term wâjib al-wujûd before Ibn Sīnā.[7] Thus Ibn Sīnā is not the first philosopher who coined the term of wâjib al-wujûd. He used first this concept in his first philosophical work entitled "al-Hikmat al-Arûziyya", he wrote it in Bukhara in 998 or 999 BC, when he was 21 years old.[8] But we know for certain that he is the creator of the concept of al-wâjib al-wujûd. Ibn Sīnā has

4 Zarkasyi (H.F.) : "Ibn Sīnā's Concept of Wâjib al-Wujûd", Journal *THAQAFAH*, Vol. 7, No. 2, October 2011, p. 376.

5 Ibn Sīnā: Risâletü'z-Ziyâra, Jâmi'i al-Badâ'i', Cairo, 1917. p. 33.

6 Goichon (A.-M.) : Vocabulaires Comparés d'Aristote et d'Ibn Sînâ, Paris, 1939, p. 37–38. See Aristotle's Metaphysics Λ 7, 1072 b 10.

7 Al-Fârâbî : Uyûnu'l-Masâil, Cairo, 1907, p. 3–9; this short treatise was traditionally atributed to al-Fârâbî. Very recently some scholars doubted the nomination of al-Fârâbî as the author of Uyûnu'l-Masâil; they have attributed it to Avicenna; but they have no convincing evidence. Fr. H. Dieterici is right to attribute it to al-Fârâbî, See his "Alfârâbî's philosophische Abhandlungen, Leiden, 1890. Al-Âmirî : al-Takrîr, ed. by S. Halifât, Amman, 1988, p. 304–308; İnkâz al-Bashar, ed. by K. Turhan, Istanbul, 1996, p. 4–6.

8 Muhsin Sâlih: al-Hikma al-Arûziyya, Beyrouth, 2007, p. 1, 12; Gohlman (W. E.): The Life of Ibn Sīnā: A Critical Edition and Annotated Translation, Albany, New York, p. 38.

frequently used these two concepts side by side in all his philosophical works from al-Shifâ' and Dânish-nâma[9] to his latest work al- Mubâhasât. Let's note here that he did not use the concept of al-wâjib al-wujûd only in his first work "al-Hikmat al-Arûziyya".

Why were these two concepts seen in the same sense before us? We try to answer very briefly to this question. There could be two reasons for this. Firstly, they have seen the Arabic formulations of the concepts as al-wâjib al-wujûd and wâjib al-wujûd as grammatically same; and as it is indicated in the quotation from Goichon above they could not see any difference between the words of al-wâjib and wâjib; as we will see below there could be difference between the worlds al-wâjib (with article al-) and wâjib (without article). Secondly, it is that Ibn Sīnā has also pointed to God with both of these two concepts.

## 1-al-Wâjib al-Wujûd: The Necessary Being

The concept of al-wâjib al-wujûd has been understood as the Necessary Being or Existence;[10] this is correct, there is no problem. But here we should emphasize that, as for Ibn Sīnā the Necessary Being is God, he means by this concept especially the necessity of God's existence. And this concept is used by him only for God; not for other beings.

## 2-Wâjib al-Wujûd: The Necessitating Existence

The concept of wâjib al-wujûd is also rendered traditionally as the necessary existence, because as we have already said that the scolars before us did not see any difference between the concepts of al-wâjib al-wujûd and wâjib al-wujûd. But we think that this is wrong. If they were same in meaning, as have been pretented, it becomes difficulte to explaine why then Ibn Sīnā used these two separated concepts for one thing one behinde the other. Secondly as we shall see, the concept of wâjib al-wujûd is used for God as well as for any possible being when it becomes cause for the existence of any other possible being. This concept is intrinsically realeted to Ibn Sina's creative causality. When it is used for God, Ibn Sīnā speaks not of the necessity of God's existence but of the necessity of God's acts or Godhead.

9 For us Ibn Sīnā himself did not composed Dânish-nâma-i Alâî in Persian; it is a free Persian translation of his al-Shifâ' by his disciple Abdu'l-wâhid al-Jurjânî.

10 For similair rendering see Hourani (G.F.) : "Ibn Sīnā on Necessary and Possible Existence", The Philosophical Forum, New Series, vol. 4 No. 1, 1972, p. 75.

For the reasons that we will explain below, we have to translate the concept of wâjib al-wujûd, whether it has been used for God or for possible existence, as Necessitating Existence, although it might not sound and seen a good expression in English. For our understanding wâjib al-wujûd must be translated and understood as the Necessitating Existence because of the following two reasons or justifications.

**a-The Causality Principle:** As it is known Ibn Sīnā's philosophy and metaphysics is basically dependent of causality. In order to understand properly why he might have used these two concepts such concepts, we have to know adequately his theory of causality; because he discussed especially the concept of wâjib al-wujûd very closely in the context of causality. Our duty here cannot be to explain his theory of causality, this is of course a long job; the scope of this problem is dauntingly broad.

We will point out just make in brief some important points. As it is known his theory of causality is Aristotelian. But, although Aristotle's causality in its essence depends closely on motion or movement, whereas Ibn Sīnā's is creatrice, sc. It depends ultimatetly on God's will.

Ibn Sina defines the efficient cause or agent as that which bestows existence to another.[11] He distinguishes the metaphysical definition of the efficient cause from that of the natural philosopher as follows: "Metaphysical philosophers do not mean by "agent" only the principle of motion, as the natural philosophers mean, but the principle and giver of existence, as in the case of God with respect to the world. As for the natural efficient cause, it does not bestow any existence other than motion in one of the forms of motion. Thus, in the natural sciences, that which bestows existence is a principle of motion."[12] So, Avicenna considers his definition of the efficient cause as a giver of being to another to encompass both natural agents and creative agents.

One striking feature of Ibn Sīnā's account of causation is the use of the modal terms "necessary" and "possible" to analyze the causal relation, which emphasize his necessitation thesis: "with the existence of its cause, the existence of an effect is necessary". But Ibn Sīnā does not employ this thesis to restrict the scope of causal power to God. Ibn Sīnā defends the necessitation thesis in order to support his coexistence thesis, which states that cause and effect coexist in time, not in being. In other words, Avicenna considers the necessitation thesis to entail that the priority of cause to effect is ontological, not temporal.[13] In the

11 Marmura (M.E.) : Avicenna, op.cit, p. 194.

12 Marmura (M.E.) : Avicenna, op.cit, p. 195.

13 Marmura (M.E.) : "Avicenna on Causal Priority", in Morewedge, P. (ed.), 1981, Islamic Philosophy and Mysticism, Delmar: NY: Caravan Books, 1981, p. 67–68.

central part of the argument for the necessitation thesis, Avicenna attempts to show that the causal relation cannot be fully understood in terms of possibility.

Avicenna ultimately concludes that, with the existence of its cause, the existence of the effect is not merely possible, it is necessary too. So, with God's existence, the existence of the first existent, the first intellect, is necessary.[14] Since for Ibn Sīnā, a cause is concurrent with the existence of its effect, the former is then a source of becoming.

**a1- God as the Necessitating Existence:** For Ibn Sina God is the Necesseary Exitence (al- wâjib al-wujûd) as well as He is the Necessitating Existence (wâjib al-wujûd). Being the creator and Necessary Existence, God creates necessarly the things. He is then the Necessitating Existence and the First Cause. That is why he defines wâjib al-wujûd as ". . ...The First Cause named among philosophers as wâjib al-wujûd (necessisating existence) ."[15]

العلة الاولى المسماة عند الحكماء بواجب الوجود . . . .

**a2- Possible Existence as the Necessitating Existence**: As we have said the concept of wâjib al-wujûd is not used only for God but also for possible being or existence. Ibn Sīnā have indicated this for example in this statement:

و كل واجب الوجود فهو حق "And every necessitating existence is then real. . ."[16] Here it is obvious that "every necessitating existence" indicates the plurality of necessitating existence. Therefore by "every necessitating existence" Ibn Sīnā could not mean God, but he meant possible beings; as we have said that according to the causality theory of him possible beings become cause for each other . Then they become necessitating existences. As it is well known that Ibn Sina subdivides the concept of wâjib al-wujûd into two kinds as wâjib al-wujûd bi-thâtihî (the necessitating existence by virtue of itself) and wâjib al-wujûd bi-ghayrihî (the necessitating existence by virtue of another).[17] The first kind is God; the second kind is possible being.

---

14 Richardson (K.): " Causation in Arabic and Islamic Thought" Stanford Encyclopedia of Philosophy (2015): http://plato.stanford.edu/entries/arabic-islamic-causation/.,

15 Ibn Sīnā: Risâla al-Ziyâra, Jâmi' al-Badâi, Cairo, 1907, p. 33. The concept of wâjib al-wujûd mentioned in this statment is translated into French as Être nécessaire (Necessairy Being) by Goichon for example: La Cause premiêre nommée chez les philosophers Être nécessaire. See Goichon (A.-M.) : Lexique, op.cite, p. 417.

16 Ibn Sīnā: al- Shifâ', ed. and English trans. by M.E.Marmura : The Metapysics of the Healing, Brigham Young University Press, Provo, Utah, 2005, p.284. Marmura's transl. of the statement is this: " And all that is a necessary existent is truth." p. 284. But for us Marmura's translation is not so correct.

17 This subdivion is to be found nearly in all his philosophical works' metaphysical sections; see for example M.E.Marmura: The Metaphysics of the, p. 30, 32, 38; Ibn

**b- Gramatical construction:** The second reason for the difference in the meanings of the concepts of wâjib al-wujûd (دوجولا بجاولا) and wâjib al-wujûd (واجب الوجود ) is their gramatical construction; although their Arabic grammatical construction is nearly the same, yet there is an important difference in meaning to be noted. As you may see with a naked eye at first, there is Arabic artical al+ before the first wâjib, that's all. Now let'us try to explain that difference.

Since there is no problem on the meaning and translation of the concept of al-wâjib al-wujûd, we won't dwell on it. Here we will focus on wâjib al-wujûd. The word wâjib is the present participle (al-ism al-fâ'il) of Arabic verb Wa+Ja+Ba (literally to oblige, to necessitate, ect.). Wujûd (existence) is the infinitive (al-masdar) of the Arabic verb Wa+Ja+Da (literally to have found, to be known, ect.). As we know that according to Arabic grammar the present participle, which is derived from the verb and shows the doer in the verb, has some grammatical functions and can be used as a verb, as a noun and as an adjective in the sentence. When it is used without the Arabic article al+, in some cases it may function as Arabic simple present or present continuous tense, of course it depends of the context. So, for our undestanding the word wâjib in the concept of wâjib al-wujûd is the present participle of the verb Wa+ Ja+ Ba (to necessitate) and functions as the simple present .

Thus from this we could conclude that the concept of wâjib al-wujûd means as the necessitating existence, not as the necessary existence or being as it has been pretented and presented. For Ibn Sīnā God is both Necessary existence and Necessitating Existence at the same time,but the possible being can be only necessitating existence, when for Ibn Sīnā it becomes cause for another possible being. In order to explain this Ibn Sīnā gives this example: "... 4 is necessitating existence not by itself but on the supposition of 2+2,..."[18]

If our understanding of the concept of wâjib al-wujûd as the necessitating existence is accepted as valid, many questions may come to mind. One of them could be: will Avicenna's already translated works need to be re-translated? For

---

Sīnā: Kitâb al-Najât ed. by M.S.Kurdî, 2nd ed., Cairo, 1938, p. 224–227, 235. Although Ibn Rushd (Averroes, 1126–1198) says that Ibn Sīnā was first philosopher who made this subdivison, See. Tahâfut, ed. by. M.Bouyges, Beirut, 1930, p. 198, this is not correct becuase we know that before him al-Âmirî had made such a division. Ibn Sīnā has been severely criticized for this by Ibn Rushd,and especially by al-Shahristânî (1086–1153) in his Kitâb al-Musâra'a, Arabic edition and English translation of this book by W.Madelung and M. Toby: Struggling with the Philosopher, A Refutation of Avicenna's Metaphysics, London, 2000.

18 Ibn Sīnā: al-Najât, ed. by M.S.Kurdî, 2nd ed., Cairo, 1938, p. 224.

us, no. What could be then? The reader can do, if he wants of course, like the example we will give below, by detecting the sentences in which the concept of wâjib al-wujûd is mentioned. This can be easily done; the concept is not very frequently used in every of his works; each work may contain maximum 20 uses at most.

Here is our example: We have chosen Marmura's edition and English translation of Ibn Sīnā's al-Shifâ' (The Metaphysics of the Healing, Brigham Young University Press, Provo, Utah, 2005) page 32. He translated the concept of wâjib al-wujûd both as necessary existent and necessary existence. We put the word the Necessitating Existence in front of these necessary existent and necessary existence words as follows:

(7) We [further] say: It is impossible for the Necessary Existent[19] --- the Necessitating Existence — be equivalent to another necessary existent --- another necessitating existence --- so that this would exist with that and that would exist with this, neither being the cause of the other [but] both, rather, being equal with respect to the matter of the necessity of existence ---the Necessitating Existence---- [This is] because, if the essence of the one is considered in itself, apart from the other, then it would have to be either [(a)] necessary in itself or [(b)] not necessary in itself.

(8) If [(a)] necessary in itself, then either it would have also a necessity with respect to the other, whereby a thing would be both a necessary existent in itself - a Necessitating Existence in itself - and a necessary existent through another - a Necessitating Existence through another- (which, as we have seen, is impossible); or it would have no necessity by reason of another and, hence, it would not be necessary for its existence to be consequent on the existence of the other, and it follows necessarily that its existence would have no relation with the other such that it exists only when this other exists.

(9) But, if [(b)] it is not necessary in itself, then, considered in itself, it must be possible in existence and considered, with respect to the other, necessary in existence. From this it follows that either the other is of the same [state] or [it is] not. [If not, then it would not be equivalent in existence.] If the other is of the same [state], then it follows that the necessity of existence of this [one] derives from that [other] when that [other] is either [(i)] within the bounds of

19 Marmura's the Necessary Existent translation is not correct; because there we have wâjib al-wujûd concept, not wâjib al-mawjûd.

possible existence or [(ii)] within the bounds of necessary existence ---- the Necessitating Existence----."[20]

The second question might be: If Ibn Sīnā's concept wâjib al-wujûd was understood as the necessitating existence, as we suggest it, was he still severely criticized for this concept?

We know that Ibn Sina was firmly criticized for that concept by many theologians and philosophers, such as, for example, al-Ghazzâlî (d. 1111), al-Shahristani (1153), Ibn Rushd (d. 1198) and Ibn Taymiyyah (d.1328) because like many others they understood it as the necessary existence or necessary existent. What is wrong for them in the concept of wâjib al-wujûd? Since Ibn Sīnā used it for both God and possible or contingent beings, they criticized him by saying how a possible being becomes necessary being? But Ibn Sīnā never seen possible being as necessary being; the thinkers who criticized him for this misunderstood his concept of wâjib al-wujûd as we have said. For Ibn Sīnā the possible being's existence remain always possible, but when it becomes a cause for another possible being, because of this causation, it is named as wâjib al-wujud; then for the actual existence of that another possible being, the previous possible being becomes necessary; without which that another possible being could not come into actual existence. To explain this, let's give again Ibn Sina's own example that we have above referred to: ". . . 4 is necessitating existence[21] not by itself but on the supposition of 2+2,. . ."[22] Thus for the existence of 4, two piece two, 2+2, are necessary. We shall give our example: Parents and child; as existence and existent all are possible beings; but for the child, the parents are necessary; because without them he or she can not come into existence. And it is in this sense that Ibn Sina says: "What is not necessary does not exist."[23] The possible existence does not actually exist unless rendered necessary by another possible existence. The possibly existent can enter the domain of the actual existence only if a factor other than itself comes with existence. During the present of this factor, the existence of the possibly existent being become necessary.

20 Ibn Sīnā: al-Shifâ', ed. and transl. By M.E. Marmura:The Metapysics of the Healing, Brigham Young University Press, Provo, Utah, 2005, p.32.

21 The concept of wâjib al-wujûd In this sentences has been translated as necessary existence or necessary of existence by Goichon (A.-M.): La Distinction de l'Essence et de l'Existence d'apres Ibn Sînâ (Avicenne), Paris, 1938, p. 159; Carame (N.): Avicennae Metaphysices Compendium, Rome, 1926, p. 66; Hourani (G.F.): "Ibn Sīnā ", op.cit. p. 79.

22 Ibn Sīnā: al-Najât, op. cit., p. 224.

23 Ibn Sīnā: al-Najât, op. cit., p. 226.

An examination of Ibn Sīnā's works demonstrates that his concepts of Necessary Being and Necessitating Existence are placed in relation to his theology, ontology, and cosmology, and they are regarded as the *axis mundo* of his system of philosophy. The concepts have been used in two senses and can be categorized into two: that which is necessary by virtue of itself and that which necessary by virtue of another, as we have mentioned above.

Finally, we hope that this study will be the basis for new studies on Ibn Sīnā' metaphysics and ontology in the future.

## Short Biography of Mehmet Bayrakdar

He was born in 1952 in Konya's Beyşehir District. He graduated from Ankara University Faculty of Theology in 1973. Between 1973-1978, he completed his master's and doctorate degrees in Philosophy and Islamic Science at Paris Sorbonne University in the field of Islamic Philosophy. He worked as a lecturer in Ankara University Faculty of Theology for many years.

He was a member of the Religious Affairs High Board of the Presidency of Religious Affairs. Visiting faculty at the University of London (1986-1987), USA Georgetown University (1988-1989), International Islamic Institute of Malaysia (1990-1993), Gregoriana University of Rome in Italy (1999-2000) and Kyoto University of Japan (2000-2001) served as a member. He is currently working in the Department of Anthropology at Yeditepe University Faculty of Arts and Sciences.

Bayrakdar, who knows Arabic, Persian, Italian, French, Spanish, English, Latin, Greek and Japanese, has some of his published works: Introduction to Islamic Philosophy, History of Science and Technology in Islam, La Philosophie Mystique chez Dawud de Kayseri, Phenomonology of Worship in Islam., Sufism and Modern Science, Islam and Ecology, Evolutionist Creation Theory in Islam, Davut from Kayseri, Idris-i Bitlisi, Freedom of Thought in Islam, Philosophy of Love in Yunus Emre, Introduction to Philosophy of Religion, History of Islamic Thought, A Christian Dogma: Trinity.

Prof. Dr. Dana Baran, M.D., Ph.D.

# Ibn Sina - Avicenna, A Medico-Historical Paradigm

*Abstract.* Ibn Sina`s work illustrates a transtemporal, transregional, transnational, transconfessional and transgenerational medical paradigm. His writings dealt with anatomy and physiology, pathology, pharmacology and therapy, epidemics and hygiene principles, obstetrics and neonatology, with both clinical and experimental medicine. Art, poetry and music, moral rules, an enriched pharmacopoeia, psychotherapy and physiokineto-therapy achieved treatment targets in the individual's body, soul and mind. Ibn Sina-Avicenna revisited outstanding Greek and Roman authors in an original manner. Transgressing limits, his medical epistemology was taught and analyzed by scholars of his time and his spiritual space, as well as by their followers throughout centuries, on a universal level. Together with Hippocrates and Galen, Avicenna became one of the three pillars - "three magi of Orient" - of medieval medical education. Concurrently, he constituted a reference point for Arabic medicine itself. Nascent modern medicine owed him a lot in the transition from the Middle Ages to the Renaissance, since Ibn Sina bridged Oriental and Occidental mentalities and practices. In medieval Princely Schools from the Romanian Provinces of Moldavia and Wallachia, Avicenna's medicine could have been taught as iatrosophia. Political connections and cultural influences the Ottoman Empire exerted until the dawn of the XIX$^{th}$ century, probably enabled the presence of Avicennian ideas in this region too.

**Keywords:** *Ibn Sina, Romanian Provinces, medicine, paradigm*

***General Background***. Whereas the Middle Ages were a "twilight zone" in Western Europe, they soon became a luminous area in the Eastern Islamic world. From the IX$^{th}$ to the XII$^{th}$ century, the Golden Epoch of the Islam facilitated the birth of Arab humanism, that assimilated the cultural and scientific traditions of many other indigenous peoples who preceded the Arab - Islamic civilisation. (Anghelescu 2009) Muslim scientists, doctors and engineers contributed to the technology of medieval Europe by preserving and greatly enriching their substantial heritage by their own inventions, innovations and expertise.

At the crossroads between Europe and Asia Minor, in the Middle East, important medical centers already existed since the Byzantine period: the academy and hospital of Edessa was one of them, while Gundeshapur (Gondishapur) turned into a flourishing city renowned for its medical school, hospital and academic erudition under the Sassanids in the VI[th] century. In 489, the Nestorian theological and scientific center in Edessa was closed by the Byzantine Emperor Zeno. The School of Nisibis (Nisibīn) resulted, where pagan, Christian, Hebrew and Arab scholars and philosophers carried out translations and original research in medicine, astronomy and mathematics. Education and training were offered in philosophy, theology, medicine and other sciences.(Hill 1993)

Greek philosophers, Nestorian Assyrian monks and lay persons fled religious persecution by the Byzantine Empire and took refuge in this region, contributing to its progress. In the VI[th] century, during the Sassanid Emperor Chosroes, Gondeshapur gained its medical and academic fame. The Sassanid ruler asked doctor Borzuya to invite also Indian and Chinese scholars to Gundeshapur in order to continue their valuable activity there.

Even though in the VII[th] century the Muslim Arab armies defeated the Sassanid dynasty, Gundishapur maintained its university status, as a place for higher learning. The tremendous translation effort was perpetuated, and the most significant writings continued to be converted from Greek to Arabic, from Syriac to Arabic, from Greek to Syriac or other local dialects. Unlike medieval Christianity, Islam proved to impose more permissive religious constraints at that time, enabling interethnic, interconfessional and multilinguistic collaboration in various fileds of the social and scientific life, including medicine, astronomy, astrology, philosophy, useful crafts. However, by and by, Gondishapur, a prominent "House of Wisdom", had to give way to Bagdad, the new brilliant academic city that arose during the Golden Age of Islam.

***Medicine, a Universal Science.*** Since man is the focus of the Universe and of every day life, medicine itself is a global science. Ibn Sina`s endeavour to master and link together various complementary aspects of human life forged a synchronic and diachronic holistic medical paradigm, engendering multifaceted "morphogenetic frames" that propitiated the progress of the healing art as a whole, in an integrative form: anatomy and physiology, but also psychology, pharmocological and non-pharmacological therapies, surgery and sports, preventive medicine, ethical and deontological behaviour, education, music- and arts- therapy. (Sufie and Sidik 2017) In good keeping with Plato (428/427 or 424/423–348/347 BC) and Aristotle (384–322 BC), from ethics to aesthetics, art treatments helped individuals achieve *mimesis* and *catharsis,* getting rid in part of their troubles.(Turker 2010) Under these circumstances, more than ever maybe, medicine revealed its unity and universal character encompassing both human and non-human living beings. Not only did the Eastern Arab world take over the impressive treasure of knowledge handed down by Antiquity, but it equally encouraged its preservation, further selection, enhancement and deepening of concepts, methods and practical knowledge that stood the test of time. It was in this proficient and stimulating cultural environment that Ibn Sina - Avicenna (980, Afshanah, near Bukhara-1037, Hamadan) lived and trained himself as a polymath, a "universal man", an encyclopedic personality. (Fig.1)

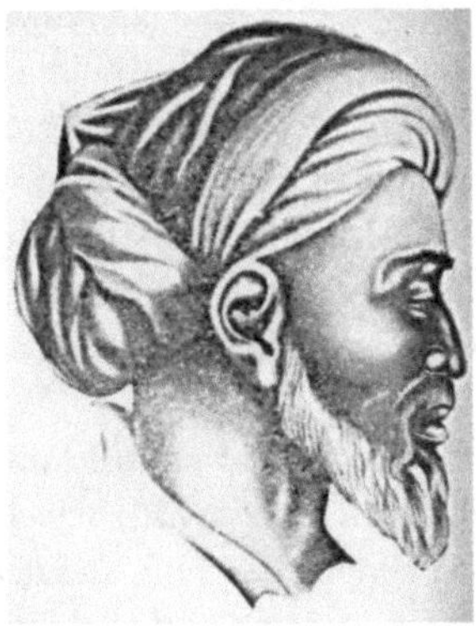

**Fig. 1.** Ibn Sina's portrait such as the Russian archaeologist and anthropologist Mikhail M. Gherasimov reconstructed it, in accordance with the size and morphology of the Persian scientist's skull.

***From the Dark Ages to the Renaissance.*** Avicenna's meandering paradigmatic destiny marked a step forward on the way towards a more rational evidence-based medicine. During a lifetime experience with ups and downs, a labyrinth pathway with many obstacles to overcome, so close to his "Hayy ibn Yaqzhan's Story" - *The story of the Living Son of the Awake One* or *Alive*, son of *Awake*. (Ibn Sina 2014) He studied and wrote in the field of mathematics, music and astronomy, law, logic, ethics and philosophy, besides medicine - anatomy, physiognomy included, physiology, clinical pathology, *materia medica*, surgery, massage and physical exercises, travel medicine and epidemiology –, alchemy, geology, geography, psychology, Islamic theology, physics, metaphysics, and poetry. Among others, Ibn Sina followed in the footsteps of Al Razi - Rhazes (c.854–925), an impressive Arab forefather, and was acquainted with the contribution of Ali ibn-Ul Abbas (930–994). To this worthy heritage he added his personal observations and conclusions reached during discussions with his own patients, while he was admiring, mastering, critically compiling and reconsidering the works of noteworthy Greek masters - Hippocrates via Galen, Galen himself and Dioscorides, along with Aristotle and Plato. Avicenna succeeded in combining these complex, yet classical medical approaches that structured the healing art over time, setting up an original theoretical and practical synthesis, an extremely useful working tool, an original all-encompassing medical paradigm.

A brilliant figure in the history of medicine, the "Preeminent Master" after Aristotle, whom Avicenna called "The First Teacher", he had "the mind of Goethe and the genius of Leonardo da Vinci". In *La Divina Comedia,* Dante placed him in the Limbo, whereas Chaucer mentioned him in *The Canterbury Tales.* Most explicable details, since, indeed, according to Manfred Ullmann: "For long the rule held that he who would be a good doctor must be a good Avicennist". (Ullmann 1978, Modanlou 2011)*Gül A.* Russell added that Western European intellectual tradition "would be difficult to imagine without Avicenna's influence on specific individuals in addition to his many-layered complex legacy in diverse areas". (Russell, 2003)

The way from Ancient Greece and Rome to Islamic Renaissance humanism had been a long and difficult one, along which scientists acquired wisdom and better understanding of the phenomena of life and death at the level of both the macrocosm and the microcosm, of soma and soul, body and mind, religion and rationality, reality and phantasy. By "error and trial" they investigated their own nature and that of the Universe, pain and happiness, mood disorders and physical suffering. As Ibn Sina used to say, from a medical point of view physicians should either conserve or recover health: "Medicine is the science by which we learn the various states of the human body, in health, [and] when not in health, the means by which health is likely to be lost, and when lost, is likely to be restored to health. In other words, it is the art whereby health is conserved and the art whereby it is restored, after being lost." (*The Canon of Medicine*) (Smith 1980) The physician should always be able to rebalance the four basic elements, the four humours, and their four properties, identifying the right cure in keeping with the patient`s peculiarities, disease and temperament or constitution.

***The Canon of Medicine.*** A fundamental book – *The Law of Medicine*, a medical authority, *The Canon* (*Al-Qānūn fī al-ṭibb*) impacted Western European medicine and was part of medical curricula of Christian universities for about 500 years, since the XII$^{th}$ almost until the XVII$^{th}$ century. (Fig.2)

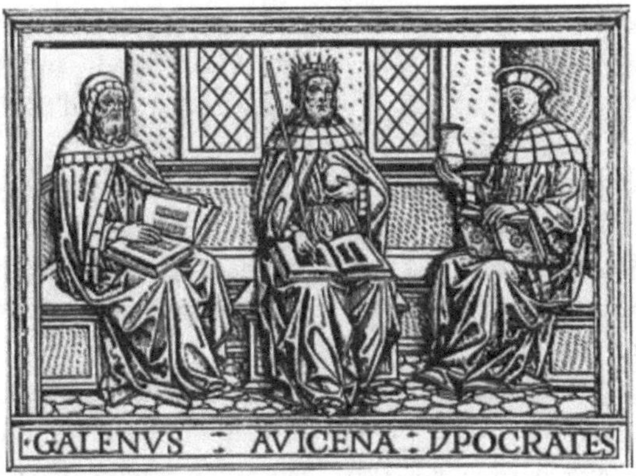


**Fig. 2.** "Sacred conversation" of the "Three Magi of Orient" in Medicine: Avicenna flanked by Hippocrates (right) and Galen (left)

Nevertheless, eventually it was severely criticized and rejected by Paracelsus (1493–1541), another outstanding contributor to clinical medicine and pharmacology.

The Canon included five books that illustrated medical knowledge from Hippocrates (c. 460 – c. 370 BC) to Galen (129–210 AD), fit into Aristotle`s natural philosophy (IV$^{th}$ century BC), and combined to ideas of that very period, the X$^{th}$ -XI$^{th}$ centuries. It was completed in 1025. Books I, III and IV were each further divided into parts *(fanns)*, chapters *(ta'līms)*, subchapters *(jumlahs)*, sections *(faṣls)*, and subsections *(bābs)*. These volumes dealt with:

*Book I* – elements, humors and temperaments; problems of anatomy, functions of physical structures; basic medical and physiological principles; course of medical treatment, diet, and/or exercise for conserving or restoring health; the importance of environmental factors on health condition – i.e. that of unpolluted air, water, soil; recognition of contagiousness of several infectious diseases; general therapeutic procedures; according to Avicenna, in medicine both the causes of health and those of diseases had to be known.

*Book II* – description of about 800 simple medical substances - herbal, mineral, and of animal origin - were listed alphabetically, followed by an essay on their general pharmacodynamic properties and their substitutes; all drugs were considered to have the same four properties as disease-heat, cold, dryness and moisture; this *Materia Medica* also comprised seven rules for experimenting with new drugs, partly inspired from Galen; "The recognition of the strengths of the characteristics of medicines through experimentation" was the earliest known treatise related to clinical trials and similarities with modern concepts of pharmacology and clinical trials were identified (Sajadi et al); Ibn Sina elaborated himself methods for assessing drug efficiency and laid the basis for experimental pharmacology.

*Book III* – diagnoses and treatments for diseases specific to each organ or part of the body - special pathology; for each disease etiology, symptoms, diagnosis, prognosis, and treatment were specified; special attention was paid to stroke, intemperaments of the brain; headache; epilepsy, paralysis, meningitis, lovesickness etc; sexual disorders.

*Book IV* – diagnoses and treatments for illnesses covering multiple body parts of or the whole body: fevers and poisoning, along with wounds and bone fractures were included; personal hygiene principles emphasized care of the hair, skin, nails, body odor, and the treatment of overweight and underweight conditions.

*Book V* – the Formulary, i.e., preparation of 650 compound drugs from Arabic, Indian and Greek sources, but original ones, too; he trusted remedies previously tested through experience, and supposed that compounds could have unexpected or stronger effects than expected from the effects of their individual components; the volume provided information about the complex forms of drugs such as powders, teas, juices, infusions, ointments, syrups, jams, oils, etc. and their application for various diseases.

***"Globalisation" of the Canon.*** Towards the end of the XII$^{th}$ century the *Canon* was translated into Latin in Toledo (central Spain) by Gerardo da Cremona or Sabbioneta (Gerardo Cremonensis Sabloneta), an Italian born representative of the Toledo School of Translators. It exerted an enormous impact on medieval medicine ever since. Ibn Sina's writings became first known and used by the medical schools of Salerno (Southern Italy), founded at the dawn of the IX$^{th}$ century, and of Montpellier (Southern France), that probably appeared as early as 1137, and where physicians trained in Salerno and in Spain already taught by then. One should equally mention that in Salerno many translations were performed as well, the first of them being ascribed to Constantine the African (he probably died before 1098/1099), a physician and a Benedictine monk. Besides, it was not haphazardly that in accordance with the legend, the School of Salerno was established by four doctors, symbols of four great medical traditions: the Latin Salerno, the Greek Ponto, the Jew Elino and the Arab Adela (Abdulah). And undoubtedly the city of Salerno was a crossroads of various peoples, religions and cultures, a real "melting pot" of humanity. In fact, medicine has always been a transnational, transconfessional and translinguistic science, transgressing barriers and setting up its own "hyper-empire of knowledge".

Ibn Sina`s *Canon* - a standard medical textbook - greatly influenced medieval and renaissance medical teaching in both Arab and Western European schools. "*The Book*" represented an important text in Unani medicine until nowadays, too. A sort of traditional Perso-Arabic medicine practiced in India, the Unani healing art derived from the teachings of the Greek physicians Hippocrates and Galen, but concurrently it was influenced by Indian and Chinese traditional medical systems and by Arabic medicine, as well. As generally admitted, Greek medicine was a source of inspiration for both Al-Razi – Rhazes and Ibn Sina Avicenna, who in turn left their mark on Unani medical theory and practice.

Unani healing art promoted a complex medical system, based on observations, methodical experimentation and deductions.Its content reflected and summed up ideas and practices from ancient Greek and Roman writings, as well as from Arabic, Ayurvedic, Persian, Indian, and Chinese ones. At the same time it assimilated influences of other East-Asian cultures.

***Iatrophysics.*** Many aspects of human anatomy, pathology and therapy ere characterised from a physical or biomechanical standpoint. Apart from details concerning disorders of ocular structures that accompany cataract formation, data concerning the operative technique were specified, together with methods for reestablishing the humoral balance. (Nejabat et al 2012) Other writings focused on biomechanical aspects of the skeleton and traumatology, the shape and mechanical forces involved in scar formation and shaping. Techniques for reducing fractures and dislocations were described, along with massage methods. Manual tasks were associated to an improved lifestyle, diet and antalgic and sedative remedies.(Choopani et al 2016) Effects of massage depended on its intensity and direction. Movements could be round, straight, or repeated; frictions could be hard, moderately hard, rough, gentle or soft. Massage diminished fat accumulation in the body, could relax or contract muscles, detoxify or enhance muscle force. Frictions either strengthened the musculature and the body, or increased blood flow rate. They were preparative for or restorative after physical exercises, able to soothe pain and repair exhaustion. Exercises called "Riazat", described in the first book of the Canon, interfered with waste material elimination, internal heat and humours. Correctly and timely used, physical exercise could help both prophyalxis and treatment of diseases. In their turn, riding and walking were recommended. Avicenna also described some illnesses possibly due to physical inactivity.(Siahpoosh et al 2012)

***Iatrochemistry.*** Ibn Sina not only prepared classic drugs and remedies, but he invented some others. His new recipes were aimed at rebalancing the four humours, elements, and their properties of being wet and dry, cold and hot, a theory that resisted centuries, since Hippocrates, passing through Galen and their followers. Alchemic procedures were applied for obtaining such remedies: calcination, dissolution, separation, conjunction, fermentation, distillation, coagulation. Even though Ibn Sina was not an alchemist and did not believe in gold production by transmutation of base metals, he authored four studies on this topic, adopting a critical, rational approach. He was particularly interested in the use of herbal medicines and biologically active points for various diseases and he described about 800 plant remedies. (Aliasl and Khoshzaban 2013)

***Experimental medicine***. Precise observation and accurate experimentation were a *sine qua non* tandem in Ibn Sina`s activity.

**A. *Psychosomatic disorders***. A classic psychological experiment Avicenna performed focused on self-awareness, consciousness and fear in animals, observing the effect on health status.(Alwishah 2016) Two identical lambs were placed in two separate cages, and a wolf was put in one side cage. Only one lamb could see the wolf while for the other the wolf remained out of sight. Months after, the lamb who saw the wolf died out of stress and fear, even though the wolf did not physically aggress him. The control lamb lived on. Two problems were studied by this experiment: one concerned animals` consciousness whereas the other bore on the negative emotions the wolf`s presence induced in the lamb who did perceive his presence and who eventually ended up in anxiety, neurosis and death.

Ibn Sina grounded his psychology on physiology. His account of the soul was in keeping with the natural science of the body and its abilities of perception. The philosopher psychologist explained connection between soul and body by his understanding of perception: bodily perception interrelated with the immaterial human intellect. In sense perception, the perceiver sensed the object by his external senses. This sensory information was then supplied to the internal senses, able to merge everything into a whole, unified conscious experience.

As a matter of fact, extrapolating the data to humans, Ibn Sina always took into account both the physical and mental status of his patients and tried to treat them not only from a materialist point of view, but also emotionally.

**B. *Pharmacological experiments***. Partly inspired by Galen, these rules and conclusions were meant to determine the pharmacodynamic features of various remedies and drugs.

Seven conditions for "The recognition of the strengths of the characteristics of medicines through experimentation" were dealt with:

1. *The drug must be free from any acquired quality*: the drug should not be submitted to other environmental influences.
2. *The experiment must be done on a single, not a composite condition*: it should not be tested on patients with multiple illnesses.
3. *The drug must be tested on two contrary conditions*: a drug may act directly on a disease and be effective against a different disease by relieving its symptoms.
4. *The quality of the drug must correspond to the strength of the disease*: it is best to experiment first using the weakest [dosage] and then increase it gradually until the potency of the drug is known, i.e., the efficient dose is defined; *drugs potency could be told in two ways, by analogy (qiyas) and by experiment (tajribah).*
5. *One should consider the time needed for the drug to take effect. If the drug has an immediate effect, this shows that it has acted against the disease itself.*
6. *The effect of the drug should be the same in all cases or, at least, in most. If that is not the case, the effect is then accidental, because things that occur naturally are always or mostly consistent*: drug specificity.
7. *Experiments should be carried out on the human body [. ].the quality of the medicine might mean that it would affect the human body differently from the animal body.* (Nasser et al 2009)

***Iatromathematics***. Traditionally, medical astrology was equally known as iatromathematics and investigated the association between various parts of the body, diseases, and drug effects with influences exerted by the sun, moon, planets, and the twelve astrological signs. The time of day, light-dark cycles, the seasaons were medically significant periodicities, too. The zodiac man perfectly illustrated this tight interrelationship connecting the human microcosm to the environmental macrocosm. Avicenna did not cultivate astrology, a foretelling ability, but astronomy. He considered that each planet had some influence on the earth, and in general, the environment had a huge impact on human health and disease contition. The same is true in today *Chrono(astro)biology*, which expresses modulating links between environmental cycles and biospheric time structures or chronomes (Halberg). (Otsuka et al 2016)

***Clinical medicine***. It was around the IX$^{th}$ century that the expanding Islamic world turned into a center of arts and sciences, medicine included. Hospitals were established, original therapies developed, and ethical principles applied. The first documented and reputed general hospital (*bimaristan*) in the Islamic territories was that in Baghdad, inaugurated in 805 by Caliph Harun al-Rashid. It was preceded in 706 by a hospital for lepers, blind and poor people, in Damascus due to the Umayyad Caliph Al-Walid, and another one possibly in Cairo.(Sayili 2006) At the same time, *bimaristans* were institutions for medical education, for hospital or bedside teaching, where the principle of associative learning functioned. (Modanlou 2011) First introduced by Ibn Sina in Book VI of the "Kitab al-Shifa" (*The Book of Healing*), it became part of scholastic educational methods, as well. Ibn Sina authored a synthetic and encompassing work where all the aspects of a diseases and a diseased person were characterised. Three states of the human body were distinguished: sickness, health and an intermediate one which was neither disease nor health. Symptoms and for the first time syndromes were defined, thoroughly analysed and correlated with the fundamental elements, humours, their basic properties, individual physiognomy and temperament. The patient`s physical examination comprised inspection, uroscopy, palpation, direct auscultation. As things happened with other doctors, like Erasistratus e.g., pulse was assessed and psycho-emotional, neuro-vegetative reactions carefully noted, e.g., in lovesickness. Knowing by causes was essential and largely supported Avicenna`s good sense of dignosis. The pathophysiological approach gave an idea of the illnesses etiology. The detailed description of signs, symptoms, and syndromes oriented the diagnosis, hence the therapy aimed at rebalancing human body and soul, as a whole. The means by which health was likely to be lost indicated how exactly it was likely to be restored. Sanogenetic reconstruction had to compensate for the pathological deconstruction.

***Preventive Medicine and Hygiene.*** In Avicenna`s opinion, medicine was not only about getting rid of pain and suffering, but equally about preserving good health. It was a sanogenetic medicine, able to prevent and cure the diseases. Medicine was the sum of hygiene and treatment. He defined four stages of life: growth, adulthood (the prime of life), elderly decline and decrepitude. Hygiene was important since the very beginning of one`s life course until old age and death: healthy eating, drinking, performing sports, sleep quality and quantity, along with various environmental factors could impact health condition differently according to age. Neonatology and pediatric medicine, together with medicine of the elderly were dealt with by this outstanding medical thinker. The newborn infant hygiene, breastfeeding and upbringing were discussed, and advice was given on physical, nutritional and psychological care of the child. (Modanlou 2011) Old age preoccupied Ibn Sina: premature aging, the relationship between age and susceptibility, vulnerability and resistance to diseases, care for the elderly were topics also addressed in his "Canon".(Hatami 2001)

As to contagious diseases, which were quite frequent at that time, he formulated criteria for differential diagnosis between plague and cholera, he understood that tuberculosis was a communicable illness and in his writings these subjects were tackled in a most specific and reasonable way. Avicenna referred to the association between rats and plague in his description of the epidemic in Mesopotamia about the year 1000 A.D. He mentioned elements predicting epidemics and four etiological factors for transmissible diseases: bad quality of air, water, soil/Earth, and impact of celestial bodies. Preventive measures during epidemics consisted in restriction of movement, social distancing, isolation or quarantene, fumigations, use of vinegar, antidotes (theriac) and diet: avoiding milk, oil, sweet, meat, and alcohol.(Alam et al 2020) To a certain extent these ideas were comparable to those Hippocrates had expressed in his book "On epidemics".

***Philosophy and medical ethics.*** Often considered an Aristotelian or a Neoplatonist, Avicenna`s rationalism and esotericism incorporated the entire Oriental thinking of his time, as *The Book of Healing* reveals, too. As far as Universalia were concerned, Ibn Sina`s formula was shared by other Arab scholars but also by Toma d`Aquino, one of Ibn Sina`s admirers. In fact, the Westen European world was quite acquainted with the ideas and interpretations of the Arab "Prince of Philosophers" and "Prince of Medicine", for whom "the intellect ellaborates universality in essence-forms". In his famous "Flying Man", he meditated on human intellect or self-awareness, on the soul and its immortality, concluding that consciousness of the self could not be denied and that it was "independent from the material body", i.e. beyond sense data (perception and memory of perception): I think – I understand / I am aware of – I am. In this respect, Ibn Sina`s epistemology was often compared to Descartes` "Cogito, ergo sum".(Black 2008)

And, similarly to Descartes, he was interested in optics and the perception of light.

Even though influenced by sufism and mysticism, Avicenna remained a rational personality with a realistic approach to medicine and sick people.

Directly linked to philosophy and theology, to universals and essences, ethics, as a scientific discipline, held a significant place in the work of prominent oriental thinkers like Avicenna, one of the most brilliant minds of the Middle Ages and Pre-Renaissance. His religious and philosophical background, his socio-humanitarian ideas helped him adopt an ethical and deontological attitude towards human beings in general, towards the poor and the diseased, in particular. Supporting the patient and mastering his own profession were two prerequisites for a good, self-confident physician. "The physician's countenance should be pleasant, and his encouraging words increase the potency of the warmth inherent in man's natural temperament." (Levy 1957) Ibn Sina's principles "On Ethics" were obviously in accordance with those of the Hipocratic Oath. Avicenna was equally concerned with the concept and reality of natural death from a psychological, medical and religious standpoint, aspects of palliative medicine that contemporary bioethics continues to investigate and apply. Maintaining the patient's faith in spiritual and moral immortality of the soul is still a complex and often contradictory topic. Avicenna's philosophy and ethics of death ensued from his moral comprehension of life.

***Ibn Sina and some of his connections to Romania.*** The fame Ibn Sina gained in the Ottoman Empire, on the one hand, and its vicinity with the Romanian Countries of Moldavia an Wallachia, could have enabled exchanges of medical information. (Fig.3) However, it is surmised that some physicians coming from the Eastern world could have been familiar with Avicenna's teachings.

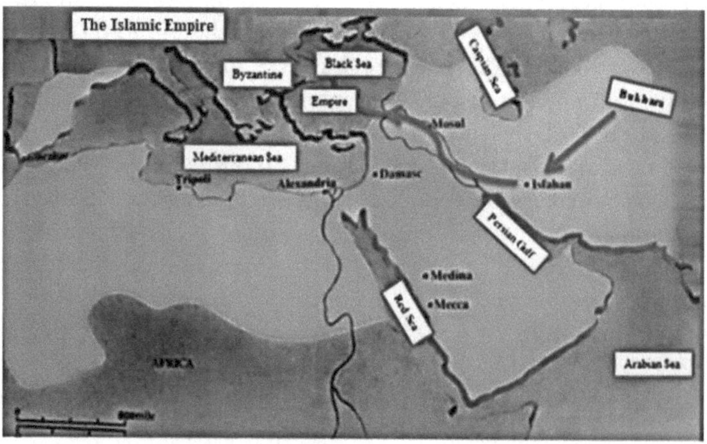


**Fig. 3.** Map of the Islamic Empire during its maximum expansion. The arrows indicate the roads from Bukhara to Isfahan, the Byzantine Empire, the Black Sea and the territories of present day Romania

One such case probably was that of Isaac Beg, a Spanish born Hebrew doctor and diplomate who came to assist Moldavia's Ruling Prince, Stephen the Great, severely ill, who in fact died in 1502[1]. (Halévy 1956) Other medical

1 Isaac Beg was not only a doctor, but a "contact man" between Persia, the Holy Seat; Venice, Hungary and Moldavia.

doctors coming to the Romanian Lands who graduated from Western European Universities, such as Padua, Ferrara, Bologna, Vienna, or Pesta, but from Oriental ones as well, knew Ibn Sina's work, even though in their writings they emphasised the importance of ancient Greek and Roman medical personalities and tradition.

On the other hand, in the XVI$^{th}$ century Academies of Sciences were established in Iasi and Bucharest where "iatrosophia", i.e. theoretical medicine, was taught, debating upon the aphorisms of Hippocrates, Galen's writings and Ibn Sina (Avicenna)'s concepts. Highly learned Greek professors, such as Nicholaos Kerameus (early XVII$^{th}$ century-c.1663), Ioannis Comnenus Molyvdos (c.1657–c.1717) and Markos Porphyropoulos (1660–1716), trained both in Eastern and Western European schools, traveled to Moldavia and Wallachia, and worked in these Princely Academies, supposedly teaching general medical ideas, too. Towards the end of the XVII$^{th}$ and the dawn of the XVIII$^{th}$ centuries, Dimitrie Cantemir (1673–1723), a famed polymath and polyglot, the philosopher Ruling Prince of Moldavia (1710–1711), became familiar with Ibn Sina's scientific, and particularly philosophical writings, during his long stay as a hostage in Istanbul. Cantemir was an excellent specialist in Ottoman music. (Karabaşoğlu 2015), But he also got initiated into medicine by the diplomat and medical doctor Alexander Mavrocordatos "the Exaporite" at the Patriarchal School of Constantinople.

He was soon replaced on the throne by a Greek born ruler of Moldavia and then of Wallachia, Nicholaos Mavrocordatos (1670–1730). Son to Alexandros Mavrocordatos "the Exaporite" - "keeper of the Secrets" in Constantinople, Nicholas was a humanist, a polyglot diplomat and physician, able to speak Arabic and Persian, as most of the contemporary intellectual elite. He refounded in Iasi the Academy of Sciences, where iatrosophia would have found its place once again. Nicholaos Mavrocordatos owned a famous library, with medical books, as well.

In 1937, on June 21$^{st}$, on the occasion of the 900$^{th}$ anniversary of Avicenna's death, the Turkish Society of History organised a congress and published a volume dedicated to Ibn Sina's life and work. The book also included a study by Dr. Victor Gomoiu, President by then of the International Society for the History of Medicine (ISHM), and honorary president of the Romanian Society for the History of Medicine, he had established in 1929. (Fig.4) Dr. Gomoiu, together with the Dr. Jean-Joseph Tricot-Royer, ISHM founding member and honorary president, supported in their lectures not only the paramount role Ibn Sina played in the progress of Western medicine, but, paradoxically, they concurrently strove to prove the Turkish origin of this scientist of Tajik–Persian descent, an erroneus hypothesis.(Gomoiu1937)Remarkably, Victor Gomoiu possessed in his valuable bibliophile collection a copy of Ibn Sina`s "Canon" in Latin, dating from the XVI$^{th}$ century (1512–1556): *"Avicennae Medicorum Arabum Principii Liber Canonis"*. (Scheau et al 2013) Due to his numerous contributions in the medical field, Avicenna was often called, indeed, the "Arabian Prince of Medicine".

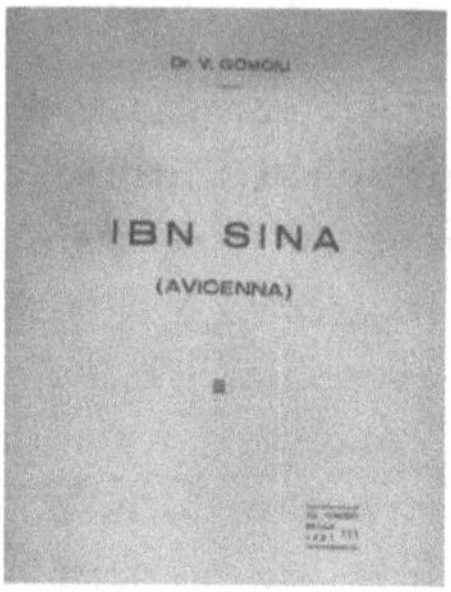


**Fig. 4.** Dr. V. Gomoiu. *Ibn Sina (Avicenna)*, Presa Publishing House, Braila, 1937

In 1962 Ibn Sina`s "Poem of Medicine" and an abbreviated version of "The Canon of Medical Sciences" were edited in Romanian language, with an introductory study by Dr. Gheorghe Bratescu.(Bratescu, 1962) (Fig.5) Other writings of this remarkable scholar appeared later and essays of him were included in various books dealing with the Arab-Islamic civilisation and its prominent personalities.(Fig.6)

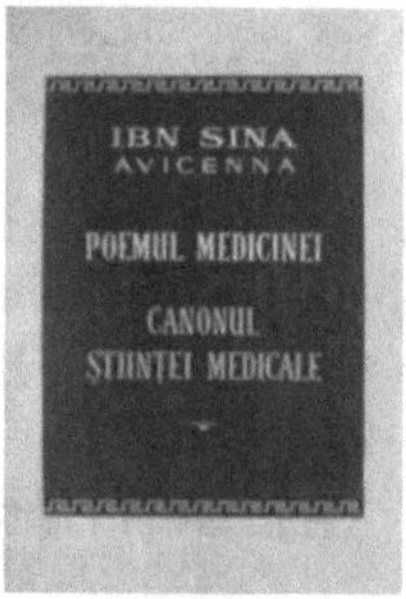


**Fig. 5.** Ibn Sina. *The Poem of Medicine. The Canon of Medical Science*, Medical Publishing House, Bucharest, 1962.

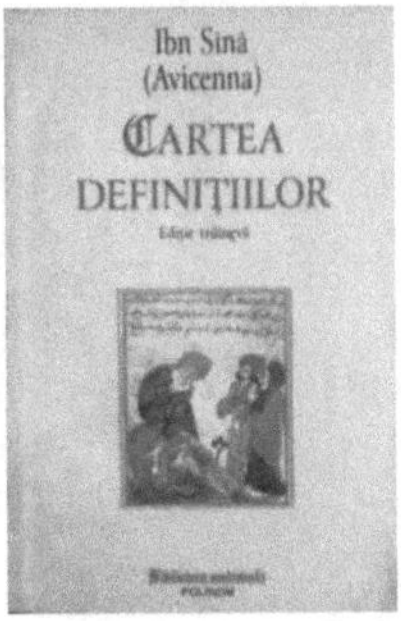


**Fig. 6.** Ibn Sina. *Book of definitions*, Polirom Publishing House, Iasi, 2012.

Lately, medical centers, clinics and computer centers were created in Romania, bearing Ibn Sina - Avicenna's name.(Fig.7, Fig.8) Established in April 2012, the "Avicenna" Profertis Clinic in Iasi, e.g., is involved in assisted human reproduction (IVF). It belongs to an international network, including centers in France, Great Britain, and Slovakia. Apart from *in vitro* fertilization (IVF) methods, specializations of this medical clinic are obstetrics-gynecology, ultrasound and plastic surgery. "Avicena" Profertis Clinic has been the only medical center in Romania to own a PrimoVision™ device for evaluating the quality of embryos in order to increase IVF success rate. Avicenna's memory is also perpetuated by devices named after him: Avicenna Robot is such an example. In 2015, in Bucharest, Professor Petrisor Geavlete used for the first time in Romania an Avicenna Roboflex system to perform flexible ureteroscopy and lithotripsy for renal calculi. This relatively minimally invasive endourological procedure, pioneered by Prof. Dr. Remzi Saglam (Turkey), revealed to be safer and with much better outcomes.(Geavlete et al 2016)

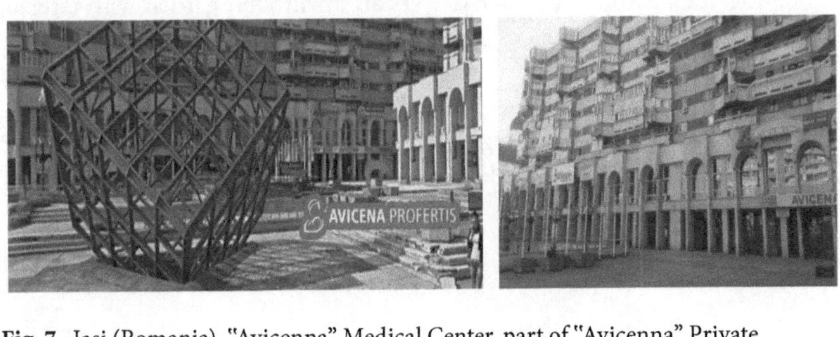


**Fig. 7.** Iasi (Romania). "Avicenna" Medical Center, part of "Avicenna" Private Hospital Network

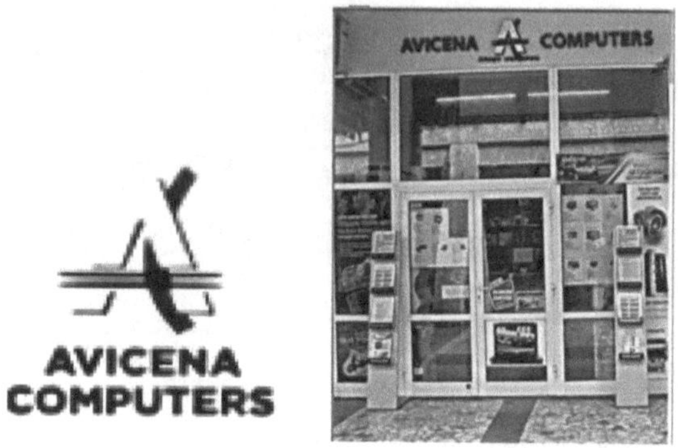


**Fig. 8.** Iasi (Romania). "Avicenna" Computer Centre (since 1996)

***Knowledge is power.*** Ibn Sina`s complex medical model undoubtedly illustrates an integrative, allopathic and homeopathic, psychosomatic and philosopical approach, able to associate evidence based practice and experimental data. For today`s modern medicine "The Canon", along with many other texts, remains a reference writing, a "nomadic" ubiquitous historic masterpiece that already turned into a handbook of complementary and alternative medicine, still inspiring traditional practices and folk directions, potentially building up a possible holistic medicine of the future. Not only did he focus on the unity of knowledge, developing an encyclopedic vision of the human world, but he demonstrated that somehow "globalisation" always existed and information has constantly been among the best shared things in the world. A wandering philosopher, Ibn Sina was constantly in search for his own and mankind`s true identity, a precondition for well-being and perfect health.

Significantly, traveling through the enchanted paradise of sciences that belong together, through the eternal Persian meditation garden with trees of life, reviving waters and lots of books of wisdom, Ibn Sina ended up his life journey in Hamadan, city of the symbolic "Silent Academy" of the immortals. His cross-cultural heritage proved originality and usefulness, as an ever since renewed transtemporal - transregional - transnational - transconfessional and transgenerational working paradigm.

## References


1. Anghelescu Nadia (2009). [*Arab Identity. History, language, culture*], Polirom Publishing House, Iasi, pp: 169–188.
2. Hill R. D. (1993). *Islamic Science and Engineering.* Edinburgh University Press.
3. Sufie S.N.M., Sidik R. (2017), *What is Medical Music Therapy in Islamic Civilization?,* International Journal of Business and Social Science, 8; 3:195–199.
4. Turker H. (2010). *A Discussion of the Aesthetic Views of Ibn Sina and Aristotle on the Basis of Aesthetic Value*, In: Tymieniecka AT., Muhtaroglu N. (eds) *Classic Issues in Islamic Philosophy and Theology Today. Islamic Philosophy and Occidental Phenomenology in Dialogue*, Springer, Dordrecht, vol 4. pp: 151–170.
5. Ibn Sina (2014). *Hayy ibn Yaqzhan's Story*, in Grete Tartler, [*Arab Wisdom. V-XV centuries*], Polirom Publishing House, Iasi, pp: 304–13.
6. Ullmann M.(1978). *Islamic Medicine [ Islamic Surveys II ]*. Edinburgh, University Press
7. Modanlou H.D.(2011). *Historical evidence for the origin of teaching hospital, medical school and the rise of academic medicine,* Journal of Perinatology, 31: 236–239.
8. Russell G.A. (2003). *Avicenna (Ibn Sina),* https://doi.org/10.1038/npg.els.0003613.Retrieved January 31st, 2021.
9. Smith R.D.(1980). *Avicenna and the Canon of Medicine: A millennial tribute.* West J Med, 133:367–370.
10. Sajadi M.M., Mansouri D., Sajadi M-R.M.(2009). *Ibn Sina Clinical Trial,* Ann Intern Med.;150:640–643.
11. Nejabat M., Maleki B., Nimrouzi M., Mahbodi A., Salehi A.(2012). *Avicenna and Cataracts: A New Analysis of Contributions to Diagnosis and Treatment from the Canon,* Iran Red Crescent Med J, 14; 5:265–270
12. Choopani R., Ghourchian Anahita, Hajimehdipoor H., Kamalinejad M.(2016). *Scientific Evaluation of Pharmacological Treatment of Osteoarthritis in the Canon of Medicine,* Journal of Evidence-Based Complementary & Alternative Medicine, 21; 3: 235–242.
13. Siahpoosh MB. Ebadiani M., Shah Hosseini GhR, Isfahani MM., A Nikbakht Nasrabadi A., Dadgostar H.(2012). *Avicenna the First to Describe Diseases which May Be Prevented by Exercise,* Iranian J Publ Health, 41;11: 98–101.

14. Aliasl J, Khoshzaban F.(2013). *Traditional Herbal Remedies for Burn Wound Healing in Canon of Avicenna*, Jundishapur J Nat Pharm Prod. 2013, 8; 4:192–196.( doi: 10.17795/jjnpp-11686).

15. Alwishah A.(2016). *Avicenna on Animal Self-Awareness, Cognition and Identity*, Arabic Sciences and Philosophy, vol. 26, pp. 73–96.

16. Nasser Mona, Tibi Aida, Savage-Smith Emilie (2009). *Ibn Sina's Canon of Medicine: 11th century rules for assessing the effects of drugs*. Journal of the Royal Society of Medicine, 102; 2: 78–80.

17. Otsuka K., Cornelissen G., Halberg F.(2016). F*rom Chronomics to Chronoastrobiology: Many Rhythms Are Control Information for Whatever We Do.* In: *Chronomics and Continuous Ambulatory Blood Pressure Monitoring.* Springer, Tokyo, 2016, pp: 53–98.

18. Sayili A., El-Gomati M., Nazir A.(2006). *The Emergence of the Prototype of the Modern Hospital in Medieval Islam*. Foundation for Science Technology and Civilisation, FSTC Limited.

19. Modanlou H.D.(2011). *Historical evidence for the origin of teaching hospital, medical school and the rise of academic medicine,* Journal of Perinatology, 2011, 31: 236–239.

20. Hatami H. (2001). *The principles of geriatrics in Avicenna's Canon*, Pathobiology Research (Modares Journal of Medical Sci.), 2001, 3; 2: 127–137.

21. Alam M A, Quamri MA, Sofi G, Ayman U, Ansari S, Ahad Mariyam (2020). *Understanding COVID-19 in the light of epidemic disease described in Unani medicine*, Drug Metabol Pers Ther (De Gruyter), 35; 4: 20200136.

22. Black L. Deborah (2006) *Avicenna on self-awareness and knowing that one knows, Individual.utoronto.ca*. Retrieved January 31, 2021.

23. Levy R. (1957). *Avicenna-His Life and Times,* Med Hist (Cambridge University Press), 1; 3: 249–261.

24. Halévy MA.(1956). *Le rôle d'Isaac Beg, médecin et ambassadeur de Yuzun-Hassan en Moldavie et dans les pays voisins*, XV-e Congrès International d'Histoire de la Médecine, Madrid.

25. Karabaşoğlu C.(2015). *Tradition of notation in the history of Turkish Music*, Procedia - Social and Behavioral Sciences, 174: 3832 – 3837.

26. Gomoiu V. (1937). *Ibn Sina (Avicenna)*, Presa Publishing House, Braila; Dr. Gomoiu. *Ibn Sina (Avicenne)* (in French and Turkish), in Turkish Historical Society (1937), *İbni Sina. Studies Regarding His Personality and Works* (Büyük Türk Filozofu ve Tıp Üstadı İbn Sina, İstanbul: Türk Tarih Kurumu Yayınları),VII. seri, no. 1, l.

27. Scheau M, Carata Ana, Nicolae Laura-Cristina (2013). [*History Pages: "Victor Gomoiu"* Museum of the History of Medicine and Pharmacy in Craiova], NOEMA, vol. XII: 291–305.
28. Bratescu Gh. (1962), [*Ibn Sina – Avicenna. The Poem of Medicine. The Canon of Medical Science* (excerpts)], Medical Publishing House, Bucharest.
29. Geavlete P, Saglamb R, Georgescu D, Multescu R, Iordache V., Sinan Kabakcic A, C. Ened C, Geavlete B., *First Romanian Experience with Robotic (Avicenna) Flexible Ureteroscopy in Renal Stones*, Romanian Journal of Urology, 2016, 15; 3: 22–25.

## Short Biography of Dana Baran

Specialisation and publications in Histology-Cell Biology, Chronobiology, History of Medicine.
Member of international and national associations:
General Secretary – International Society for the History of Medicine
Vicepresident – Romanian Society for the History of Medicine
Herald – Pan-Hellenic Society for the Dissemination of the Hippocratic Spirit (Athenes)
Member – European Academy of Sciences, Arts and Letters (Paris)
Member – Executive Committee - Balkan Medical Union - Romanian National Section
Honorary Member – Romanian Society for the History of Pharmacy
Member – History of Medicine Commission (History of Sciences Commission) of the Romanian Academy
Scientific councillor – Society of Physicians and Naturalists (Iaşi, Romania)
Member – Romanian Society of Physician Writers and Publicists
National and international medals, honorary and excellence prizes, awarded for scientific and editorial activities by national and international institutions (International Society for the History of Medicine, Balkan Medical Union, Romanian Societies for the History of Medicine, and History of Pharmacy, "Grigore T. Popa" University of Medicine and Pharmacy, Iasi, "Apolonia" University, Iasi, Romanian Society of Biomaterials; Romanian Society of Algesiology, among others)
Active professor emeritus.
e-mail: dana_baran@yahoo.com

Ömer Faruk Erdoğan[1], Assoc. Prof.

# Why was Avicenna Declared an Infidel? An Analysis within the Frame of al-Ghazzāli's Tahāfut al-Falāsifah

**Abstract:** Among the important discussions of Islamic thought is the debate around *Tahāfut al-Falāsifah* (*Incoherence of the Philosophers*) between al-Ghazzālī and the Muslim Peripatetic (*Mashshā'ī*) philosophers. In the presence of all the criticism process, which started with al-Ghazzālī's *Tahāfut al-Falāsifah* and continued with many alternative commentaries on *Tahāfut al-Falāsifah* in the later stage, I mainly focus on the correspondence of al-Ghazzālī's accusations and claims in Avicenna's philosophical system. This study is limited to the issues of eternity, knowledge and resurrection, which are the topics containing takfīr accusation by al-Ghazzālī and will be discussed from the perspective of Kalām and Philosophy. From this view, this study aims to present the reality in the way it has been manifested in *Tahāfut al-Falāsifah* discussions rather than the one it ought to be.

**Key words:** Avicenna, al-Ghazzālī, Tahāfut al-Falāsifah, Takfīr.

## INTRODUCTION

*Abū 'Alī* al-*Ḥusayn* Ibn *Sīnā* (d. 428/1037) is a dual citizen of the Hellenistic and the Islamic World. The impact Avicenna has created on the philosophical thought as a result of his intellectual and spiritual accumulation contains the synthesis of Platon (427–347 B.C), Aristotle (384–322 B.C), Neo-platonism, and even the Islamic Kalām tradition. Despite being influenced by the Greek philosophy, Avicenna didn't establish anything contrary to the Islamic belief. He has prescribed how to reconcile the revelation with reason. (Karlıga, 1999, pp. 3–4; Okumus, 2000, p. 341)

Acknowledged as one of the important theologians of Islamic thought, *Abū Ḥāmid al-Ghazālī* (d. 505/1111), through the course of *Tahāfut al-Falāsifah*,

1 Associate Prof. Kütahya Dumlupınar University, Faculty of Theology, Department of Islamic Philosophy. email: omerfaruk.erdogan@dpu.edu.tr / ORCID ID: https://orcid.org/0000-0003-4131-3532

declared Abū Naṣr al-Fārābī al-Turkī (d. 339/950) and Avicenna -being closest to the time he lived and being the most competent philosophers of their times- his adversaries. According to al-Ghazzālī in *Tahāfut al-Falāsifah*, the philosophers have been mistaken in twenty philosophical doctrines. They have fallen into infidelity on the first, thirteenth, and twentieth of these doctrines, and on the others, they have committed heresy and have sinned. As for the reason of falling into infidelity of philosophers, who strive to base every issue on reason, al-Ghazzālī beholds that their views contradict the Qur'ān and the prophetic tradition while in three doctrines, they have been in complete disagreement with all Muslims. (al-Ghazzālī, 1998, p. 67)

Although al-Ghazzālī in *Tahāfut al-Falāsifah*, based on their wrong views on topics regarding metaphysics, accused these philosophers of infidelity and heresy, the word "infidelity" here should be given, rather than its religious terminology, a different sociologic meaning signifying the digress of Muslim philosophers from the Islamic society with their new thoughts and mentality, which contradicted the existing tradition. (Deniz, 2012, p. 435)

Al-Ghazzālī in the introduction to *Tahāfut al-Falāsifah*, links the main reason for the Muslim peripatetic philosophers' deviation to disbelief to the fact that they had been influenced by philosophers such as Socrates (469–399 B.C), Hippocrates (460 (?)-375(?)), Plato, Aristotle. (al-Ghazzālī, 1998, pp. 2–3, 1998, pp. 45–46) According to al-Ghazzālī, peripatetic philosophers have fallen into disbelief in their judgments about the creation of the universe, attributes of God, and the resurrection of the corpses. (al-Ghazzālī, 2009, p. 8) Inclusion of the issue of God's attributes in the list of reasons for their infidelity, and on the other hand not mentioning the issue of God's inability to know the particulars in it, is remarkable. Because al-Ghazzālī, in substantive issues of *Tahāfut al-Falāsifah*, accuses the philosophers of falling into heresy when it comes to the attributes of God. (al-Ghazzālī, 1998, pp. 55–56, 2009, pp. 97–110)

In the first discussion of *Tahāfut al-Falāsifah*, al-Ghazzālī claims that the philosophers have fallen into infidelity by accepting the universe as eternal, however where this issue is discussed he does not put this claim into distinctive sentences. Here, al-Ghazzālī discusses the issue of eternity with the reflex of a theologian, taking the infidelity claim to the third issue. In the third discussion of *Tahāfut al-Falāsifah*, he accuses Avicenna of rejecting Islam's principle of oneness of God by accepting the emergence of plurality from God and following the views of Materialist and Naturalist philosophers and some views of Mu'tazila. (al-Ghazzālī, 2009, p. 39,71–72,77–78)

In the thirteenth discussion, which is based on the claim that God cannot know particulars, al-Ghazzālī once again claims that the philosophers have fallen into infidelity. He holds that philosophers say that God does not know the details about people like Zaid, Amr and Halid, however, He, with his undivided knowledge, only knows the universal human, the details about him, his qualities, and that his body is made up of many organs and that each one of these organs has a function, and such other things. (al-Ghazzālī, 2009, p. 136) In al-Ghazzālī's view, the first part of the claim in *Tahāfut al-Falāsifah*'s thirteenth discussion is the one which the philosophers have put forward on this topic. The second part of the claim consists of al-Ghazzālī's interpretation of what philosophers have tried to explain.

In the introduction to the twentieth discussion, where al-Ghazzālī once again declares them infidels, he writes that philosophers' views on the resurrection of the corpses have damaged Muslims' beliefs and have contradicted Islam. (al-Ghazzālī, 2009, p. 207) However, if examined carefully, this accusation of infidelity is not pointed towards their refusal of belief in the hereafter, but to their explanation of its circumstances related to the resurrection of corpses and the explanation of afterlife events through depiction and use of metaphors. (Erdogan, 2020, p. 26) Accusations of infidelity by al-Ghazzālī in this part are directed towards the concepts of negation of resurrection with bodies, and linking soul-body relation to the theory of causality. In the twentieth discussion as well, being a pattern of *Tahāfut al-Falāsifah*, al-Ghazzālī has quoted the philosophers' views first and then interpreted them. (al-Ghazzālī, 2009, pp. 218–220) Takfīr allegations, in this case, are further extended to the rejection of some Qur'ānic verses by philosophers. ("Does he promise you that once you are dead and reduced to dust and bones, you will be brought forth ⌜alive⌝? Impossible, simply impossible is what you are promised! al-Mu'minūn 23/35–36 "Philosophers denying the mystic knowledge and the miracle have come face to face with even greater denial than the denial of atheists who say 'even after we have been reduced to decayed bones?') (al-Nazi'at/11) (al-Ghazzālī, 2009, p. 222)

In the conclusion of *Tahāfut al-Falāsifah*, al-Ghazzālī answers a question regarding whether the philosophers have fallen into denial. This part, rather than summarizing the *Tahāfut al-Falāsifah*, is like a short letter where it is asked whether the philosophers can be accused of denial or not. Likewise, one more importance of this part is the presence of essence of al-Ghazzālī's allegations against philosophers regarding their falling into denial due to three issues altogether and its being the only part where these have been expressed explicitly. (al-Ghazzālī, 1998, pp. 55–56, 2009, pp. 225–226; Erdogan, 2020, p. 28) As a result of the above-mentioned evaluations, the first, thirteenth, and the twentieth discussions of *Tahāfut al-Falāsifah*, where the topics of eternity, knowledge and resurrection have been discussed and some other related issues will be discussed below in these headings.

## 1. Eternal Universe is not the ontological equal of Etnernal God.

Thoughts put forward regarding the existence of the universe have been evaluated under the title of problem of ontological principle in philosophical literature. The problem of ontological principle, about which lots of philosophers have produced many ideas, discusses the root or the source of the universe or its ultimate and the highest cause. When viewed from the perspective of Avicenna, the two most basic points that should be discussed about the explanation of existence seem to be the theory of causality, whose roots systematically are found in Aristotle, and can be extended to the neo-platonism in its theory of emanation. (Kılıc, 2009, pp. 80–81)

The problem discussed under this heading is this: "while the existence of 'First Principal' is necessary, eternal and everlasting, is the existence of universe, which necessarily comes from it, necessary, eternal and everlasting as well?" Being a general and inclusive, according to al-Ghazzālī, this question creates suspicion: If God's precedence over universe is in respect of its being (self), we would be obliged to talk about a universe which gets its existence as a co-existent and existing at the same time as God. This too is a sign of universe's being eternal and not having a beginning for its being.

According to al-Ghazzālī, philosophers don't agree with each other about the existence of universe and its coming into being. Most of them think that the universe is eternal. This universe has existed extratemporally with God as its work and in the very way the effect exists with its cause and the light exists with the sun. God's precedence over universe is the same as the precedence of cause over cause. This precedence is not in terms of time, but self and position. Universe is eternal and can't come out of God without a mediation, who has existed without any created cause. (al-Ghazzālī, 2009, pp. 14–16) In this regard, Avicenna accepts the existence of universe, not as something created, but as something coming into being from its eternal possibility.

From philosopher's views 'there is no timewise beginning of universe' al-Ghazzālī reaches a new conclusion that 'God and universe have existed together', however, Avicenna doesn't have any such claim. Furthermore, despite everything, he thinks that universe has its particular beginning. (Avicenna, 2013a, p. 238)

According to al-Ghazzālī, philosophers have evaluated all the possibilities of existence of universe and have come to the conclusion that it is eternal. In our opinion the main point that needs to be taken into consideration regarding the debate of eternality of universe or its creation is this: we need to determine the correpondence in the system of Avicenna of a claim put forward by al-Ghazzālī as a quotation from him that universe is eternal. Al-Ghazzālī thinks that philosophers believe in universe's eternity and by this he thinks that they refer to the fact that a created being cannot emanate from God. While talking about this topic, philosophers, contrary to their above-mentioned claim, find the emanation of a created one form God as possible, not because of the fact that universe is eternal but from the fact that God is eternal. It becomes much clearer when studied in light of the works of both these thinkers. Avicenna discusses the relation between God and universe from the theories of causality and self-time precedence, rather than its (universe's) being eternal. For instance, according to Avicenna's understanding of causality, God and universe are neither categorically, nor as self and time together. In addition to this, it is obvious that neither universe nor anything emanating from the First Principle (such as imntellect, *nafs* or sphere) have been held equal to him in respect of being. Therefore, in the system of Avicenna, God is the only cause of the existence of everything and his existence is only due to himself. (Erdogan, 2020, p. 39)

> "It is known that the existence of a possible existent is connected to its cause and that it does not possess its own existence. Its existence is due to another thing. That is what is known as coming into being. Similarly, we had already mentioned that other intellects end with the Necessary Being. There is only one necessary being. In this case, we can say that the universe has its unique beginning, which does not resemble the universe. The existence of the universe is due to God. His existence is due to himself. His existence comes from himself. In fact, he is the absolute being and everything else's existence is due to God."(Avicenna, 2013a, pp. 238–239)

As can be seen in the expressions above, Avicenna separates the existence of God and the existence of the universe very clearly. (Kutluer, 2002, pp. 97–104) According to the philosopher, the universe has its own particular beginning. However, this is not in terms of time, but it is in terms of contingency. (Avicenna, 2013a, pp. 238–240)

On this topic, *Abū* al-*Walīd* Ibn Rushd (Averroes) (d. 595/1198) and *Abū* al-Fazl Fakhr al-Dīn al-Rāzī (d. 606/1210) support Avicenna too. Averroes thinks that what philosophers understand from 'eternity' is different from what al-Ghazzālī meant by it. From this point, there is no legitimate reason to declare them infidels. (Averroes, 1994, pp. 104–107) According to al-Rāzī, the term 'eternity of universe' corresponds to God's eternal act and not to the universe's being ontologically eternal. In the system of Avicenna, only the First (God) is eternal. (Fakhr al-Dīn al-Rāzī, 1990, p. 228; Fakhr al-Dīn al-Rāzī, 2005, pp. 342–343; Kutluer, 2002, p. 105; Altas, 2015, p. 375) The common point here is that the universe's being a creation is not in terms of time (Mutahharī, 2003, p. 208)

Eventually, Avicenna refers to two different meanings from eternal and being created. According to the philosopher, the eternal can be divided in two ways: 1. Being older of one thing from another in terms of time i.e. "Precedence based on syllogism". 2. Absolute eternal which is further divided into two: a. Eternal due to itself. b. Eternal in terms of time. Eternal in terms of time is the one which does not have a temporal beginning. Eternal due to itself is the absence of anything which can be responsible for a thing's self-existence. In other words, it means that it does not have any beginning which is related to it. It is indeed the only truth the God himself. (Deniz, 2009, p. 64) Therefore, a thing, which does not have a cause for its existence and whose existence is before the existence of time, is called eternal. The same goes for the created one. It means that a thing having a cause for its creation is called the created one, and also the one which is created within time -the beginning of existence-, is called the created one. When applied to the relation of God and universe, these definitions show that God, the creator, is eternal both from the point that he exists without a cause and also from that he hasn't come into being within the limits of time. The universe, on the other hand, is eternal from one side due to its existence before time -the beginning of creation-, and it (being the first one to be created uniquely) is the created one from the other side because of its need for a cause, i.e. the creator for its existence. (Ozdemir, 2012, p. 91) Now, let's explain these points in the headings below.

## 1.1. Eternal Being

The main question of this heading is this: "Do God and universe both exist together as eternal entities?" The explanation of the difference in terms of time and place between God and creation is necessary from the point of ontic as well as epistemic and must be elaborated. In the second evidence of the first issue in *Tahāfut al-Falāsifah*, al-Ghazzālī begins this topic as follows:

> "According to the philosopher's claim, one who says 'universe is after God, and God is before the universe', must have referred to the notion that God is before universe not in terms of time, but in terms of his being. This is exactly similar to the precedence of a cause before its effect in the same way as the precedence of 'one' over 'two', the motion of a person over the motion of his shadow, and the motion of hand over the motion of water, which despite being able to exist at the same time are not so due to the requirement of their nature." (al-Ghazzālī, 2009, pp. 31–32, 2015, p. 48)

As already claimed, according to Avicenna, God is before the universe not in terms of time, but in terms of his being, rank, and status. These questions are answered in order to further elaborate this issue: By what are the actions coming into being of the First preceded? By its being or by time? If preceded by his being, even if together, 'one' for 'two' and again if together, in the example of the motion of something that moves with the effect of a motion by its source, both the eternal First and all the actions coming out of it must be created ones. (Avicenna, 2004a, p. 122) According to Avicenna, God is the one that does not exist on the basis of time, which is the subject of precedence and subsequence, and He is the one who cannot be thought to be compared in terms of being and time with the things that have emanated from him. There is no precedence or subsequence for the one who exists by itself (Avicenna, 2004b, pp. 145–146)

> "If the existence of one of two things is not from the later one, but from itself or the third source, in terms of being, it is before the second one. Therefore, the intellect never finds these words odd such as 'When Zaid moved his hand, the key also moved' or 'Zaid moved his hand, and then the key moved'. But, although the intellect admits understanding the sentence "When the key moved, Zaid's hand also moved', it finds this sentence odd 'when the key moved, Zaid also moved his hand'. Because although both the movements happen at the same time, the intellect accepts one as the first and the other as the second. Because, the cause for the existence of the motion of first is not the motion of the second, but the motion of the first is the cause for the motion of the second". (Avicenna, 2004b, p. 147, For more see 2005, p. 138)

As we have already understood that the above-mentioned cause and effect relation between hand and key was given to explain the relationship between God and the universe. Now, we can clearly conclude that although the universe exists necessarily from God, being a necessary entity due to an outer cause, it is a possible entity in terms of its existence. In reality, Avicenna does not declare the universe a necessary entity, but he claims that its coming into existence is a necessity. To him, the universe's being eternal is due to the fact that it gets its existence from God. Not that it got its existence or the cause of its existence from itself. (Kaya, 2011, pp. 253–254)

## 1.2. Eternal Time

According to al-Ghazzālī, if Avicenna thinks that the precedence of God over the universe is not due to its being but due to the time, it means that there is a time when there was no universe before the existence of universe and time. In this case, the absence of the universe is before the existence of it, which means that God existed a very long period, that begins with the creation of the universe and goes back to eternity. Saying that there was an infinite time before the creation of time would be a contradiction. This is the reason why Avicenna finds the creation of time impossible. In this way, when he finds time, which is nothing but a measurement of movement, as an eternal entity, he necessarily accepts the movement and the movement that contributes to the continuity of time by its movement, eternal as well. (al-Ghazzālī, 2009, p. 32)

Al-Ghazzālī's allegation of Avicenna of repugnance in this topic is due to the fact that he has judged him from the perspective of some kind of theologians. It is obvious that Avicenna thinks differently from Aristotle on the issue of time's eternity. Aristotle thinks that time was created but at the same time it is eternal and everlasting. However, Avicenna on the other hand, when he says that time is eternal, he does not mean that the time was eternal beside the existence of God and being equal to his existence. Contrarily, time's being eternal is due to the fact that it cannot be given a beginning in terms of time. (Rahman, 1990, p. 43) However, from the point of existence, the time has a beginning and it is in the hands of God. (Atay, 1974, pp. 80–81)

## 1.3. Eternal Contingency

When the issue of eternity is concerned, discussions about "contingency" are very important. In my opinion, what al-Ghazzālī and Avicenna understand of this term is different from each other. Instead of accepting contingency as an ontological fact, al-Ghazzālī prefers to identify it with the might of the perpetrator. Besides thinking that the universe is a created being, he thinks that it is possible to fix the time for this contingency (i.e the creation of the universe). That is the point where al-Ghazzālī criticizes the philosophers. Whereas, the quality of being created later automatically disappears when the universe, from the view of philosophers, is accepted as eternal. (Kaya, 2011, p. 257) In this respect, according to Avicenna, the contingency expresses the passage of creation from its potential state to an active one. The option of non-existence is not true for a philosopher.

> "Every created one, before being so is contingent or not contingent in itself. One that is impossible to exist cannot exist. The contingent one has been preceded by its possibility of existence. In such a way, the possible is a meaning both the current one and the one that is in a topic and is connected to it. We call the contingency of existence the potential of existence. The carrier of this potential of existence is named as a subject, matter, or phantasm. It means every created one is preceded by matter (but the necessary one is never preceded by matter)". (Avicenna, 2004b, pp. 162–163)

In the system of Avicenna, the theory of causality is grounded by contingency. In this respect, being necessary in the sense of having existence is before contingency. However, it comes after the term "contingency" in the sense of emerging as a result of creation, the self of the present one or its nature, and therefore in the sense of being continuous. In this way, Avicenna elaborates the existence and contingency of tangible objects and struggles to arrive at the term "necessity" through "contingency". (Turker, 2009, pp. 318–319) In addition to it, Avicenna thinks that the universe has always been contingent without being impossible because it is not reasonable for an impossible in the beginning to turn into a contingent later.

### 1.4. Eternal Matter

As a result of the discussion of God's precedence over the universe in terms of self and time, the claim that the body is eternal is also present in al-Ghazzālī's critic of Avicenna:

> "According to philosophers, 'matter that every created has is before that thing'. Because the created cannot be without matter, and in this case as well matter would not be created. Even the created itself is a collection of different forms, attributes, and properties of matter. (Hence matter is the essence of creation)". (al-Ghazzālī, 2009, p. 41)

In this claim of him, al-Ghazzālī has compared philosophers and theologians. In Avicenna 's definition of substance, there is no claim of eternity for it. He wants to say that the potential power that has been given to a substance is eternal, not the substance itself. By talking about a substance having eternal potential, he actually proves that the substance is mortal. This makes it very clear that the powerful one cannot move any substance other than itself, and in the wheel of movement, the source of the power does not come within itself unless it is supplied by an eternal outer source of power. (Erdogan, 2020, p. 133)

## 2. Divine Knowledge: God Knows Particulars in a Universal Way

Al-Ghazzālī, especially in the thirteenth discussion of *Tahāfut al-Falāsifah*, has transformed the philosophers' view "God knows particulars in a universal way" into a claim "God does not know particulars, He only knows the universals." When he begins explaining this issue, he quotes philosophers' words "God knows particulars in a universal way" rightly. However, in the explanation part, he reaches a different conclusion; "God does not know particulars, He only knows the universals". When Avicenna's writings are taken into consideration, one can see him expressing clearly that God knew everything, nothing and not even a single particle could be hidden from his knowledge. Insomuch that beyond saying that God knows particulars, he goes on to explain the way He (God) knows them. (Acar, 2006, p. 99) When looked at Avicenna's metaphysical system as a whole, the thing that comes out is "God knows the universals, and within universals, He also knows the particulars". This expression is enough to show the invalidity of al-Ghazzālī's takfīr allegations. Yet, al-Ghazzālī said that Avicenna's God was not Omnipotent and All-knowing and going beyond, he alleged that he and all those who follow him had fallen into disbelief. (Deniz, 2010, p. 78)

Based on the texts in *Tahāfut al-Falāsifah*, while al-Ghazzālī thinks that some philosophers say that God only knows Himself, Avicenna claims that God not only knows Himself but other than Himself, He also knows all the things He has created. (al-Ghazzālī, 2009, p. 134) Avicenna writes: "Necessary Being, knows everything as they are along with their causes. He does not know things by the help of things, but also, emerging from him, He knows all of them and their causes. Therefore, in this sense He is wise. His wisdom in the meantime is His knowledge. A necessary being is the existing one, who is the cause of all the creation and gives necessity to all the creation." (Avicenna, 2013a, p. 262. For more see. 2005, p. 165, 2013b, p. 228, 1335, pp. 9–14) By saying this, Avicenna makes it absolutely doubtless that God not only knows himself but also all that is out of him.

> "Necessary Being is the one who knows by His self. He knows others with all their details. Necessarily Being and his oneness, that the whole that is made from him, its coming into being and knowing His self, is all very obvious. From the fact that he knows His self, His knowledge matches reality, and His being the principle of all the creation and all the realities, it can be said that in heaven and the earth nothing is hidden from him. Furthermore, everything that comes into being is so due to him. He is the cause of all causes. Therefore, the Necessary Being knows the cause and effect and all that he has created." (Avicenna, 1335, pp. 8–9)

While man gets his knowledge from the objects of information, God does not get His knowledge of things out of Him from them. On the contrary, things exist due to God's knowledge of them. Regarding the simplicity of God's knowledge, Avicenna maintains that His knowledge does not involve time and ontological series. (Marmura, 1962, p. 301; Acar, 2006, p. 108; for comparison see. Terkan, 2009, pp. 348–349) Thus according to Avicenna, this verse also points to this state: "Not even an atom's weight is hidden from Him in the heavens or the earth." (Saba', 34/3) (Avicenna, 2004a, pp. 104–105, 2013b, p. 225; Averroes, 1999, p. 135; Durusoy, 1993, p. 73)

> "In that case, there is a difference of knowing between knowing the changing particular things with timely knowledge and knowing with universal knowledge. Necessary Being knows everything with a universal knowledge; nothing big or small is hidden from him."(Avicenna, 2013a, p. 352)

Following expressions of al-Ghazzālī in the sixth discussion of the *Incoherence* are regarding Avicenna's claim that God cannot know the particulars:

> "According to him (Avicenna) God knows everything as a whole without an aspect of time. But, He does not know the particulars because in that case, it would mean that a change has occurred in His knowledge." (al-Ghazzālī, 2009, p. 102)

Since the concept of God's knowing particulars has been evident, now we need to introduce the relationship between time and the particular and universal knowledge. According to Avicenna, since God is simple and unchangeable, the tenses of past, present, and future cannot be applied to Him. For this reason, God's knowledge is named as universal knowledge in Avicenna's philosophy. (Yavuz, 2009, p. 338)

> "It is imperative for the Necessary Being that His knowledge of particulars is not in the way of timely knowledge involving past, present and future. Or otherwise, a change in His attribute of self would occur. Furthermore, His knowledge must be in a sacred way of time and timely love. And yet again his being the knower of everything is necessary."(Avicenna, 2005, p. 168)

Al-Ghazzālī argues that Avicenna's premises such as God's knowledge is in a universal way and it is independent of time and that He knows the timely events through their causes, do not support the knowledge of particular events. Rather he thinks that the knowledge of particulars requires a temporal relation between the knower subject and the known object. Because without temporal relation events that occur actively cannot be known. We cannot know if they have happened or not, or before their time of happening. Again we cannot know if they are likely to happen or their state of being happened if they have happened. Thus holding God away from this temporal relation, al-Ghazzālī thinks Avicenna has rejected God's knowledge of particulars. (Acar, 2006, p. 104)

> "Actually, philosophers have wished to say that: God does not know the announcement situation even when Prophet Muhammad (p.b.u.h) declared his prophethood. God does not know each prophet one by one, but he knows that there are some among humans and that they have some kind of qualities. He does not know the prophethood of a particular individual. Since this is something that is known with the help of senses, God does not know things coming through the help of senses. For knowing the changing condition of an individual in terms of time, requires a change in that individual."(al-Ghazzālī, 2009, p. 137)

Whereas according to Avicenna, since all the creation gets its existence from God and have emanated from him, God knows their existence and also the causal relationships among them. (Yavuz, 2009, pp. 338–340) Avicenna asserts that he has based his above-mentioned claim on the Qur'ān and in this way holds that God's knowledge is above all and encompasses everything. Therefore, Avicenna's aim is not to exclude any information related to time from God's knowledge but to put forth the fact that his knowledge is clean of all the flaws caused by temporal procedures. (Erdogan, 2020, p. 224)

> "The First (God) knows the things at once, however, this knowledge does not create a plurality in His essence or in the reality of His being, it does not cause Him to have a form with the form of things. Contrarily, forms of things overflow from the First intellectually." (Avicenna, 2004a, p. 108)

In conclusion, saying that 'God doesn't know particulars' and 'God does not know things the way divisible beings do within the limits of time and place' are two different expressions. The first postulate suggests that God can never know any particular knowledge in any way of acquiring knowledge. Moreover, He cannot even know what knowledge it is. Such a claim about God for al-Ghazzālī is a prove of philosophers' blasphemy. Also in Averroes' opinion, the philosophers say that God does not know the particular with the new knowledge that has to appear along with the creation of a thing or being. The verse 'How could He not know His Own creation? For he alone is the Most Subtle, All-Aware' (al-Mulk, 67/14) explains this case. (Averroes, 1999, pp. 125–126)

## 3. Will The Resurrection be in the Form of Soul Only?

Involving the discussion about the relation of the soul with the body, this topic is more about circumstances emerging with death than their unity in the world. In this respect, al-Ghazzālī's first objection is that the philosophers' claims regarding the afterlife that descriptions of happiness and haplessness were all symbolic, and that the resurrection in the afterlife will be in the form of soul, is against the basic laws of religion. This view is present in Avicenna in the same way as claimed by al-Ghazzālī.

> "When the intellectual power reaches its level of perfection, the soul leaves the body in order to reach its maximum capacity of perfection. This is the same as a situation when the most delicious and appetizing food is presented before him, a benumbed (or a diseased individual as al-Ghazzālī calls him) remains unaware of it, but when he gets round he perceives that great taste."(Avicenna, 2011b, p. 51; for comparison see. al-Ghazzālī, 2009, pp. 209–211)

The reason philosopher thinks so is because people find it difficult to accept God and the afterlife when expressed in completely intangible terms especially in the concepts of oneness and exoneration (*tanzīh*) and is also due to the concern that they will have to prefer distancing themselves from religion. Therefore, ordinary people can't understand it with intangible things. Religion must explain the said life the way God's existence and His attributes are explained through metaphors. (Capku, 2015, pp. 137–138) Al-Ghazzālī's objection here is directed to the claim by philosophers that this concept can only be known by the mind. This point should also be noted that Avicenna has explained this issue by showing several proofs with examples from religion (the Qu'rān and Hadith) (Erdogan, 2020, p. 259) Finally, al-Ghazzālī's claim; "soul-body relation, collection of bodies, resurrection and that afterlife enjoyments involve similes and depictions", is not in the way that Avicenna had denied afterlife, but that it must be understood as a way of expression regarding the circumstances of the afterlife.

Al-Ghazzālī's second objection is directed towards the affairs of bodies' resurrection in the afterlife. There are three different views on this topic. 1. The view of some theologians that man is just a body and its resurrection will also be in the form of the body. 2. This is a view of those who say that soul exists and will continue its existence even after death, and the same body will come up by a combination of its parts, which will then be given its soul. 3. Return of the soul to either the first body or any other made up of other parts will happen. It does not matter as long as the soul is the same. Man is so not by its matter, but by his soul. (al-Ghazzālī, 2009, p. 214; For comparison see, Avicenna, 2011a, pp. 4–6) Al-Ghazzālī, while evaluating these three views, criticizes Avicenna and even declares him an unbeliever for not accepting the third view, which expresses that resurrection will be with both soul and body. (al-Ghazzālī, 2009, p. 218)

Avicenna, regarding the nature of the resurrection, finds the view of those who argue that the afterlife will only be with the body, the least reliable among the three views. For him, the soul is the thing that makes a man. From Avicenna's view, if we accept the situation as; When thought about the resurrection of human bodies that have mixed up with soil and disappeared, the same essence, the same atmospheric conditions and hence in any way the same material body cannot be made, instead of human form or human soul that has come up with divine essences, consistency of accepting that the body, which has come into being by integrating with essences from the soil and which is only made up of matter, will be punished or rewarded is debatable. For if punishment and reward were to the matter only, even in the case when matter which is soil came up with the same essences in the same person, the superiority of matter over the soul would be accepted. (Erdogan, 2020, p. 281) Therefore, Avicenna's verified view, also accepted by virtuous philosophers, is his opinion that resurrection will be spiritual.

As can be seen, al-Ghazzālī's criticism of Avicenna regarding resurrection in the form of the soul has its answer in the philosopher's views. According to Avicenna, most fertile lands are made up of decomposed bodies of living beings. Well, how will it be possible to resurrect matter containing the form of two persons who lived at different or the same time without distinguishing them from each other? If someone asks 'what kind of soil, air or such a thing will be used to resurrect a body for a soul? and says that 'the body doesn't need to have the same particles as it had in its life', it would be a clear reincarnation. Moreover, since the body at the time of the second resurrection would not be the same as the human body at the first resurrection and also this human soul would enter a second body after the first one, once again the thing called reincarnation would have occurred. (Avicenna, 2011a, p. 15) If this is the case, the human body at the second resurrection would not be the same as the one at the first resurrection and this soul would enter the second body after the first one, which is again reincarnation.

Al- Ghazzālī's third objection in his argument about the resurrection is Avicenna's attribution of this issue to the principle of causality. According to him philosophers who do not accept bodily resurrection, do not find suitable the causes that create a human body to be in the form of 'when He says it to be so it becomes' without going through a process. Because for philosophers soil cannot be addressed. Without going through these stages, soil can't turn into a human. And without these causes, it can't go through the said stages. (al- Ghazzālī, 2009, pp. 219–220) The fact here, as already known, is that the expression "كُنْ فَيَكُونُ" in Quranic verses regarding this topic is used by al-Ghazzālī in his allegations of blasphemy against philosophers. Al- Ghazzālī, related to this topic, accuses philosophers of denying resurrection for their lack of acknowledgement of God's power because they hold that God does not know the cause behind magnets's pulling of iron. (al-Ghazzālī, 2009, p. 222) However, Avicenna's view on this topic, is not the denial of things' creation on God's command. On the contrary, there is an emphasis on the fact that God knows the cause behind all his creation. And also, that every created thing has a cause and an unknown cause and that everything created has a cause for its creation. (Erdogan, 2020, pp. 294–296)

Finally, in the eye of al-Ghazzālī, such views by Avicenna and other philosophers who think in the same way, are completely contradictory to the fundamental resources of religion and also to the Muslims' beliefs. (Kuyel, 1956,

p. 107) However, in the end, Avicenna does not deny the afterlife, but he has some different thoughts regarding the circumstances of the afterlife, which he presents by way of interpreting some verses from the the Qur'ān. Therefore, al-Ghazzālī's takfīr allegations cannot be taken as getting out of religion.

## Conclusion

Al-Ghazzālī has accused philosophers in general and Avicenna in particular of blasphemy on three occasions in his book called *Tahāfut al-Falāsifah*. These are the discussions of eternity, knowledge, and resurrection. In the discussion about eternity, Ghazali thinks that philosophers, after evaluating all the possibilities of the universe's coming into being, have concluded that it is eternal. For al-Ghazzālī, this view of Avicenna is a sufficient justification in declaring him an infidel. However in Avicenna's perspective, the eternal in real terms is only the First Principle. He has found the emanation of the one coming into being later as possible, not from the fact that the universe was eternal, but that God is eternal. Avicenna explaining this point with the example of hand and key. According to this, the universe exists necessarily from God. On the other hand, the universe, being a necessary existent due to an outer source, is a possible entity in terms of existence. Therefore, Avicenna does not give necessity to the universe's existence by itself, but he gives necessity to its coming into being. The universe is eternal because its existence comes from God.

In the discussion about knowledge, al-Ghazzālī thinks philosophers have claimed that "God does not know particular events happening in time, but He universally knows them." From this reasoning of philosophers, al-Ghazzālī has concluded that God does not know particulars. This again is the right justification for philosophers' blasphemy. However, when Avicenna's writings are considered, this is clearly stated that God knows everything, nothing, and not even a particle can remain out of his knowledge.

In the discussion about the nature of the resurrection, al-Ghazzālī has objected to the philosopher on three points. First is about depictions of happiness and haplessness in the hereafter that they are nothing but symbols. The second is about the details of the resurrection of bodies in the hereafter. Al-Ghazzālī thinks that in the hereafter the event of resurrection in the form of the soul only is against the basic laws of religion. The third is the subjection of this issue to the principle of causality by Avicenna . Despite objections leading to his takfīr allegation by al-Ghazzālī, Avicenna does not deny the afterlife, he only carries out different reasoning about the circumstance of the afterlife. Even in that case, he wishes to prove his arguments by interpreting the Qur'ānic verses.

## References

Acar, R. (2006). Allah'ın Cüz'îleri Bilmesi: Klasik İbn Sînâ Yorumunun Değerlendirilmesi. *Divan İlmi Araştırmalar Dergisi (Journal of Interdisciplinary Studies)*, 20 (1).

Altas, E. (2015). *Fahreddîn Râzî'nin İbn Sînâ Yorumu ve Eleştirisi*. Iz Yayınları.

Atay, H. (1974). *Fârâbî ve İbn Sînâ'ya Göre Yaratma*. Ankara Üniversitesi İlahiyat Fakültesi Yayınları.

Capku, A. (2015). *İbn Sînâ, Gazzâlî ve İbn Rüşd Düşüncesinde Ahiret*. Kayıhan Yayınları.

Deniz, G. (2009). *Kelam-Felsefe Tartışmaları/ Tehâfütler Örneği*. Fecr Yayınları.

Deniz, G. (2010). *İnsan Hürriyetinin Metafizik Temelleri*. Litera Yayınları.

Deniz, G. (2012). Ebû Hâmid el- Gazzâlî ve Tehâfüt'ü. In. B. A. Cetinkaya (Ed.), *İslâm Felsefesi Tarihi* (Vol. 1). Grafiker Yayınları.

Durusoy, A. (1993). *İbn Sînâ Felsefesinde İnsan ve Âlemdeki Yeri*. Marmara Üniversitesi İlahiyat Vakfı Yayınları.

Erdogan, O. F. (2020). *Tehâfütte Tekfir Tartışmaları*. Çizgi Yayınevi.

al-Ghazzālī, A. H. (1998). *Dalâletten Hidâyete* (Y. Pakis, Trans.). Umran Yayınları.

al-Ghazzālī, A. H. (2009). *Filozofların Tutarsızlığı Tehâfütü'l-Felâsife* (H. Sarıoglu & M. Kaya, Trans.). Klasik Yayınları.

al-Ghazzālī, A. H. (2015). *Mişkâtü'l-envâr Nurlar Feneri* (S. Ates, Trans.). Bedir Yayınevi.

Ibn Rusd, A.-V. (1994). *Tehâfütü't-tehâfüt* (M. el-Arıbi, Trans.). Daru'l-Fikri'l-Lübnani.

Ibn Rusd, A.-V. (1999). Damîme. In. Bekir Karlıga (Trans.), *Faslu'l-makâl* (pp. 117–127). İşaret Yayınları.

Ibn *Sīnā*, A. A. (1335). *Risâletü'l-arşiyye fi tevhîdi Teâla ve sıfâtihî*.

Ibn *Sīnā*, A. A. (2004a). *Metafizik* (E. Demirli & O. Turker, Trans.; Vol. 2). Litera Yayınları.

Ibn *Sīnā*, A. A. (2004b). *Metafizik* (O. Turker, Trans.; Vol. 1). Litera Yayınları.

Ibn *Sīnā*, A. A. (2005). *İşaretler ve Tenbihler, el-Işârât ve't-tenbîhât* (A. Durusoy, Trans.). Litera Yayınları.

Ibn *Sīnā*, A. A. (2011a). El-Adhaviyye fi'l-me'âd. In M. Kaya (Trans.), *Felsefe ve Ölüm Ötesi*. Klasik Yayınları.

Ibn *Sīnā*, A. A. (2011b). Eş-Şifâ/el-İlâhiyât. In. M. Kaya (Trans.), *Felsefe ve Ölüm Ötesi*. Klasik Yayınları.

Ibn Sīnā, A. A. (2013a). *Dânişnâme-i alâî Alâî Hikmet Kitabı* (M. Demirkol, Trans.). Türkiye Yazma Eserler Başkanlığı (Manuscript Institution of Turkey) Yayınları.

Ibn Sīnā, A. A. (2013b). *En-Necât* (K. Senel, Trans.). Kabalcı Yayınları.

Karlıga, B. (1999). İbn Sînâ, Etkileri. In. *Türkiye Diyanet Vakfı İslâm Ansiklopedisi* (Vol. 20, pp. 345–353). Türkiye Diyanet Vakfı Yayınları.

Kaya, C. (2011). *Varlık ve İmkân, Aristoteles'ten İbn Sînâ'ya İmkânın Tarihi.* Klasik Yayınları.

Kılıc, M. F. (2009). İbn Sînâ'da Varlığın İlkesi. *Şarkiyat İlmi Araştırmalar Dergisi (Journal of Oriental Scientific Research)*, 3 (2).

Kutluer, I. (2002). *İbn Sînâ Felsefesinde Zorunlu Varlık.* Iz Yayınları.

Kuyel, M. T. (1956). *Üç Tehâfüt Bakımından Felsefe-Din Münasebeti.* Türk Tarih Kurumu (Turkish Historical Society) Yayınları.

Marmura, M. E. (1962). Some Aspects of Avicenna's theory of God's Knowledge of Particulars. *Journal of the American Oriental Society*, 82 (3).

Mutahharî, M. (2003). *Felsefe Dersleri* (A. Celik, Trans.; Vol. 1). İnsan Yayınları.

Okumus, M. (2000). Gazzâlî'nin Kur'an Yorumlarına İbn Sînâ'nın Etkileri. *İslâmî Araştırmalar Dergisi (Journal of Islamic Research )*, 13 (3–4), 341–353.

Ozdemir, M. (2012). *Gazzâlî'nin Tehâfütü'l-Felâsife Adlı Eserinde Üç Meselenin Ele Alınışı ve İbn Sînâ'nın Görüşlerinin Mukayesesi.* Marmara Üniversitesi.

Rahman, F. (1990). *İbn Sînâ's Teory of God and Creation an World Realitionship.* University of Notre Dame Press.

al-Rāzī, Fakhr al-Dīn. (1990). *el-Mebâhisü'l-meşrikıyye* (M. M. el-Bağdâdî, Trans.; Vol. 1–2).

al-Rāzī, Fakhr al-Dīn. (2005). *Şerhu'l-İşârât ve't-tenbîhât* (A. R. Necefzâde, Trans.). Ercümen-i Âsâr.

Terkan, F. (2009). *İbn Sînâ, Zorunlu Varlık'ın Cüz'iyyatı Bildiğini Tutarlı Olarak İddia Edebilir mi?* (M. Mazak & N. Ozkaya, Ed.; Vol. 1). İstanbul Büyükşehir Belediyesi Yayınları.

Turker, O. (2009). *İbn Sînâ Düşüncesinde Nedensellik İlkesinin Temellendirmesi ve Metafizikteki İşlevi* (M. Mazak & N. Ozkaya, Ed.; Vol. 1). İstanbul Büyükşehir Belediyesi Yayınları.

Yavuz, Z. (2009). *İbn Sînâ, Ezelîlik ve Özgür İrade* (M. Mazak & N. Ozkaya, Ed.; Vol. 1). İstanbul Büyükşehir Belediyesi Yayınları.

## Short Biography of Ömer Faruk Erdoğan

He was born in 1980 in Isparta. He completed his bachelor masters and PhD degrees at Ankara University, Turkey. In 2014, he joined the Dumlupınar University as an assistant professor where he served as head of the Islamic Philosophy department. Currently he holds an associate professor position at the Department of Islamic Philosophy under the faculty of Islamic Sciences in the above-mentioned University. His master's degree dissertation's title is "Khojazada's philosophy books" and He worked in his PhD on "al-Ghazzālī's criticism of Avicenna in Tahāfut al-Falāsifah".

His research is situated in the field of Religion-philosophy relation, with a special focus on Islamic Kalām-philosophy discussions, Muslim Peripatetic (Mashshā'ī) philosophers, Tahāfut al-Falāsifah and the commentaries on this book, celestial spheres, eternity-beginning in time, universal-particular knowledge, existence-absence and time-space discussions. In addition, he authored two books named "Philosophy of The Celestial Spheres" and "Takfīr Discussions in Tahāfut al-Falāsifah". Besides this, he has published several scholarly articles both national and international journals, book chapters, conference proceedings and projects.

email: omerfaruk.erdogan@dpu.edu.tr
ORCID ID: https://orcid.org/0000-0003-4131-3532

Engin Erdem, Assoc. Prof.

# Ibn Sīnā's Critique of Deism: A Debate on God's Creation and Sustaining

## Introduction

Ibn Sīnā's (d. 428/1037) metaphysical views on causality and the God-universe relationship have brought new dimensions to the philosophical and theological debates in many ways. After the criticisms and accusations of the later theologians, such as al-Ghazālī, about him, the very original aspects of Ibn Sīnā's conception of creation and causality have remained under the shadow of the debates on the eternity of the universe. In the discussions between Muslim philosophers and theologians, Ibn Sīnā is admitted on the side who advocates the eternity of the universe, while al-Ghazālī and his followers advocate the creation of the universe. From al-Ghazālī's point of view, Ibn Sīnā admits that the universe is eternal and he rejects God's act of creation. Leaving these discussions aside, in order to understand the views of Ibn Sīnā and what he actually wants to do, it is necessary to formulate the real context of the discussion between Muslim philosophers and theologians on the matter of creation. The Muslim theologians emphasize the attribute of God's creation and argue that there must be a temporal gap between God and the universe. For them, God is *the cause of origination* and the universe was created a finite time ago in the past (al-Ghazālī 2000). But, for Ibn Sīnā, holding that there is a temporal gap between God and the universe means that the need of creatures for God ceases after the first moment of creation. Since, in this understanding the role of God in creation is to bring something into existence and when the created being came to existence God's act of creation ends. Just as a child is no longer in need of her/his father to survive after being born, the universe can survive independently from God after it came into existence. This means that the view of temporal creation leads to some kind of deism (Ibn Sīnā 2005, 2014; Erdem 2016). According to Ibn Sīnā, God is not only a creator but also a sustainer of the universe. Ibn Sīnā's aim is not to advance an argument that the universe is eternal, but, to overcome deism by developing a *causal* or *analytical priority* relationship between God and the universe. This paper seeks to offer a new perspective on Ibn Sīnā's metaphysics of creation by interpreting his views on the nature of the timeless causality as an effort to overcome deism.

## Formulating the Problem

Ibn Sīnā has established a unique metaphysical system by critically analyzing the legacy of the ancient Greek philosophy and the early Islamic theological tradition. He has criticized the blind devotion of the Muslim Peripatetics to Aristotle by comparing it to the Hanbalīte attitude in Islamic tradition, which sees all kinds of new views as a heresy (Ibn Sīnā 1910). On the one hand, he benefited from the intellectual heritage of early Islamic theological tradition, on the other hand, he did not hesitate to criticize the Muʿtazilites' and Ash'arites' conceptions of God for containing anthropomorphic elements. In the post-Avicennian era, it is extremely important that the pure Aristotelian philosopher, Ibn Rushd, as well as the Ash'arī theologians such as al-Ghazālī, and Muʿtazilī theologians, such as al-Malāḥimī, have criticized Ibn Sīnā, showing how broad the spectrum of his metaphysical system is. Ibn Sīnā's metaphysical views about causality, creation and the relationship between God and the universe were heavily criticized in late Islamic thought, especially by the Muslim theologians. Looking at these discussions, especially the first chapter of al-Ghazālī's *al-Tahāfut*, it is seen that the most important criticism is focused on the beginning of the universe, and on the issue of creation.

According to al-Ghazālī's interpretation, Ibn Sīnā holds that the universe is eternal, there is no temporal beginning for the universe; since the universe has existed with God from all eternity, in such an understanding it cannot be said that God is the creator of the universe. For al-Ghazālī, in order to say that God created the universe, it is necessary to accept that only God existed in the beginning, but the universe did not exist. At the beginning there was God but nothing else, and then God created the universe (al-Ghazālī 2000). However, according to Ibn Sīnā, as we will see below, the real cause coexists with its effect and there cannot be a temporal priority between God and the universe. Since Ibn Sīnā does not accept a temporal gap between God and the universe, at first glance, the criticism of al-Ghazālī and of those who think like him about Ibn Sīnā may be seen as rightful.

However,- it should be noted that one of the most important obstacles to understand the views of Ibn Sīnā, as it would be like any other philosopher, is to address his metaphysical views through the formulation of his opponents. As Wittgenstein (1953: 255) says "the philosopher's treatment of a question is like a treatment of an illness". The aim of philosophy is to solve the philosophical problems by changing our way of thinking about those problems. In other words, to solve philosophical problems, we need to realize the problems arising from our approach to those philosophical problems. Addressing Ibn Sīnā's views on causality and creation in the context of the debates on the eternity of the universe is one of the most important reasons why his views are not understood correctly. To consider Ibn Sīnā's views on God-universe relationship under the title of *On the Eternity of Universe* is to put him in the chair of the accused. The opponents of Ibn Sīnā interpret his view as the eternity of the universe and they are therefore convicting him religiously. But is this really the case? In order to understand to what extent the criticisms about Ibn Sīnā are justified, it is necessary to examine Ibn Sīnā's own views on causality and God-universe relationship on its own. While doing this, the basic questions to be answered should be the following: Does Ibn Sīnā really deny God's creation, or does he defend a theory of creation superior to understanding of the theologians? Does he dismiss temporal creation because he does not care about religion as his opponents claim and is blindly attached to Greek philosophers such as Aristotle and Plotinus, or is there another reason? What kinds of problems arise if it is accepted that there is a temporal priority between God and the universe? If God is the creator of the universe, what kind of priority, if it is not temporal, is there between God and the universe?

If we want to find satisfiying answers to these questions, we have to address the issue through Ibn Sīnā's own texts, not in terms of the criticism and formulations of his opponents. Only having done this can we identify the true context of the discussion between Ibn Sīnā and the the Muslim theologians. Thus, the main purpose of this study is to develop a new approach related to the disputations between Ibn Sīnā and the Muslim theologians about God-universe relationship and to reformulate the the problem with respect to Ibn Sīnā's point of view. In doing so, I will first analyze Ibn Sīnā's metaphysical theory of causality, especially his conception of the efficient cause, which forms the basis of his doctrine of creation. Secondly, I shall tackle his criticisms related with Aristotle's concept of efficient cause and the views of Muslim theologians on temporal origination. Lastly, I will examine how Ibn Sīnā tries to overcome deism with a conception of timeless causality.

## Metaphysics of Causality

For Ibn Sīnā, the aim of the metaphysics is to prove God's existence; the True God (al-Ilāh, Allāh) is a Necessary Existent that does not need anything, but everything needs him (Ibn Sīnā 2005, 2014b). So, he is very aware of the fact that it requires to lay down the metaphysical foundations of causality, both to prove the existence of God and to explain divine creation and sustaining. First of all, when Ibn Sīnā speaks of the cause and the effect in metaphysics, he does not mean a phenomenon that is found in the physical world. In a way, he predicted Hume's criticism beforehand, saying that causality cannot be proved through sense experience. According to Ibn Sīnā, when we make observation in natural sciences, we can only detect that two events come one after another. No matter how often two events occur after each other, this does not indicate a causal relationship between the two.

> Again, knowledge of absolute causes comes about after the science establishing the existence of causes for those things that have causes. For, as long as we have not established the existence of causes for those things that are effects (by establishing that the existence of [the latter] has a relation to what precedes them in existence), it does not become a rational necessity that there is an absolute cause and that there is here some cause. As for sensation, it leads only to concomitance. And it is not the case that, if two things concomitants, it then follows necessarily that one of them is the cause of the other. (Ibn Sina 2005: 5-6)

In accordance with this passage, until now, we may have observed that when a piece of fire touches cotton, it burns, the sun is always rising from the east and sinking from the west. Based on these observations, we cannot say that the former is the cause and the latter is the effect and there is a causal relation between them. So, it is not possible to establish a cause-effect relationship between two things through sense experience. By means of sense experience, it can be determined that there is only succession or concomitancy between two things. Based on our many experiences with one after another, we may suppose that fire causes burning, and ginger causes heating. But, in order for this to be true, as Mullā Ṣadrā says, we must first assume the following rational proposition: *there must be a causal relation between frequently successive things.* It means that the causality that is tried to be proved by the sense experiences between the two things is based on an idea of *absolute causality* that preceded it. However, it is not an apodictic knowledge that there is absolute causality between things, it is only a *famous* knowledge but a famous knowledge does not reveal the truth, because it is not based on demonstration, that is scientific knowledge. Therefore, the fact that some of the existents are causes in an absolute sense can be proved by demonstration only in metaphysics (Mullā Ṣadrā 2007). Gaven Kerr's explorations on Aquinas' metaphysics of causality is very helpful to understand Ibn Sīnā's approach to the same issue. According to Kerr (2012), causality is a one-way dependency relationship; there is an asymmetrical relationship between cause and effect. The existence of the effect depends on the cause, but the opposite is not true. So, causality is a relationship between two things, one that exists on its own and has the power to bestow existence to someone else, and another that does not exist on its own and needs someone else to exist; the thing which is the cause here is not necessary to be material. As Kerr (2012:543–44) says, "Construing causality in terms of a relation between events undermines the very real relationship and connection between cause and effect that is at the heart of the causal relation."

Ibn Sīnā does not only say that the nature of causality cannot be proven by sense experience, but he also points to where the issue should be held. According to him, the nature of causality can only be explained in metaphysics (Ibn Sīnā 2005). To better understand what Ibn Sīnā means, it is necessary to examine the contexts in which the subject of causality is related in his metaphysical system. Topics such as the subject matter of metaphysics, the terms of necessary and possible, and the distinction between essence and existence are the context of discussion to which causality is deeply related. Ibn Sīnā, in the fourth chapter of his book *The Metaphysics of Healing*, in which he talks about *on the totality of matters in this science,* he lists cause and effect among the topics that this science comprises. According to Ibn Sīnā, every science has a subject matter and every science investigates the necessary accidents of the subject it deals with. For instance, the subject matter of medicine is the human body and the subject of music is voice. Medicine investigates the necessary accidents of the human body, such as illness and well-being; the music investigates the voice in terms of its harmony or disharmony. Similarly, the subject matter of metaphysics is being qua being and its necessary accidents. For him, cause and effect, like unity and multitude, necessity and possibility, are the necessary accidents of being qua being, which is the subject matter of metaphysics. So, it is the duty of metaphysician to demonstrate the nature of causality (Ibn Sīnā 2005).

For Ibn Sīnā, unlike the particular sciences, which studies only one region of being, such as mathematics, physics, and biology, metaphysics is a universal science and it deals with being qua being in its most general sense. Our knowledge on existence is self-evident; there is no doubt that something exists (Ibn Sīnā 1982). When a metaphysician analyzes the nature of existence he apprehends that whatever exists is either necessary in itself or necessary by another. Any existent, when considered by mind just itself, it is seen that there are three modalities: necessary, possible, and impossible. It is not permitted to say that it is impossible after it was supposed existing. So, any existent considered just itself is either *necessary in itself (wājib al-wujūd bi-dhātihī/necesse esse per se)* or *necessary by another (wâjib al-wujûd bi-ghayrihi/ necesse esse per aliud).* (Ibn Sīnā 2005; Richardson 2013)

> Every being, if considered from the point of view of its essence and without consideration of other things, is found to be such that either existence necessarily belongs to it in itself or it does not. If existence belongs to it necessarily, then it is the truth in itself and that whose existence is necessary from itself. This is the Independent Reality. If, on the other hand, existence does not belong to it necessarily, it is not permissible to say that it is impossible in itself after it was supposed existing. But if, in relation to its essence, a condition is linked to it, such as the condition of the nonexistence of its cause, it becomes impossible or, such as the condition of the existence of its cause, it becomes necessary. If no condition is linked to its essence, neither existence nor non-existence of a cause, then there remains for it in itself the third option, that is, possibility. Thus, with respect to its essence, it would be a thing that is neither necessary nor impossible. Therefore, every existent either has necessary existence in essence or has possible existence in essence. (Ibn Sīnā 2014a: 122).

For Ibn Sīnā, whatever exists is necessary in some sense of *necessary.* God is the only being necessary existence in itself, whose non-existence is impossible, wheras the creatures are possible in themselves, but, their existence is necessary through another, that is by God. These basic concepts of Ibn Sīnā's metaphysics, *necessary in itself, possible in itself* and *necessary by another,* reveals also the meanings of cause and effect. What is necessary in itself does not need to anything to exist apart from itself. What is possible in itself is, by definition, needs the cause both to come into existence and to survive its existence. This shows that when we grasp the meaning of necessity and possibility in metaphysics, whereby we can understand the meaning of cause and effect too. Since, there are parallelisms between the necessary and the cause and between the possible and the effect. The role of the efficient cause is to bestow existence to whom who has not existence in itself. "The agent" says Ibn Sīnā (2005:196), "bestows from itself an existence upon another thing, which this latter did not possess." But, when the possible in itself came into existence thanks to grace of necessary existence in itself, its neediness to him does not cease, but it needs him at every moment of its existence. Only God exists by itself, all other creatures exist thanks to an act of existence granted to them by God. So, it has become evident that everything other than the necessary existence in itself is possible in its existence and it acquires existence from another. "This is the meaning of a thing's being created." (Ibn Sīnā 2005: 272). After explaining the metaphysical basis of causality in this way, Ibn Sīnā, examines the problems encountered in the understanding of causality of Aristotle and of the Muslim theologians. Now, let's look at his criticism closely.

## Critique of Deism: The Principle of Existence, Not of Movement or Origination!

Ibn Sīnā criticizes both Aristotle's conception of the *cause of movement* and of the *cause of orgination* of the Muslim theologians. According to him, in the former, God's attribute of creation is excluded, and, the latter can not explain divine sustaining or conservation after the first act of creation. To begin with Aristotle's cause of movement, the conception of four causes is common between Aristotle and Ibn Sīnā, but there is a fundamental difference in two philosophers' understanding of the efficient cause. The disagreement between the two philosophers can be seen as a natural result emerging from the difference of point of view about whether the issue of causation is a subject matter of physics or metaphysics. For Aristotle, who moves from physics, the efficient cause is the cause of movement or tranquility; for example, the decision maker is the cause of the action and the father is the cause of the child (Aristotle 2016). Unlike Aristotle, Ibn Sīnā makes a fundamental distinction between *the natural efficient cause* and *the metaphysical efficient cause*. According to him, the natural efficient cause is the agent of movement or change, as Aristotle said. For example, the father, as a natural efficient cause, is the agent of the movement of the sperm required for the child to be born into the mother's womb; but it is not the cause for the child's existence. For Ibn Sīnā, who refers directly to the the Qur'anic term *al-ibdā*ʿ in explaining the efficient cause in metaphysics, it is incompatible with theistic concept of God to see him solely the cause of movement. Thus, to him, the fact that God is the creator of the universe means that he is the efficient cause of its existence, not just its movement (Ibn Sīnā 2005). Ibn Sīnā explicitly expresses the difference between metaphysical philosophers like himself and natural philosophers such as Aristotle about the meaning of the efficient cause:

> This is because the metaphysical philosophers do not mean by "agent" only the principle of motion, as the naturalists mean, but the principle and giver of existence, as in the case of God with respect to the world. As for the natural efficient cause, it does not bestow any existence other than motion in one of the forms of motion. Thus, in the natural sciences, that which bestows existence is a principle of motion. (Ibn Sīnā 2005: 195).

In this passage, Ibn Sīnā contrasts the the natural efficient cause and the metaphysical efficient cause. The causal efficiency of God on the universe can not be explained in terms of natural science. We can explain God's creation only by considering the meaning of the efficient cause in metaphysics (Lizzini 2020). As a matter of fact, events in the universe can be explained by natural causes;

however, the coming into existence of the universe itself can not be explained by natural causes, but only by metaphysical causes. So, the most important flaw in Aristotle's understanding of efficient cause, from Ibn Sīnā's standpoint, is that he only tackled the issue in terms of natural science. Whereas in metaphysics the efficient cause has a more comprehensive meaning than in natural science (Ibn Sīnā 2005). According to Duns Scotus, who adopts Ibn Sīnā's view exactly on this matter, *efficiency* can be treated as either a metaphysical or a physical feature; in metaphysics efficiency means *to give existence to someone else*, which is wider than the meaning of *efficient* in physics; therefore, efficiency in metaphysics offers a stronger way to prove the existence of God than in physics (Scotus 2004).

It is seen that, Ibn Sīnā revised Aristotle's concept of efficient cause by pointing out to the metaphysical dimension of the issue and introduced a new concept of efficient cause that is the principle of existence. It is very likely that, Ibn Sīnā might have been inspired by the Qur'anic concept of God in developing such kind of very original concept of efficient cause, in the sense of *the giver of existence*, namely the creator of the world. However, on paying attention the debates in the early Islamic theological tradition on God's attribute of creation, one might argue that the creative concept of God that Ibn Sīnā advocates against Aristotle was not original to him, and that was already a view previously held by the Muslim theologians.

It is a well known fact that, the early Muslim theologians mainly focused on the problem of beginning of the universe to argue against the naturalist philosophers and developed a new kind of proof for the existence of God by arguing that the universe was created a finite time ago in the past. This proof is called in the literature of modern philosophy of religion *Kalām Cosmological Argument* (Craig 2000). It is clear that Ibn Sīnā and the Muslim theologians stand in the same rank in the face of Aristotle with regard to holding God's attribute of creation. Although, Ibn Sīnā shares the same view with the theologians about the creativity of God, he has a different approach of how it should be understood. As I said above, the disagreement between Ibn Sīnā and Aristotle is about whether God is the principle of movement or the principle of existence. In contrast, the conflict between Ibn Sīnā and the Muslim theologians is concerned with the question of temporal creation and eternal creation. Both sides agree that everything other than God is in need of him. But, they differentiate in answering the question what is the reason for the neediness. For the theologians, the cause of neediness is origination (ḥudūth); whereas, according to Ibn Sīnā, the creatures' neediness to God depends on the possibility (imkān) (Ibn Sīnā 1982). The conflict on this issue also led to the emergence of two different versions of the cosmological argument. *The Kalām Cosmological Argument* that the Muslim theologians hold aims at proving that the universe had a temporal beginning. However, according to *the contingency argument* or *the metaphysical proof* that Ibn Sīnā advocates, God's existence can be proven, even if the universe does not have a temporal beginning.

For the adherents of the view of the temporal creation, the history of the universe in the past is not infinite; it was created a finite time ago. To prove that the universe was created, it is necessary to put forth that it was not infinite in the past. Their proof for the existence of God is based on the impossibility of an infinite temporal regress of events and it can be formulated as below:

1. Everything that begins to exist requires a cause for its origin.
2. The world began to exist.
   (a) There are temporal phenomena in the world.
   (b) These are preceded by other temporal phenomena.
   (c) The series of temporal phenomena cannot regress infinitely.
      (i) An actually existing infinite series involves various absurdities.
   (d) Therefore, the series of temporal phenomena must have had a beginning.
3.Therefore, the world has a cause for its origin: its Creator (Craig 2000: 48,49).

The theologians claim that the creativity of God and the createdness of the universe depend on the existence of a temporal gap between the two. According to them, the non-existence of the universe, when it was not created, precedes its existence. God created the universe from out of nothing; at the begginning there was only God, but nothing else. Then the universe has existed with him later on. In this understanding, God is *temporally prior* to the universe; there is *a temporal gap* between God and the universe, just as the father was before the child and the builder was before the building. For the theologians, there is a parallelism between temporal creation and creation from nothing; denying temporal creation also means denying the creation *ex nihilo*. There are two options in the minds of the theologians about the creation of the universe: existence and non-existence. For these theologians who cannot go out of these two options, there is only one option left for a person who does not agree to creation ex nihilo: creation from something, that is, the eternity of the universe. Accordingly, from their point of view, since Ibn Sīnā denies the temporal creation this leads to the conclusion that he accepts the eternity of the universe. Whoever defends the eternity of the universe he denies also God's creation and gets out of religion (al-Ghazālī 2000; al-Malāḥimī 2008).

Above, we have seen that Ibn Sīnā criticized Aristotle's view of efficient cause for not icluding a concept of creation. Why did he criticize the view of the temporal creation of the Muslim theologians at the expense of blasphemy? To answer this important question, it is necessary to find out the problems that Ibn Sīnā sees in temporal creation. According to Ibn Sīnā, God is not only creator, but, He is also the sustainer of all creatures at every moment of their existence; accepting that there is a temporal gap between the cause and the effect, that is between God and the universe, poses important problems both in explaining the nature of causality and the neediness of the creatures to God after his first act of creation. In discussing the problems faced by the theologians about explaining the divine sustaining, Ibn Sīnā puts forward the distinction between *the cause of origination (ḥudūth)* and *the cause of existence (wujūd).* In the former, held by the theologians, the role of the efficient cause is to originate something and the cause is temporally prior to its effect. In this understanding, the relationship between God and the universe is similar to the relationship between the builder and the building, and between the father and the child. Just as there is no child when there is a father or there is no building without a builder, in the same way, there was only God in the beginning and there was nothing with him. God's creation of the universe means that while it did not exist. He did originate it later (Ibn Sīnā 2005; 2014a).

But, for Ibn Sīnā, if the efficient cause is considered to be the cause of origination, it becomes very difficult to explain God's keeping creatures in existence after the first act of creation. Their conception of cause of origination involves God's creation, but not his sustaining. Because in this understanding, the creatures are in need of God for their origination, not for their existence. Because of the fact that the sole function of God is just origination, once the created thing originates thanks to God's act, its neediness to God ends there. Just as the child can exist independently of the father after it exists, the universe can also exist independently of God after it was created.

> Someone may think that the agent and the cause are needed only for a thing to have existence after nonexistence and that, once a thing is brought into existence, the thing would [continue to] exist as sufficient unto itself [even] if the cause is no longer present. Thus, someone has thought that a thing is in need of the cause only for its origination, but that, once it is originated and comes to exist, it no longer needs the cause. For such a person, the causes are thus only the causes of origination, being [temporally] prior [ to their effects], not simultaneous with them. This is a false belief. (Ibn Sīnā 2005: 198)

The fact that the theologians use the term *the Maker* (al-Ṣāni') for God and the *the made* (al-Masnu') for the universe is a clear proof that they see God as a

*Builder* and the universe as his *building.* Anyway, the method that theologians follow to prove the existence of God is to go from work to artist, from building to the builder. However, according to Ibn Sīnā, neither the builder is the cause of the building nor the father is the cause of the child. As Kara Richardson says, Ibn Sīnā identifies both the builder and the father as causes of motion: "Builders and fathers are causes of houses and children in the sense that they are causes of certain motions, which are terminate in certain combinations: brick arranged house-wise or sperm conjoined with the matter of womb. Builders and fathers are not causes of existence of houses and children to which they are temporally prior" (Richardson 2013: 231).

From Ibn Sīnā's point of view, an agent that originates something but can not keep it in existence is not a real cause, it is only an *accidental* or *auxiliary* cause. To explain this crucial point, he examines the modality of the the originated thing after its origination. The existence of the originated thing (let's call it *X*), after its origination is either necessary or not necessary. If *X*'s existence is necessary, then it's necessity is either through its essence or not. If it is through its essence, then its origination is impossible, since the origination of the thing that is necessary in its essence is impossible. If *X*'s existence is necessary not through its essence, then, the cause if its necessity must be either the origination, or one of the attributes of its essence or something external. Ibn Sīnā, by using *a reductio ad absurdum* argument, eliminates the options and concludes that the necessity of *X*'s existence after its origination must be due to an external cause (Ibn Sīnā 2005).

It is understood that the creatures do not only need God to come into existence from non-existence, they also needs an external cause to sustain their existence. Given that the universe came into existence, how is God's maintenance of the universe realized? The originated thing after its origination needs an external cause to stay in existence; but, the conception of agent of the theologians is far from meeting this need. Since, the role of the cause of origination in creation is just to bring something into existence. When the universe originates, it does not need God any more. Because in terms of their definition of agent, the causal efficacy of the agent ceases when he performs its action.

> They may also say that if a thing is brought into existence, the need for the agent disappears; so that if the agent is missing it is permissible that the effect remains in existence. This is exemplified in their observation of the missing of the builder, while the building still subsists. Many of them do not hesitate to say that if nonexistence were permissible for the Creator, the exalted, his nonexistence would not harm the existence of the world. For the world, according to them, needs the Creator, the exalted, only to bring it into existence, that is, to bring it out of nonexistence into existence.

> By doing so, he is an agent. But if the world is caused and acquires existence after nonexistence, then, after that, how could it come into existence after nonexistence in a manner in which it would need an agent? (Ibn Sīnā 2014a:132)

To understand what Ibn Sīnā means here, we need to consider his distinction regarding the series of causes. As we said before, theologians advocate temporal creation, while philosophers advocate eternal creation. Accordingly, there are two types of series causes depending on this distinction: *accidentally ordered series* and *essentially ordered series*. When it is accepted that there is temporal priority between cause and effect, then, this means that the series of causes must be an accidental type. As an example of the accidentally ordered series, we can consider the fathers-sons series. The grandfather is temporally prior to the father. There is no father when the grandfather exists, then the father exists with the grandfather. But the death of the grandfather does not prevent the father from surviving. Even after the grandfather's death, the father may cause the grandson to be born. There is an *intransitive* causal relation between them; as Kerr (2017:157) says, "since in that series there is no dependence of the effect to on the cause for causality, rather, a single cause brings about a single effect, but it is not in virtue of the cause that the effect can itself be a cause in the same respect." However, as we will see below, according to Ibn Sīnā , it is necessary to hold an essentially ordered series including a transitive concept of causality to explain divine creation and sustaining.

In addition, according to Ibn Sīnā, the conception of agent of the theologians is self-contradictory. An agent, by definition, is to be in action. For the theologians, the condition for an agent to be an agent is to accept a situation where it was not acting. Since for them, at the beginning there was God, but nothing else; God had been inactive until to the moment of creation. However, if only God is the agent in a full sense, there can be no time in which he did not act. If God's will to create the universe could bring itself into existence, why had it not done this before? If there is a situation where a cause exists but its effect does not exist, this means that it is not a real cause. That is because, the real causes coexist with their effects. In a full sense the only real cause is God and exists with all his effects in a timeless manner. The real cause gives existence to the creatures and sustains their existence at every moment. It is possible to hear that the verses of the Qur'an echo on the background of these metaphysical explanations of Ibn Sīnā: "Indeed, Allah sustains the heavens and the earth, lest they cease. If they should fail, there is none can sustain them thereafter: Verily He is Most Forbearing, Oft-Forgiving" (35/41).

From Ibn Sīnā's point of view, when God is seen as a cause of origination, it is possible to say that God did bring the universe into existence, but, he cannot prevent it from falling into non-existence. Thus, this understanding fails to explain God's causal efficiency on the creatures after his first act of creation. This means that, God is a Creator, but he is not a Sustainer (al-Qayyūm). If we express Ibn Sīnā's criticisms above in modern philosophical terms, we can say that this is a kind of *critique of deism* (Erdem 2016). Here, by the term deism, I mean a belief in a God who created the world but has since remained indifferent to it. Of course, there is no clear statement of deism in the texts of the early theologians and their modern followers may reject it. However, when Ibn Sīnā analyzes their conceptual framework on causality, he argues that, even if they oppose it, such a conclusion will inevitably arise. As a historical fact, Ibn Sīnā's criticism of the early Muslim theologians precedes the criticism they directed towards him. But, the fact that the later theologians preferred to criticize Ibn Sīnā instead of responding to his criticisms may be an expression of their efforts to avoid Ibn Sīnā's criticisms. In other words, the criticism of the theologians against Ibn Sīnā may be seen as an effort to cover the criticism that Ibn Sīnā had previously directed at them. Because of the fact that Ibn Sīnā was labeled as a philosopher who defends the eternity of the universe, his criticisms of theologians has been overshadowed by these charges against him.

## Overcoming Deism: A Creating and Sustaining God

Above, we have seen why Ibn Sīnā criticized the views of cause of orgination and cause of movement. Now, we can dwell upon *the cause of existence* that he advocates. In the remainder of this paper, I want to touch upon some interesting aspects of the relationship between Ibn Sīnā's theory of causality and his conception of divine sustaining. While developing his metaphysical theory of causality, Ibn Sīnā's main aim is to establish a concept of God that both creats and sustains. According to him, a metaphysically consistent theory of causality should set forth a concept of divine creation and conservation. To overcome the shortcomings he sees in the conceptions of causality of Aristotle and of theologians, Ibn Sīnā enhances a new theory of *timeless causation.*

According to Ibn Sīnā, above all, the fact that the universe is temporally beginningless does not mean that it was not created. Accordingly, the belief of the theologians that creation is synonymous with temporal beginning of the universe is not a warranted assumption. In order to explain this, Ibn Sīnā points out the two different meanings of the term of eternal (al-qadīm): *eternal in itself* and *eternal in time.* What is eternal in itself is that its existence does not depend on a a cause; i.e., it does not owe its existence to someone else. The only being that is eternal in itself is God, who is necessary in itself. What is eternal in time has no beginning in time. The angels, celestial intellects are eternal in time, are not eternal in themselves, but they are created in themselves. It is true that Ibn Sīnā holds that the universe is eternal in temporal sense, that is eternal in time; but it does not mean that the universe was not created. The meaning of creation, for him, is to be owing existence to someone else, not to have a beginning in time. Hence, creation and temporal beginning do not coincide with each other (Ibn Sīnā 1982).

According to Ibn Sīnā, the fact that two things are simultaneous does not mean that one is not prior to the other. Two things can be simultaneous, but one of them may precede the other *causally* or *analytically*. Here, if we mention the interesting examples Ibn Sīnā gives, when I shake my hand, my ring moves with my hand; similarly, when I turn the key, the door lock moves simultaneously with the key. When considered temporally, the movement of the hand and the movement of the ring, similarly, the movement of the key and the movement of the lock of the door are simultaneous. But, the movement of the hand is causally prior to the movement of the ring, and the movement of the key is prior to the movement of the lock door. So, there is a difference between two kinds of priority: causal priority and temporal priority. The true cause coexists with its effects, that is, God and the creatures exist simultaneously, but, God is causally prior to it. There is no temporal gap between the cause and effect, but the cause is prior to effect due to itself (Ibn Sīnā 2014a).

While explaining the issue of priority, Ibn Sīnā also draws attention to two meanings of the term *created*. The created is a thing that comes into existence while it was non-existent and, the term created (*ḥādith*), like eternal, has two meanings: Created due to itself and created due to time. The existence of created due to itself is preceded by non-existence (*laysiyyah*), but the existence of created due to time is preceded by time and matter. If we express the same issue in terms of posteriority, the existence of the created due to itself is posterior to its non-existence. Whatever is created due to itself is firstly non-existent; then, it gets existence due to its cause. Every effected thing (*mā'lul*) is created, since it gets its existence while it was non-existent. Thus, every effected thing, although it might have been in existence at all times, is created due to itself. It is not created only in one moment of time, but it is created all moments of time. But, what is created due to time must be preceded by time and matter. Because of the fact that the existence of created due to time must have a temporal beginning, *before* its coming into existence there must be a time in which it was non-existent. But, thinking of a beginning for time requires accepting another time that precedes it, and, the idea of temporal creation leads paradoxically to the infinity of time (Ibn Sīnā 1982). The following statements of Ibn Sīnā comparing the understanding of creation of theologians with his own understanding are quite remarkable:

> Immediate [absolute] creation *(al-ibdāʿ)* is a thing's giving existence to another that depends on nothing other than it—without the mediation of matter, instrument, or time. That which is preceded by temporal nonexistence, on the other hand, cannot dispense with an intermediary. Immediate creation is in a nobler rank than material production *(al-takwīn)* and temporal production *(al-iḥdāth)*." (Ibn Sīnā 2014a: 139).

According to Ibn Sīnā, denying temporal creation, contrary to the claims of the theologians, does not mean refusing to create from nothing. On the contrary, accepting temporal creation leads to such a conclusion. Since explaining this point requires a wider discussion, I am not going into more details here.

If return to the issue of priority again, to better understand what Ibn Sīnā meant by causal priority, we must remember how he explained the relationship between cause and effect. I have already said that Ibn Sīnā explains causality as a relationship between *necessary existence in itself* and *possible existence in itself*. For him, every existent is either necessary existence in itself or possible existence in itself. What is possible in itself does not come into existence due to its essence; since, inasmuch as it is possible, existence by its essence is not more preferential than non-existence. Thus, if it comes into existence, this is only because of something else. It shows that the existence of every possible thing in itself is from another. When the necessary existence in itself gives existence to the possible in itself, the latter gets the status of necessary existence through another. Because of the fact that a possible thing can not come into existence unless getting necessity from *the necessary existence in itself*, creation does not only mean to give existence, but it is also a transferring of the necessity through necessary in itself to the possible in itself. Thus, the created thing with respect to its essence is possible in itself, but, with respect to its cause it is necessary (Ibn Sīnā 1982; 2014a). "Hence the Necessary Existent is one, nothing sharing with Him in His rank, and thus nothing other than Him is necessary existent. Since nothing other than Him is a necessary existent, He is the principle of the necessitation of the existence of everything" Ibn Sīnā 2005: 273).

When Ibn Sīnā ascribes necessity to the creatures, he does not want to say that they are autonomous, but rather he wants to emphasize that they are in need of God at every moment of their existence. After coming into existence, the modal status of the creature still remains the same: possible in itself. For Ibn Sīnā, divine creation and sustaining is one act. The true efficient cause, that is the cause of existence, bestows existence to the others, prevents them falling into non-existence, and co-exists simultaneously with its effects. Ibn Sīnā's conception of timeless causation involves an essentially ordered series. To him, the first cause is, no matter how long the series of causes, cause of all causal series. All intermediate causes need the first cause for causal efficiency (Ibn Sīnā 2005). So, in this sense, the only real agent is God, who does not need anything, but everything needs him. Since the theologians explain divine creation in terms of time, it is necessary to go to the beginning of the universe to explain the neediness of creatures to God. However, because of the fact that, Ibn Sīnā sees creation as a timeless causal relationship between the Creator and the creatures, the creatures, even if they had no beginning in time, are in need of God at every moment of their existence.

## Conclusion

Here we have pointed to a different dimension of the debate between Ibn Sīnā and the theologians on the nature of creation and made a new suggestion whether it is possible to reformulate the problem from a different perspective. It can be said that it is not justified to interpret Ibn Sīnā's critique as deism, because the theologians defend the doctrine of *continuous creation* to overcome deism. It seems to me that, Ibn Sīnā's aim is not to ignore the theory of continuous creation, but just to point out that the conceptual framework they base on to explain the God-universe relationship might lead to deism. What this article tries to do is just to draw attention to a neglected aspect of the discussion between the philosophers and the theologians. Treating the debate between Ibn Sīnā and the theologians not only in terms of the eternity of the universe, but also in terms of deism, may be helpfull to better understand the conflict between the two sides. On remembering the criticisms Ibn Sīnā made against theologians about the issue of creation and the criticisms that theologians directed against Ibn Sīnā at the same issue, it is more appropriate to consider the conflict between the philosophers and the theologians as two different models of creation. Seeing the conflict from this point of view, hopefully, can contribute to put the debate on a more balanced ground and inspire to get closer to the truth. Ultimately, what is more appropriate from a philosophical point of view is not to pay attention to the accusations of two sides about each other, but to investigate which model of creation provides a stronger and simpler explanation. It should not be overlooked that Ibn Sīnā prefers to say that his view is *stronger* and *nobler* rather than saying that the views of his opponents are wrong.

## References

Aristotle, (2016) *Metaphysics*. translated with introduction and notes by C.D.C. Reeve, Indiana: Hackett Publishing Comp.

Avicenna (2005). *The Metaphysics of The Healing*: A Parallel English-Arabic Text, M.E. Marmura (ed. and trans.). Provo (Utah): Brigham Young University Press.

Craig, William Lane (2000). *The Kalām Cosmological Argument*. West Brodway: Wipt and Stock Publishers.

Erdem, Engin (2016). *Varlıktan Tanrıya: İbn Sina'nın Metafizik Delili*. Istanbul: Endülüs Yay.

Al-Ghazālī (2000). *The Incoherence of the Philosophers/Tahāfut al-falāsifa*. A parallel English-Arabic Text, M. E. Marmura (ed. and trans.), 2nd. ed., Provo (Utah): Brigham Young University Press.

Ibn Sīnā (1910). *Manṭiq al-Mashriqiyyīn. ed. M. al-Khaṭīb and ʿA. al-Qatlā. Cairo: Al-Maktaba al-Salafiyya*.

Ibn Sīnā (1982). *Kitāb an-Najāt*., ed. Mājid Fakhry, Beirut.

Ibn Sīnā (2014a). *Ibn Sīnā's Remarks and Admonitions*: physics and metaphysics: an analysis and annotated translation/ Shams C. Inati. New York: Columbia University Press.

Ibn Sīnā (2014b). *İhlas Sûresi Tefsiri*. Trc. Ahmet Hamdi Akseki, haz. Ahmet Faruk Gü- ney, 2. Baskı, Ankara: DİB Yayınları.

Kerr, Gaven (2012). Essentially Ordered Series Reconsidered. *American Catholic Philosophical Quarterly* 86/4: 541–555

Kerr, Gaven. (2017). Essentially Ordered Series Reconsidered Once Again. *American Catholic Philosophical Quarterly* 91/2: 155–174.

Lizzini, Olga (2020). Ibn Sina's Metaphysics. *The Stanford Encyclopedia of Philosophy* (Summer 2020 Edition), Edward N. Zalta (ed.): https://plato.stanford.edu/archives/sum2020/entries/ibn-sina-metaphysics/>.

al-Malāḥimī (2008). *Tuḥfat al-mutakallimīn fī al-radd ʿalā al-Falāsifa*. eds. Hassan Ansari –Wilferd Madelung. Tehran: Iranian Institute of Philosophy – Institute of Islamic Studies Free University of Berlin.

Mullā Ṣadrā (2007). *Sharh al-Ilāhiyyāt min Kitāb al-Shifāʾ* [Commentary on the Metaphysics of the Cure]. Ed. Najafqulī Habībī, vol. I-II, Beirut.

Richardson, Kara (2013). Avicenna's Conception of the Efficient Cause. *British Journal for the History of Philosophy* 21/2: 220–239.

Scotus, John Duns (2004). A Treatise On God As First Principle. Montana: Kessinger Publishing.

Wittgenstein, Ludwig (1953). *Philosophical Investigations*. translated by G.E.M. Anscombe. Reprint, Oxford: Blackwell, 1997.

## Short Biography of Engin Erdem

He is Associate Professor of Philosophy of Religion at Ankara University, Faculty of Divinity. His doctoral dissertation is about the problem of divine eternity and creation (2006).

His main research areas include topics such as Ibn Sina's metaphysics, Kant's later philosophy, natural law theory and theological utilitarianism in the early Hanafi law tradition.

He took part as a researcher in the Turkish Dictionary of Scientific Terms of Turkish Academy of Sciences, 2011.

In addition to numerous articles, he is the author of the book From Existence to God: Ibn Sina's Metaphysical Proof (Endulus, 2016) and The Dictionary of Theological Terms (Grafiker, 2019), with Mahmut Ay. Currently, with Necmettin Pehlivan, he has been working to translate Ali Qushji's Commentary on Tajrid al-Aqaid.

Glen M. Cooper, Ph.D

# Avicenna and the Contest of Healing: Medical Crises and the Body Politic Metaphor in the *Canon of Medicine*

## 1.1 Introduction

These remarks are drawn from a close comparison between Avicenna's discussion of fevers and medical crises in the *Canon*, and the Greek physician Galen's discussion of the same. Since Galen was the ultimate source for many of Avicenna's medical ideas, it is useful to note how differently the latter expresses them in the *Canon*. Of particular interest is Avicenna's use of an ancient metaphor for the relationship between patient, disease, and doctor that has connections with a long tradition of political thought—the "Body Politic" metaphor. The present remarks build upon and extend my prior research in Greek and Arabic medicine and philosophy.[1] Furthermore, Galen presented a healing scenario that he framed dramatically, which Avicenna develops in his medical writings. As I shall show, the Body Politic metaphor provided Avicenna with the body as a stage where the drama of healing takes place. The plot of the story of healing is adapted from Galen, whose four stages of the patient's fever provide a temporal framework for the healing narrative.

## 2.1 The Combat Metaphor and the Body Politic

It has long been accepted that Avicenna in the *Canon* expressed a version of the Galeno-Hippocratic system of medicine in a more concise and much more user-friendly format than his Greek sources. Many of Galen's medical writings were polemical, and one must extract his meaning from extended rhetorical arguments, which is not easy to do. Avicenna in the *Canon* has already done that for the reader, adding abundant useful observations, as well as corrections and extensions, from his own practice and experience. As an example of a clarification, Avicenna elaborates a combat metaphor that is only hinted at by

1 See: Cooper (2011) and Cooper (2018).

Galen,[2] in order to explain better the roles of doctor and patient in the healing context. There, the patient is conceived of as being locked in mortal struggle with the disease. In addition, whereas Galen assigns the primary role in healing to the doctor, Avicenna gives more of a role to the patient's suffering body.

In connection with this "combat metaphor", Avicenna invokes the "Body Politic" metaphor. By this metaphor, the patient is compared to a city that is under siege by the disease.[3] Elements within the patient—organs, faculties, and his natural strength—all rally to fight the attacker. These correspond to the internal elements of the city or state that are employed to defend the city from the invading disease. Different philosophers, from Plato on, have described the comparison of body to city in various ways. This metaphor, although hinted at in Galen's writings, does not appear there is any developed form. Avicenna has elaborated it masterfully to illustrate the context of healing, by showing the essential role that each factor—doctor, nature, and patient's body—plays in it.

## 2.2 Ancient Origins of the Body Politic Metaphor

The Body Politic metaphor did not originate with Avicenna, but has a long history in the philosophical tradition, extending back to Plato, where its most familiar expression appears in the *Republic*. In order to discover the meaning of the concept of justice, which is a condition of the individual human soul, Plato has Socrates imagine the individual body to be the size of a city—with corresponding structures between body and city—in order to examine better how the parts function.[4] He concludes that justice for both the city and the individual follows from having a well-ordered soul, where all the parts perform their functions properly. The best-known feature of his ideal state is the rulership of the "Philosopher Kings," who know best what justice, truth, and the Good are for the state.[5] These Rulers correspond to the head, which is the seat of rational thought. The two other classes of citizens, the army and the craftsmen, correspond to the chest and the abdomen respectively. Plato drew upon physiological features to describe the attributes of these classes: the army corresponds

2 Galen, *Critical Days* k 9,920,16–921,2 (Cooper ed., pp. 354–355).

3 Avicenna (1593), *Kitāb al-qānūn fi al-ṭibb*, Book 4, Part 2, Treatise 1, Chapter 1, p. 41 (Doostdar transl., pp.58–59).

4 Plato (1997), *Republic*, Book 4, 434e ff.

5 Plato (1997), *Republic*, Book 5, 473d ff. For such an ideal community to ever come into being, "philosophers [must] become kings. . .or those now called kings [must]. . . genuinely and adequately live the philosophical life."

to the spirited part of the body, namely, the chest where the heart is, and the craftsmen correspond to the region below the diaphragm, where baser desires originate. In Avicenna's use of the metaphor, Nature corresponds to the wise Ruler, who knows what's best for the state, and who must defend his city. This image was suggested by Galen, but not developed by him, when he characterized favorable critical days as benevolent kings, and the bad critical days as evil tyrants.[6] However, for both Galen and Avicenna, the Ruler cannot be victorious on its own, and must rely on the doctor's superior understanding of the natural laws of healing.

So, Avicenna had much to draw upon from Greek and Arabic traditions for his use of the Body Politic and combat metaphors in his description of healing. Avicenna no doubt learned of this metaphor from the philosopher al-Fārābī (d. 950), whose writings he relied on in his study of Aristotle's *Metaphysics*.[7] Al-Fārābī's grand formulation of the Body Politic metaphor in the Arabic tradition appeared in his magisterial treatise on political philosophy, *Mabādi ʾ ārāʾ ahl al-madīna al-fāḍila* ("The Principles of the Views of the Citizens of the Excellent City") (Al-Fārābī 1985), which is an adaptation and development of Plato's *Republic*. This work makes an explicit comparison between parts of the ideal state and the human body—something that was of less interest to Plato in his discussion. Al-Fārābī combined the political body with medical ideas in a way that had not been done before.

In the process of explicitly comparing the human body to a city, al-Fārābī introduced a number of Greek scientific ideas, not discussed in the *Republic*, which we might suppose were derived from Plato's *Timaeus*. Thus, al-Fārābī combined the themes of the *Republic* and the *Timaeus* into one work, drawing upon the Galenic medical tradition for the details, thus linking the political body and medicine more closely. Consistent with his Aristotelian leanings, instead of making the head the ruling organ, as did Plato, al-Fārābī makes the heart the ruling organ (*ʿuḍwu raʾīs*).[8] He is, however, careful to make the brain

6 Galen (2011), *Critical Days*, 9,786,17–787,7 (Cooper ed., pp. 128–129). See also Plato (1997), *Republic*, 6.488d: The "true captain must of necessity pay attention to the seasons, the heavens, the stars, the winds, and everything proper to the craft [of navigation] if he is really to govern a ship."

7 See Gutas (1988), pp. 238–54, where he describes how Avicenna's metaphysics derives from his reading of a brief treatise by Fārābī on the purposes of metaphysics, his *Aghrāḍ mā baʿd al-ṭabīʿa*, (full references there).

8 al-Fārābī (1985), Bk 4, Ch. 15, sect. 4 (Walzer ed., pp. 231–232).

the heart's steward (*ṣāḥib dār al-insān*),[9] and thus kept the brain in the highest circle of power in the state. His reformulation of Greek thought in Arabic, and Platonic ideas in particular, formatively shaped the Greco-Arabic philosophical tradition, in the Islamic, and later in the Christian world.

## 2.3 The Ancient Narrative Model of Healing

Avicenna inherited the dramaturgical model of the healing scenario from Galen. The coming of the disease and its eventual outcome were framed in terms of a story. While the healing accounts of the Hippocratic *Epidemics* are very spare, with no stated plots, Galen described several of his healings and anatomical demonstrations in dramatic terms, usually making himself the hero.[10] These dramatic elements, which were very useful for teaching medicine, Avicenna has skillfully worked into his own medical textbook, the *Canon*. His dramatic characterization of healing is especially clear, a feature that may partly explain why the *Canon* had such an extended lifetime as a major medical textbook, in both East and West.

## 3.1 The Drama of Medicine in the *Canon*

My observations are drawn from Book 4 of the *Canon*, where Avicenna discuses fevers and other systemic diseases, namely, diseases that afflict the body generally and are not localized to a specific part. To begin with, in *Canon*, Book 4, fever is characterized as an "alien heat" (*ḥarāra ḫāriǧa*) that kindles in the heart.[11] From the heart it is transmitted to the rest of the body by the arteries. This alien heat is contrasted with the Innate Heat (*ḥarāra ġarīziyya*), which represents the patient's innate defense against the former alien heat. The Innate Heat is also connected with the patient's healthy nature. Although it is not obvious how an alien heat could kindle a fever in the region of the heart, as we shall see it becomes clearer after Avicenna explains that, if the body as City fails to defend its perimeter, the disease as Enemy can penetrate into the interior, where the heart is located. In what follows, I shall describe Avicenna's use of the

9 al-Fārābī (1985), Bk 4, Ch. 11, sect. 1 (Walzer ed., pp. 174–175).

10 Galen (1979). See, for example, several such episodes that Galen relates in his *On Prognosis*, especially his amazing cure of the philosopher Eudemus (p. 84).

11 Avicenna (1593), Book 4, Fen 1, Maqala 1 (Part 23), p.1 (Doostdar transl., Bk 4, pp.58–59).

combat metaphor in healing as found in the *Canon* in terms of Galen's temporal scheme, as found in his *De crisibus* ("Crises").

## 3.2 Stages of the Fever

Avicenna follows Galen's four-fold division of the times of the disease, and uses this as a background for the combat metaphor.[12] These times (*kairoi*; *awqāt* or *azmān*) are: Beginning (*arkhē*; *ibtidā*ʾ); Intensification (*auxēsis*; *tazayyud*); Climax (*akmē*; *muntahā*); and Resolution (*parakmē*; *inqiḍā*ʾ).[13]

In the Beginning stage (*ibtidā*ʾ), the Enemy alien heat has attacked and has attempted to conquer and suffocate the patient's Innate Heat. The signs of combat are discernible to the doctor through indicators in the struggling patient's body, such as discomfort, sleeplessness, etc. Invoking yet another metaphor—life is like a burning candle—when the Innate Heat has been suffocated, then like a snuffed out candle, the patient will die.

In Stage 2, Intensification (*tazayyud*), the Innate Heat rallies, and confronts the Enemy alien heat as it attempts to occupy the patient's body. This phase is crucial, for if the patient's body fails to drive off the disease, it will penetrate into the City, and its alien heat will occupy the patient's heart, and from there spread throughout the patient's entire body (as City), through the arteries.

Stage 3, Climax (*muntahā*), is when the opposing forces engage in deadly man-to-man combat. The patients' healthy nature struggles to prevent the disease from completely overcoming the heart and vital organs. Whichever way the battle is going, whether in the patient's or the disease's favor, this is discernible through the patient's cries, or shaking, or relaxing, etc. There may be several rounds of battle in a disease that has periodic fevers, with each round either strengthening or weakening the patient. The metaphor of invasion reminds us that the ancients conceived of infection as occurring from outside of the patient. Unlike today, where infection is understood to be caused by microscopic vectors, infection was then thought to be the result of inhaled miasmas, or corrupted air.

---

12 Avicenna (1593), Book 4, Fen 1, Maqala 1 (Part 23), p.2 (Doostdar transl., Bk 4, pp.61–63).

13 These are listed and described at *De crisibus* Alexanderson ed. (1967), 69, ll.7–12; (K.550–551).

## 3.3 The Medical Crisis as Dramatic Turning Point

One important indicator that the patient has the upper hand is the appearance of the critical signs—sediments in the urine, thicker substance in the sputum, changes in the stools, or excessive sweating.[14] These signs indicate that the disease-producing substance is in the process of being neutralized by the Innate Heat. The substance of the disease appears as coalesced within the normal bodily secretions and excretions, as it is expelled from the body. The metaphor for this neutralization is "concoction" or "cooking" (*pepsis*; *naḍǧ*), and derives from the Hippocratic and Aristotelian writings (Lloyd 1996). The Innate Heat does the cooking in a process similar to digestion.

A successful crisis leads to Stage 4, Resolution (*inqiḍā'*), when the Innate Heat has overcome the alien, occupying Enemy force, which then retreats from the battlefield. In the patient's body, this is observed as the fever's heat moves from the interior of the body—the place of the vital organs—to the extremities, before being destroyed (i.e. fading away). An unsuccessful crisis leads to death.

The crisis, which Avicenna does not explicitly mention here, postponing its discussion until Book 4, Fen 2, is a sign that the combat has reached a climax.[15] If it is a favorable crisis leading to recovery, this indicates that the patient has been victorious in his combat with the disease. Galen devoted two treatises to the discussion of crises and their associated critical days, which Avicenna summarizes in the *Canon*. I am currently preparing a trilingual Greek-Arabic-English critical edition of Galen's treatise *Crises*,[16] which is why Avicenna's discussion of this topic is of particular interest to me.

Avicenna introduces the concept of crisis, and elaborates it via the body-as-city metaphor, which is then developed in greater detail. He employs the same four stages of the disease as before, but describes them as phases of warfare in slightly different terms than he did earlier. The combat has become not just hand to hand, but a full-blown siege. The patient's body is like a city being attacked by an alien invader.[17] The patient's healthy nature, including his Innate

---

14 These are described in detail throughout Galen's *De crisibus* (see Galen, Alexanderson ed., 1967) and *De diebus decretoriis* (see Galen, Cooper ed., 2011).

15 Avicenna (1593), Book 4, Fen 2, Maqala 1 (Part 24), pp.41–44 (Doostdar transl., Bk 4, pp.297–315).

16 My edition of Ḥunayn ibn Isḥāq's Arabic translation of Galen's *De crisibus* will appear in Brill's *Studies in Ancient Medicine* series. It will contain Alexanderson's 1967 Greek edition in a facing page format, with translations, and a Graeco-Arabic glossary.

17 This is discussed in: Cooper (2018).

Heat, is like the Ruler of the City, a benevolent and protecting power (*sulṭān*), who must rally his forces to defend it. The main struggle is not between the body and the enemy—although the body is the battleground—but between the Ruler of the City, and the besieging illness. As far as I know, neither Galen nor any other ancient Greek medical author uses the image of the body as city in this way.

So, in terms of the siege imagery, Stage 1 of the disease comprises marginal skirmishes between these opposing forces. The City is not yet seriously threatened. If these skirmishes lead to full-blown warfare and carnage, Stage 2 is reached, and the signs of victory or defeat will gradually appear, via the patient's symptoms, including cries of pain and bleeding. The Ruler strives to prevent the enemy from penetrating the walls of the city by battling it on the outskirts.

If the Ruler is unable as yet to defeat and expel the disease from the environs of the City, Stage 3, deadly combat, is reached. This is a mortal struggle for the patient's body and life, as the disease threatens the inner parts of the city, namely, the vital organs. Victory of the disease means the City and its Ruler have been wiped out, leading to the patient's death. On the other hand, victory of the Ruler and the City means the complete destruction of the enemy, and his expulsion, leading to the patient's full recovery.

There is a third possibility: incomplete victory. In this situation, which is very common, the Ruler has cast the enemy out of the City, but the disease remains lurking in the vicinity of the City, from where it could launch another attack in the future. The doctor must be especially careful that he doesn't relax the patient's regimen, or else the disease will return with a vengeance.

How will the doctor know for certain that the Ruler and the body have defeated the disease? Here's where the crisis comes in. A good crisis is the result of the patient's healthy nature (the Ruler of the City) expelling the disease-causing substance from the inner parts of the body, where the vital organs (i.e. the heart and other vitals) are housed, and have been under attack. Moreover, the Ruler has pushed the disease to the extremities (i.e. the outskirts of the city), e.g. the hands and feet. The crisis is decisive if the enemy's strength has been overcome to the point that the power of the disease fades, and it is unable to return.

## 4.1 Conclusion

The dramaturgical analysis of healing is receiving increasing attention in recent medical literature (Bleakley 2017). According to these scholars, modern medicine, which has emphasized the clinical to the neglect of the doctor-patient relationship, needs to return to the ancient conception of healing as combat. One problem is that the patient is often identified as a passive observer (or "battlefield") on which the physician and the disease are the combatants, instead of the more helpful model, which accepts the patient as full participant in her own suffering and healing. Ancient models of this drama are being consulted and adapted to modern practice in the hope that the healing process can be improved for all parties, but especially for the patient. Avicenna's lively use of this metaphor in the *Canon*, and its continuing tradition in Traditional Persian Medicine testifies, to its usefulness.

The Body Politic metaphor in medicine, on the other hand, has not yet caught the attention of many scholars. Avicenna's use of it will no doubt form an important episode in that medical history that is yet to be written. I am in the process of exploring the many medical dimensions of this metaphor through selected periods and cultures in a book-length project.

## References

Avicenna (Ibn Sīnā) (1593). *Kitāb al-Qānūn fī al-ṭibb li-Abū ʿAlī al-Šayḫ al-Raʾīs Ibn Sīnā*. Rome: Typographia Medicea.

Avicenna (n.d.). *The Canon of Medicine (al-Qanun fi'l-tibb): Volume 4: Systemic Diseases, Orthopedics, and Cosmetics*, Translated by Hamidreza Doostdar. Chicago: Kazi Publications.

Bleakley, Alan (2017). *Thinking with Metaphors in Medicine: The State of the Art*. London: Routledge.

Cooper, Glen M. (2018). "Medical Crises and Critical Days in Ibn Sīnā and Ibn al-Nafīs: Insights from the Commentary Tradition." *Intellectual History of the Islamicate World*. 6.1–2: 27–54.

Al-Fārābī (1985). *Al-Farabi on the Perfect State: Abū Naṣr al-Fārābī's Mabādi ʾ ārāʾ ahl al-madīna al-fāḍila. Edition and Translation by Richard Walzer.* Oxford: Oxford University Press.

Galen (1825). *De crisibus, Claudii Galeni opera omnia*, ed. C.G. Kühn. Leipzig; repr. Hildesheim, 1964–1965, vol. 9, pp. 550–768.

Galen (1825), *De diebus decretoriis, Claudii Galeni opera omnia*, ed. C.G. Kühn. Leipzig; repr. Hildesheim, 1964–1965, vol. 9, pp. 769–941.

Galen (1967). *Peri Kriseon: Überlieferung und Text.* Edited by Bengt Alexanderson. Göteborg: Elanders Boktryckeri Aktiebolag. (Edition of the *De crisibus*)

Galen (1979). *On Prognosis. Edition, Translation, and Commentary, by V. Nutton*. Berlin: Akademie-Verlag.

Galen (2011). *Galen, De diebus decretoriis, from Greek into Arabic: A Critical Edition, with Translation and Commentary, and Historical Introduction of Ḥunayn ibn Isḥāq, Kitāb ayyām al-buḥrān, edited, translated, and commented by Glen M. Cooper.* London: Ashgate.

Gutas, Dimitri (1988). *Avicenna and the Aristotelian Tradition*, Leiden: Brill.

Lloyd, G. E. R. (1996). The Master Cook. In *Aristotelian Explorations*, ed. G. E. R. Lloyd, Cambridge: Cambridge University Press, pp.83–103.

Plato (1997). *Complete Works.* Cooper, John M., and D. S. Hutchinson, eds. Indianapolis / Cambridge: Hackett Publishing Company.

## Short Biography of Glenn M. Cooper

Glen M. Cooper (Ph.D. Columbia, 1999) teaches history of science at Brigham Young University. Recently, he was a research fellow at Freie Universität, Einstein Center Chronoi, Berlin. He has taught at Claremont Mckenna College and Pitzer College.

### Selected Publications

*Galen,* De diebus decretoriis, *from Greek into Arabic: A Critical Edition, with Translation and Commentary, and Historical Introduction of* Ḥ*unayn ibn Isḥāq,* Kitāb ayyām al-buḥrān. (London: Ashgate, 2011).

"Medical Crises and Critical Days in Ibn Sīnā and After: Insights from the Commentary Tradition." *Intellectual History of the Islamicate World* 6, nos.1–2 (2018): 27–54.

"Astrology: The Science of Signs in the Heavens." In *The Oxford Handbook to Science and Medicine in the Classical World*, edited by P. T. Keyser and J. Scarborough. (Oxford: Oxford University Press, 2018): 381–407.

"Ḥunayn ibn Isḥāq's Galen Translations and Greco-Arabic Philology: Some Observations from the *Crises* (*De crisibus*) and the *Critical Days* (*De diebus decretoriis*)." *Oriens* 44 (2016): 1–43.

"Traditions and Practices in the Medieval Eastern Christian World." In *Prognostication in the Medieval World*, eds. Klaus Herbers, et al. (Berlin: de Gruyter, 2020): 561–578.

Prof. Dr. Yavuz UNAT

# The Versatile Scientist of the 11th Century: Ibn Sīnā (Avicenna) His Astronomy Studies and its Effects

As it is known, while the Middle Ages was a dark period in the fields of science, philosophy and thought, the Muslims who adopted the heritage of Ancient Greek science and philosophy contributed to science and philosophy after the 8th and 9th centuries, after which these contributions and studies with Latin translations were transferred to the West following the 11th and 12th centuries and triggered the Renaissance of the 15th century. The names of several scientists who dealt with and contributed to science and philosophy after the 9th and 10th centuries are mentioned. One of them is Ibn Sīnā (980–1037), also known as Avicenna in the West. Ibn Sīnā is a versatile scientist from Bukhara, whose works cover medicine, physics, astronomy, chemistry and mechanics.

He is known as a doctor above all. In the 5,000-year history of medicine, Ibn Sīnā, mentioned with Hippocrates who lived in the 5th century BC and Galen who lived in the 2nd century AD, played a major role in the development of modern medicine with both his works and his medical understanding. Ibn Sīnā is also a pioneer scientist in physics and mechanics. In the field of mechanics and philosophy of nature, Muslims, following the footsteps of Aristotle, accepted Aristotle's understanding of cosmology with its main lines. However, some problems in the cosmology and mechanical model of Aristotle did not escape from the attention of Ibn Sīnā, and especially Aristotle's understanding of motion was criticized by him. The course of the motion theory in the Middle Ages and its transition to the modern period were determined by these discussions.

Ibn Sīnā is also an important philosopher. He reworked the rich philosophical tradition that reached his time and evaluated it as a great collection and left strong marks especially in the field of metaphysics. Ibn Sīnā was able to express and interpret philosophy with the terms of Islam's own system, thereby achieving a flawless synthesis of the philosophies of Plato and Aristotle. Thanks to these contributions, he was nicknamed "al-Shaikh al-Rais", which means the Philosopher of Philosophers. When Ibn Sīnā died from stomach disease in Hamadan in 1037, he left behind about 200 works.

## Ibn Sīnā as an Astronomer

One of the most prolific writers among Islamic thinkers and scientists, Ibn Sīnā has many works related to disciplines such as logic, philosophy of nature, astronomy, mathematics and metaphysics. His works on astronomy are as follows:

1. *On the Earth* (al-Arshiyya)
2. *On the Needlessness of Astrology* (Ibtâli Ahkâm al-Nücûm)
3. *Evidence to Prove the Falseness of Astrology* (al-Ishârât ilâ Fasâdi Ahkâm al-Nücûm)
4. *On the Celestial Bodies* (al-Acrâm al-Ulviyye)
5. *On the Astronomy* (al-Hay'a)
6. *The Observations Tools* (al-Alat al-Rasadiyya)
7. *On the Vacuum* (al-Vus'a al-Fazâ)
8. *Reasons for the Earth to be at the Center of the Universe* (Illati Kıyâmi al-Ard fî Vasat al-Samâ)
9. *On the Visibility of the Stars at Night and not at Daytime* (Sababi Ru'yat al-Kavâkib bî al-Layl lâ fî al-Nahâr)
10. *The Origin and the Ending* (al-Mabda va al-Maâd)
11. *Correction of Jurjans's Longitude* (Risâla fî Tashih Tulû al-Curcan)

Ibn Sīnā regards astronomy as belonging to the theoretical sciences in the classification of sciences. In his work *Parts of Mental Sciences* (*Aqsam al-'ulum al-'aqlīyah*), he divides the sciences into two as Theoretical and Applied sciences. He then divides theoretical sciences into three: 1. Natural sciences, 2. Riyaziyyat (Mathematical Sciences) and 3. Divine sciences. Riyaziyyat is divided into four sections: 1. Arithmetic, 2. Geometry, 3. Astronomy and 4. Music Astronomy is included among the mathematical sciences. However, some parts of astronomy and astrology are listed within the natural sciences in this science classification. Natural sciences fall into natural philosophy category, and according to Ibn Sīnā, it is divided into two as primary and secondary. Matter, four elements, creation and distortion, the situations occurring in the Sublunary region under the influence of the heavens are considered primary natural philosophy. Astrology, on the other hand, belongs to the secondary part along with the science of chemistry (Ünal, pp. 46–47). Ibn Sīnā did not give credence to pseudo sciences such as astrology and alchemy. In his works called *On the Needlessness of Astrology* and *Evidence to Prove the Falseness of Astrology*, he argued that celestial bodies had no effect on human body organs, and he did not consider these methods in diagnosis and treatment. According to him, astrology has no scientific basis. It is wrong to describe the heavenly bodies as good, bad, auspicious and ominous. Also he did not attach importance to alchemy, which is the attempt to obtain precious metals such as gold from base metals. He defended that in his experiments he had found that each element had its unique characteristics, and therefore, it was impossible to obtain precious metals from base metals (Sayılı, 1984, p. 175 and continuous).

As Ibn Sīnā expressed his views on astronomy and cosmology in the above works, his philosophical works include opinions on this subject. The main reason for this is that the Ancient and the following Medieval cosmology is ontological in that it contains metaphysical characters and, much as the Christian cosmology and astronomy, Islamic cosmology and astronomy were influenced by the works of Aristotle (385–323 BC) and Ptolemy (150s AD) on the subject. Therefore, it is necessary to first understand Aristotle's cosmology and Ptolemy's mathematical astronomy.

Aristotle explained his views on astronomy in his works *Physics, Metaphysics* and *On the Heavens*; because, according to him, astronomy and physics were inseparable. The sphere was the perfect form; therefore, the universe must have been spherical, and this was the form most suitable for its existence. The universe was finite because it was the centre of a sphere. The earth was at the centre of the universe; therefore, the centre of the universe was also the centre of the earth; it was motionless and spherical. The earth was surrounded by a series of layers of spheres, like an onion's skin, whose centres were joint. First came the spheres of the three earthly elements, namely the spheres of water, air and fire. The fire sphere was surrounded by transparent, crystalline spheres, and the planets that were fixed on these spheres were transported in the order of the Moon, Mercury, Venus, Sun, Mars, Jupiter and Saturn. Outside, there was a fixed sphere of the stars. These spheres were like physical parts of a large machine through which celestial bodies moved. Whether their forms of being were perfect or not varied according to their distance from the centre of the Earth. The further away an entity was from the Earth, the more perfect it was. For this reason, while the earth in the centre was not perfect, the Stars Sphere that was farthest from the centre was the perfect sphere. This perfect sphere was also God, that is, the primum mobile.

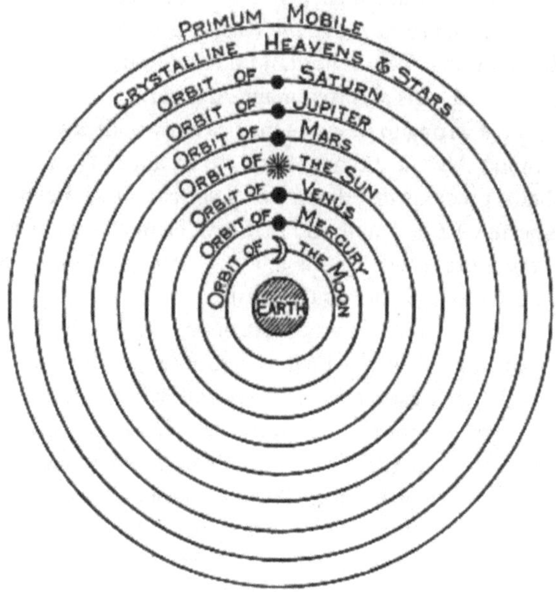


**Aristotle's universe**

Aristotle also divided the universe into two different regions. The part from Earth to the Moon was the sublunary region, and the part from the Moon to the sphere of fixed stars was the superlunary region. These two universes were very different in structure. In the superlunary region, movements were circular and consisted of the fifth element, ether. The sublunary region, on the other hand, consisted of four basic elements that were lined upwards from the centre of the Earth, namely earth, water, air and fire. In these two universes with different structures, different laws of physics applied. The celestial bodies in the superlunary region were moving in smooth circular orbits. The linear motion was dominant in the sublunary sphere, where all kinds of change took place. This view of his included a physical interpretation of the universe. However, for the science of astronomy in a universe with such a cosmological structure, there must also be mathematical determinations regarding the movements of celestial bodies. This shortcoming in Aristotle's cosmology was later completed by Ptolemy. Ptolemy made a synthesis of astronomy information that reached his time and collected these in his book *Almagest*, or with its original name

*Mathematike Syntaxis* (The Mathematical Synthesis). In this work of his, in order to make sense of the heavenly phenomena, he introduced the geometric theory based on Aristotle's physics and his mathematical model gave satisfactory results until the beginning of the 17$^{th}$ century.

Aristotle's Earth-centred physics and universe vision (Concentric Spheres System),[1] and then the mathematical model of Ptolemy changed to some extent and was dominant for many years. Especially the acceptance of the spheres used to explain planetary movements as concrete objects and the idea that they have a transparent, crystalline structure started with Aristotle, and this thought continued until the 17$^{th}$ century in the history of astronomy. This cosmological theory would also be adopted by prominent philosophers of the Medieval Islamic World, such as Farabi and Ibn Sīnā *and* would be tried to be reconciled with the understanding of God and Universe depicted in the Holy Quran.

This system established by Ptolemy was more successful than the concentric spheres system in determining the location of the planets. However, the models used in the system were always discussed throughout the history of astronomy. To some, these models were strange as they were not compatible with Aristotelian physics and were criticized especially by physicists; planetary movements are not only geometrical but also dynamic. Thus, three views emerged in the field of astronomy especially in the Middle Ages, and astronomers adopted one of these three views.

1. According to the first one, astronomical assumptions are simple mathematical constructions and their tasks are *saving the appearances (or the fact)* and the system of Ptolemy did this best.
2. Those who accepted the second view either put another system against Ptolemaic astronomy and adopt the system of concentric spheres introduced by Eudoxus and Aristotle in this direction, or proposed new systems (especially by al-Bitruji) similar to the system of concentric spheres.
3. In the third view, the system of Ptolemy was considered as sphere layers in accordance with Aristotle physics, and eccentric and epicycle models used by Ptolemy were considered as concrete objects.

1 In fact, the theory of concentric spheres was first introduced by Eudoxus (390–337 BC) before Aristotle. However, it was Aristotle who made the theory physical.

| | |
|---|---|
| 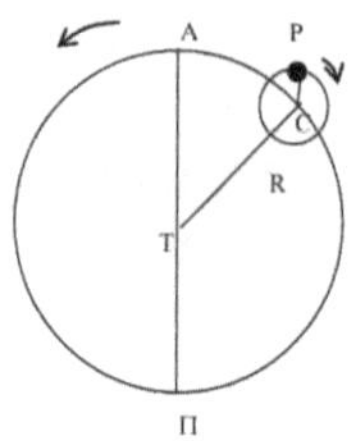  | 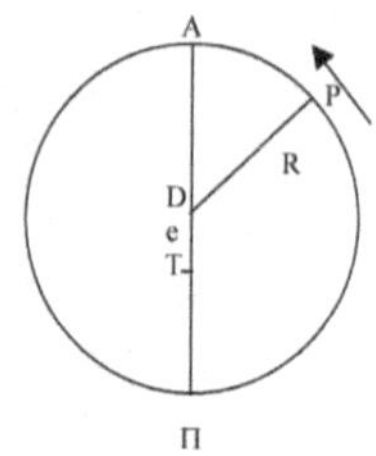  |
| **Epicycle (outer circle) model used by Ptolemy to explain the forward and backward motion of the planets** | **Eccentric (eccentric) model used by Ptolemy to explain the distance differences of planets and apparent velocity changes** |

Astronomical assumptions can be considered as geometrically constructed mathematical constructions to account for celestial motion or as real movements of concrete objects. In the first case, these assumptions cannot go beyond simple mathematical fiction and only take on the task of *saving the appearances.* In the second case, the person who designs the assumptions will want to know the essence of the diversity of movement in the sky and will feel a need to explain these assumptions. Ptolemy and the Hellenic thinkers who came after him accepted the first view and therefore were able to construct their geometric theories without adhering to different views of physics. In the same way, some of the Western and Islamic astronomers preferred to be contented with mathematical theory in the Middle Ages, finding the geometric structure of the Ptolemaic system sufficient and disregarded its fundamental physical side. According to these astronomers, the descriptive but quantitative Ptolemaic system can accurately give the movements of the celestial bodies and the location of a planet at certain times. This is the purpose of astronomy. Therefore, this fundamental problem of physics should be left to physicists or natural philosophers.

On the other hand, some astronomers argued that planetary movements were not only geometrical, but that they must also have a dynamic character, and therefore insisted that astronomy needed a physical foundation. This thought developed after Sabit Ibn Kurra and Ibn al-Haytham, and after these two astronomers, astronomers either wanted to combine the geometric assumption of Ptolemy with the real movements of solid objects and tried to make the geometric system of Ptolemy compatible with the laws of physics, or especially after the 12[th] century, with the impact of Andalusian astronomers who were under the influence of Aristotle's physics, opposed the Ptolemaic theory and adopted the system of Aristotle's concentric spheres.

According to this understanding, the Ptolemy system, which is mathematically perfect, was tried to be placed on a physical basis. One such system is the sphere layers system that makes the Ptolemaic system mechanical. Thus, this system both had a physical structure and was compatible with the Ptolemaic system (Sayılı, 1984, pp. 197–199).

In this system, the universe is designed as a set of intertwined spheres. Each planet has its own intertwined spheres. In the concentric sphere, which is the centre of the central universe and of a certain thickness, a spherical eccentric sphere (deferent) is placed in a bed shaped like a belt. The planet on the epicycle rolls in this slot along with the epicycle. These spheres are solid bodies and transparent; they are not subject to any change; they are empty; they are made of ether; they are neither heavy nor light; they are placed inside each other in the form of a layer with the radius of each being smaller than the next one (Gökmen, 1937, pp. 13–14).

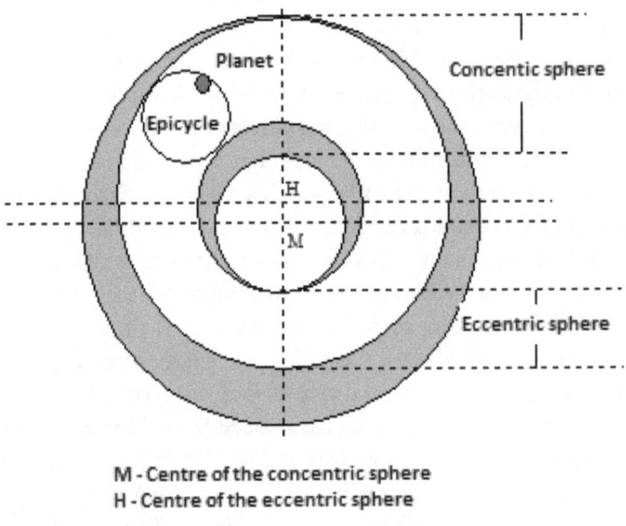


**Concentric spheres systems**

As I mentioned before, this idea was probably first developed by Ibn al-Haytham. Sayılı addresses the issue in terms of Ibn Sīnā's being contemporary with Haytham and says that Ibn Sīnā probably also adopted this idea (Sayılı, p. 199). Especially after these criticisms of Haytham, this system would be handled widely by Islamic astronomers. In contrast, Islamic astronomers would adopt Aristotle's model of the universe in a slightly modified way, in accordance with the religion of Islam, and would abandon the idea of accepting Aristotle's final sphere, the Sphere of Fixed Stars (the Sphere), that surrounds the universe as God (Primum Mobile). On the other hand, the order of spheres is compatible with Aristotle's cosmology. Ibn Sīnā also advocated the same order. The earth is in the centre of the universe. Next comes the Moon Falak (Sphere), Mercury Falak, Venus Falak, Solar Falak, Mars Falak, Jupiter Falak, Saturn Falak, Signs Falak, and finally the Sphere of spheres that covers all universe (Falak al-Aflak). According to Ibn Sīnā, every sphere is formed as a result of understanding its own essence; thus, the mind of the spheres emerges and whenever the mind emerges, it gives falak existence (body). The first reason for minds is that they have information about God. The first mind has only one power: the information it receives from God's command. The first mind forms the essence and body of the first sphere (Falak al-Aflak). As a result of the realization of the second mind, it forms the essence and body of the second sphere and this continues until the last one (Nasr, 1985, pp. 230–231). Later on, the hierarchy of the entities formed in the sublunary sphere is formed. In this context, Ibn Sīnā handled this order in accordance with the monotheistic view and at the same time, he tried to explain the multitude of the universe. Thus, he approached the idea of Neo Platonism rather than Aristotle, which led him to a theory of emergence (sudur) similar to the cosmology of Neo Platonism (Nasr, 1988, p. 129).

It is seen that the interest in astronomy was higher when compared to many disciplines in the Islamic World. Apart from approaches that share many traditional conceptions, there were those who advocated the original universe design of Aristotle, as well as those who adopted its improved version or developed different views. It is understood that one of the people who adopted the Aristotelian universe model, which was developed by making additions in various ways, was Ibn Sīnā (Topdemir, 2016, p. 126). On this subject, in his work titled *Evidence to Prove the Falseness of Astrology*, Ibn Sīnā says:

*"The star clusters called Nebula, the Milky Way and similar dense clusters contain a very large number of objects that the eye cannot select, and not only the planets but also the effect of each star and each celestial sphere on incidents on earth is known. That is what the astrologers ignore and hesitate to mention in their books. They generally do not accept the effects of the celestial spheres.*

*However, they limit themselves by talking about the effects of only seven planets, and they do not know that the number of celestial spheres detected by the help of observations reinforced by examples is sixty, and some of them surround the earth's circle, while others exclude the universe. Although they are not perceived, it is possible that the number of these spheres may be well over sixty.*" (Sayılı, 1984, p. 18).

As we mentioned above, Eudoxus was the first who proposed the idea that celestial bodies were carried by the spheres and Eudoxus designed 34 spheres to explain the movements of the planets. However, Aristotle added 22 spheres to these spheres, giving the number of spheres as 56 (Unat, 2013, p. 36). The fact that he stated the number of spheres as approaching sixty shows that Ibn Sīnā was trying to explain the movements and changes in the sky with complex models and was aware of the difficulties this situation created. For Ibn Sīnā, who thought that a simpler model was needed, the most reasonable way was to use the Ptolemaic model as the base. Ibn Sīnā also embraced the opinion that Earth is naturally in the center of the universe, and all celestial objects, including the Sun, orbit around it. However, some "disturbing" details of this model from the perspective of the Aristotelian physics need to be addressed. Ibn Sīnā's establishment of an observatory in order to obtain the correct knowledge of the sky, his invention and development of new observation tools show that he had extensive knowledge of astronomy (Topdemir, 2016, p. 127).

In this understanding of cosmology, much like that of the Middle Ages at large, Ibn Sīnā assumed that the earth was at the center and motionless. About the subject, in his work titled *Reasons for Earth to be at the Center of the Universe*, he addresses this view. According to him, every object has a natural location and preserves its location. It changes its condition when it is exposed to an external factor or by a moving force. Like Aristotle, Ibn Sīnā accepts natural and unnatural movement. In the sublunary universe, motions are linear and every linear motion is finite. Because the natural movement of an object is proportional to the force that moves it. An object left to fall from above moves naturally towards the centre of the Earth. This is proof that Earth is at the centre of the universe. Ibn Sīnā also made mention of the views that accepted the motion of the Earth. However, he ultimately accepted that the Earth was at the centre and immobile (Tandoğan, pp. 341–343).

In his work titled *On the Visibility of the Stars at Night and Not in Daytime*, Ibn Sīnā answers the question of why the stars do not appear during the day. Ibn Sīnā points out that some issues must be known first while answering this question. First of all, the air called space (faza) is transparent. Everything transparent is neither bright nor dark. Space (faza) is not bright with the presence of the Sun or a light source, nor is it dark with the absence of them. The bright things are only the dark objects that are struck by light. Visibility is achieved by passing through a transparent object like air. This is the same in daytime and at night. Though a human being cannot see his/her hand in the dark of the night, he/she sees a flaming fire at a long distance from where he/she is. All these explanations show that the eye will perceive bright objects. The luminous body is seen directly. Secondly, space which is composed of air is not absolutely pure but mixed with water and soil types such as water vapour, smoke and dust. This mixture increases on cloudy, foggy and windy days and prevents visibility from penetrating the air. Since the air is more or less always in this state, it is never fully transparent. Finally, the sky is a transparent object like air. It is not illuminated by light hitting it, and it is not darkened by being deprived of light. The apparent colour of the sky is an unreal imaginary colour. Carefully looking at a transparent object that extends to a fairly distant distance, the same colour appears, as the ability to see farther will decrease. The appearance of the fixed stars on the other side of the seven layers of the sky, the thickness of each is known, clearly shows that the sky is transparent. If the sky had not been transparent, the stars that are not seen behind a thin layer would not have been seen from the other side of the sky. In fact, when looking at the sky through a pure crystal as thick as a shield, no star is seen even though the crystal is transparent. Thus, we have to admit that the transparency of the sky, the thickness of which is so great, is extremely good. It is now well understood that a transparent and luminous body is only a medium between the visible object and the eye. It neither gives off light, nor is it dark. So, the fact that the stars are not seen during the day is, even though the soil and protrusions that have been bathed in light from the sun are soiled with dust and smoke, due to the mixed space busying our gazes (Tandoğan, pp. 344–346).

Ibn Sīnā also worked in the field of practical astronomy. He was aware that the old astronomical tables were inadequate and deficient, and these deficiencies had to be corrected. For this purpose, he established an observatory in Hamadan with the support of Ala al-Dawla. İbn Sīnā was a friend of the Amir of Asfahan, Ala al-Dawla. One day he tells him that the old astronomical tables are inadequate and incomplete. Ala al-Dawla orders him to set up an observatory in Hamadan to prepare a new astronomical table. İbn Sīnā and his student Abu Ubayd al-Juzjani (d. 1070) start the necessary studies and establish the Hamedan Observatory in 1023/24 (Sayılı, 1988, pp. 156–158). Together with Juzjani, they make an instrument measuring azimuth and height (Zat al-Samt va'l-İrtifa, Azimuthal Quadrant). The details of this instrument, which is considered to be the pioneer of theodolite, was given in Ibn Sīnā's work *Kitâb al-Lâwahik* (Tekeli, 1958, pp. 328–329). This tool is an instrument that measures the height of the stars from the horizon and their azimuth. It is placed at the tip of the round column at the midpoint of the horizontal cylindrical wall as mobile (Sezgin, p. 26–27).

A part of this tool resembles micrometre (a device for measuring very small angular positions between two celestial bodies, invented in 1670). The diameter of the azimuth ring is around 7 meters. This tool provided a very significant precision in angle measuring. We do not have any information about the preparation of any zij (astronomical table) in this observatory. This observatory was well ahead of its era in terms of the tools used and the observations made, and in many ways, it affected future astronomical studies (Unat, 2008, pp. 64–69).

There is not much information about the tools used in the Hamedan Observatory. However, besides Zat al-Samt va'l-Irtifa, some tools used by Ibn Sīnā are mentioned in the sources. One of them is the *solstitial armil* which was used for determining tropics. Ptolemy made the first description of the instrument. Abu al-Wafa developed this tool and used it to measure the slope of the ecliptic and called it the Two Targeted Tool. Ibn Sīnā also mentions this device (Tekeli, 1958, p. 344).

Another astronomical tool used by Ibn Sīnā is the equinoctial armil (Halka al-Ustuwa). Its main part consists of a large ring with a scale and has been used for determining equinox points. Ptolemy refers to Hipparchos (c. 190–120 BC) as the inventor of this tool. According to the description given of this instrument in the *Almagest*, this tool consists of a ring fixed to the equatorial plane. When the sun comes to one of the equinox points, the concave part of the ring is illuminated. According to the sources, since the bottom face of the ring was not fully enlightened, Ibn Sīnā and Muayyad al-Din al-Urdi (d. 1266) added a second ring and both eliminated this problem and facilitated error control (Tekeli, 1958, pp. 345–347).

Ibn Sīnā also wrote a work called *Correction of Jurjan's Longitude*. In this work, Ibn Sīnā determined the longitude of Jurjan to Baghdad as 9 degrees 20 minutes by measuring the height of the Moon at noon. Although al-Biruni said in his work *Taḥdīd Nihāyāt al-Amākin* that this method was wrong, the value determined by Ibn Sīnā is less erroneous than that of al-Biruni (al-Bîrûnî, p. 128; Tandoğan, p. 339).

We know that Ibn Sīnā and al-Biruni exchanged letters between 998–999. These letters included questions related to metaphysics and cosmology directed by al-Biruni to Ibn Sīnā. These answers are also interesting. Al-Biruni posed some problems on Aristotle's *Physics* and *On the Heavens* and provoked Ibn Sīnā, as it were. For example, al-Biruni, who argued that the celestial bodies had volumes and weights, shared his views with Ibn Sīnā, but Ibn Sīnā defended the opposite and remained loyal to Aristotle. Al-Biruni also claimed in his letters that void may exist, but Ibn Sīnā once again remained loyal to Aristotle and refused the existence of void. Al-Biruni also claimed that the movements of the celestial bodies did not have to be circular, and Ibn Sīnā opposed this argument as well. In another letter, they also discussed the arguments about the multitude of worlds that Aristotle definitely refused and neither of them saw a plausible reason for us to be alone in the universe (Starr, 2019, pp. 336–339).

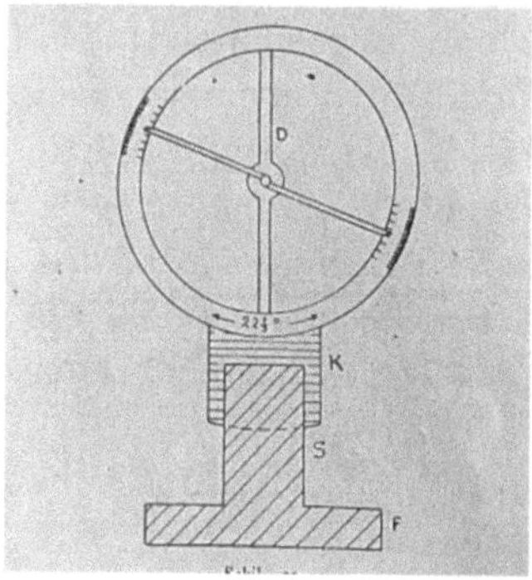


**Abû'l-Wafa's Solstitial Armil**

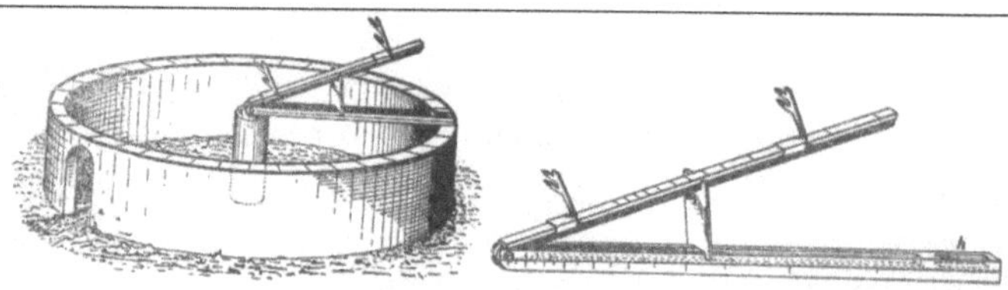

**Azimuthal Quadrant similar to micrometre used by Ibn Sinâ, considered the pioneer of the micrometre and measuring the azimuth and heights of the celestial bodies.**

In a short article written in 2011, it is stated that Ibn Sīnā witnessed a supernova explosion in 1006. This supernova, which is the remnant of a star named SN 1006, exploded in 1006 and was observed as a new star, probably exploded during Ibn Sīnā's journey to the cities of Nishapur, Marw and Kath.

Ibn Sīnā shares the information about this event not in his astronomy books but in the fifth section on meteorology of the second part of his work *Kitâb al-Shifa'*. However, it is not clear whether Ibn Sīnā made this observation himself or whether he heard it from someone else and wrote about it in his book (Neuhäser, Ehrig-Eggert ve Kunitzsch, 2011, pp. 789–791).

## Conclusion

Ibn Sīnā's work on astronomy has changed the works to come and the perspective on astronomy and especially attracted interest in observational astronomy. His observatory and his work on practical astronomy, both in the observatory and on his own, would affect subsequent astronomers. According to the sources, Ibn Sīnā also observed the passage of the Sun in front of Venus, and this observation later helped determine that Venus was sometimes under the Sun. Ibn Sīnā also worked on astronomical instruments and stated that more precise instruments increased reliability and criticized Ptolemy and astronomers of that period.

Ibn Sīnā's cosmological writings are also dominated by the philosophy of nature rather than mathematical astronomy, which allowed him to develop his physics studies and criticize Aristotle's physics. As a result of these studies, he is also one of those who advocate that the physics accepted in Ptolemaic models violated Aristotle physics and is therefore aware of the need to reconcile physics with mathematical astronomy in the Ptolemaic system.

Ibn Sīnā also played an important role in redefining and classifying astronomy and distinguished mathematical astronomy from astrology.

## References

El-Bîrûnî (20113). *Tahdîdü Nihâyâti'l-Emâkin*. Trans: Kıvâmeddin Burslan, Ed: Melek Dosay Gökdoğan and Tuba Uymaz. Ankara: Türk Tarih Kurumu.

Gökmen, Fatin (1937). İbni Sina'nın Heyet ve Riyaziyesi. *Büyük Türk Filozofu ve Tıb Üstadı İbni Sina, Şahsiyeti ve Eserleri Hakkında Tetkikler.* İstanbul.

Nasr, Seyyid Hüseyin (1985). *İslâm Kozmoloji Öğretilerine Giriş*. Trans: Nazife Şişman. İstanbul: İnsan Yayınları.

Nasr, Seyyid Hüseyin (1988). *İslam'da Düşünce ve Hayat*. Trans: Fatih Tatlıoğlu. İstanbul: İnsan Yayınları.

Neuhäser, R, C. Ehrig-Eggert, P. Kunitzsch (2011). An Arabic Report about Supernova SN 1006 by Ibn Sînâ (Avicenna). *Astron. Nachr.* 999/88: 789–795.

Ragep, Sally P. (2007). Ibn Sīnā: Abū ʿAlī al-Ḥusayn ibn ʿAbdallāh ibn Sīnā. *The Biographical Encyclopedia of Astronomers*. Thomas Hockey et al. (eds.). New York: Springer: 570–572.

Sayılı, Aydın (1984). İbn Sînâ'da Astronomi ve Astroloji. *İbn Sînâ, Doğumunun Bininci Yılı Armağanı*, 161–201.

Sayılı, Aydın (1988). *The Observatory In Islam*. Ankara: Türk Tarih Kurumu.

Sezgin, Fuat (2008). *İslam'da Bilim ve Teknik, Vol. II. Astronomi*, İstanbul: İstanbul Büyük Şehir Belediyesi.

Starr, S. Frederick (2019). *Kayıp Aydınlanma, Arap Ferihlerinden Timur'a Orta Asya'nın Altın Çağı*. Trans: Yusuf Selman İnanç. İstanbul: Kronik.

Tandoğan, Yusuf Ali (1984). İbn Sina'nın Matematik ve Astronomi Cephesi. *İbni Sina, Gevher Nesibe Sultan Anısına "İbni Sina Kongresi" Tebliğleri*. Kayseri: 334–346.

Tekeli, Sevim (1958). *Nasirüddin, Takiyüddin ve Tycho Brahe'nin Rasat Aletlerinin Mukayesesi*. Ankara: Türk Tarih Kurumu.

Topdemir, Hüseyin Gazi (2009). *İbn Sînâ*. İstanbul: Say.

Topdemir, Hüseyin Gazi (2016). *Felsefe*. Ankara: Pegem Akademi.

Ünal, Halit (1984). İbn-i Sina'da İlimler Tasnifi. *İbni Sina, Gevher Nesibe Sultan Anısına "İbni Sina Kongresi" Tebliğleri*. Kayseri: 42–49.

Unat, Yavuz (2008). *Tarih Boyunca Türklerde Gökbilim*. İstanbul: Kaynak Yayınları.

Unat, Yavuz (2013). *İlkçağlardan Günümüze Astronomi Tarihi*. Ankara: Nobel.

## Short Biography of Yavuz Unat

He was born in Istanbul in 1965. He had completed high school in 1982 and entered to the Department of the History of Science at the Faculty of Letters in Ankara University. He graduated from this department in 1987 and he began to work as an assistant at the same department in 1988. He obtained his master degree with a thesis untitled *"A Study on Fourth and Fifth Books on Heavenly Spheres of Risalât al-Fathiyyâ of Ali Qushchu"* in 1990 and his Ph. D. with *"Al-Farghânî and his Kitâb al-Fusûl (The Elements of Astronomy)"* in 1996 under the direction of Professor Sevim Tekeli.

He is still a lecturer at Kastamonu University, Faculty of Arts and Sciences. He was elected to the Board of Directors of the Turkish Philosophical Association (2000-2003), the Turkish History of Science Foundation (starting from 1990), the Editorial Board of the Journal of Philosophy World (2000-2003), the 2009 Astronomy Year - UNESCO Astronomy Specialization Committee. He is editor-in-Chief of the Dört Öge journal with mainly philosophy and science history articles.

He actually continues his studies on the fields of history of Islamic astronomy and technology.

Prof. Dr. Ahmet Hakkı Turabi

# The Musical Philosophy of Ibn Sīnā

**Abstract:** Ibn Sīnā assigned special sections for music in his books, *Kitab el-Shifa, Kitab al-Najat*, and *Danish-namai Alai*. He also gave some important information on music in his other books in several subsections. His Works were welcomed because of their scientific and artistic value, not because of his personal fame. The subjects in his Works and his operational method made him a progressivist theorist. Ibn Sīnā's works are also important in that he revitalized the theories of music that the Greeks omitted for centuries. And the musicians who came after him benefitted from his Works widely.

Ibn Sīnā's final goal in his musical Works is to form a theory of music. According to him, music is one of the four mathematical sciences along with arithmetic, geometry, and astronomy. He embraced and improved the thoughts of al-Farabi on music. Then, he created new theories on music by following al-Farabi. To him ,music is an instrument that always leads humans to the more beautiful as it gives them personal pleasure. The beauty in Ibn Sina's language is nothing, but "perfection".

## 1. Ibn Sīnā's Musical Works

The works written by Ibn Sīnā, who is called "Shayh al-Rais (Şeyh ul-Reis)" by medieval scholars and "Prince of Philosophers" by western thinkers, did not remain in the shadow of his works on science and philosophy. Because although his works on music were few in number, he attracted all the eyes in terms of science and art. These works XI. It is very valuable in terms of reflecting the understanding of music of the century.

The information of Ibn Sīnā, who is alleged to have written his works related to music in Isfahan (Şa'rânî; 1987), where he stayed for ten or twelve years at the end of his life; The Arab, Persian and Greek music systems should not be thought of as cutthroat. Considering the science and performance of the period in which Avicenna lived, Greek scholars such as Aristoxenes, Euclid, Ptolemy and Pythagoras; Yunus al-Katib (d. 765?), Ibnü'l-Müneccim (d. 912), İshak el-Mevsili (d. 850), Ihvan-ı Safa, el-Kindi It is possible that he studied the works of Arab and Turkish scholars such as İshak, al-Kindi (d.874) and Farabi (d. 950) and benefited from their views. Although it is possible to find Ibn Sīnā's musical thoughts and theories as a whole in the music section of the book Şifa, there are also information about music in the other works we have written: *Kitabü'ş-Şifa "Cevamiu İlmi'l-Musika", Kitabü'n-Necat "Muhtasar fi*

*İlmi'l-Musika", Daniş-name-i 'Alai, Risale fi'l-Huruf, Risale fi'n-Nefs, Fi Beyani Aksami'l-Ulum li-Hikemiyye ve'l-Akliyye, al-Kanun fi't-Tıp.*

In his works on the science of music, Ibn Sīnā used a pure scientific method, which, in his own words, was far from various delusions and imaginations, and that he used some traditional scriptures of the previous ones. He did not compliment the stories and tales that were given before him, regarding the relations established between music and celestial bodies, as well as the invention of instruments, and stayed away from contradictory narrations that are not based on historical and scientific evidence.

Ibn Sīnā continued the musical system of a kind of Farabi in his works. Ibn Sīnā accepts and applies the thoughts briefly explained by Farabi in music; It examines, develops and turns them into assertive theories by expanding them further within its own systematic. This is the reality of "musical thought", which is the actual field of our topic.

## 2. Ibn Sīnā's Thought of Music

Music science in the classification of sciences by Avicenna; it is mentioned as the fourth science after arithmetic, geometry, astronomy. For this reason, he named his work on music as "Music Science, the Third Branch of Mathematical Sciences" (Yusuf 1962). The same theory has been accepted by Kindi and Farabi before. Because, with the translation of the works of Euclid, Ptolemy, Phythagoras and other Greek masters into Arabic, this classification became the common custom of Muslim scholars.

According to Ibn Sīnā, music is ***"a job based on what is always better; because it is the expression of personal pleasure"***. What he means is beauty, perfection. In other words, the commonality in music must include numerical principles and proportions and these must be sound (compatible). Human is always in a development in terms of knowledge and culture. Music will also evolve with the development of these two elements. In this context, Ibn Sīnā points out that the work of a person who is developing in terms of knowledge and culture will be better than the previous one.

Avicenna takes the Farabi side against the Muslim Pythagoreans in terms of the proper study of music based on theory. Like Aristoxenes, who lived before him, he reexamined the science of music as an auditory phenomenon. Although Ibn Sīnā focuses his ideas about music around the nature of music itself; he claims that it should have priority in Islamic thought. At the same time, this does not prevent Avicenna from approaching music with the "*Pythagoreans approach that considers numbers as an essential key to understanding music*". It really is; It confirms, for example, that intervals and ratios can be thought of in their own time. What he affirms here is the truth of the musical ranges, which is essential for the musical element as an auditory experience (Shehadi 1993).

Farmer introduces Ibn Sīnā with his extreme fondness for Greek science. According to him, Ibn Sīnā attaches great importance to Euclid especially. He even reconsidered the problems that the Greeks threw aside. But whatever happens, the musical information in his works titled al-Shifa and al-Najat, XI. It provides us with valuable information about the musical performance of the century. Although his students Ibn al-Haitham (v. 1039) and Hüseyin b. Zayla (v. 1048) followed their teachers on many issues, they still could not reach the level of their teachers (Yekta 1985).

After studying all the sciences of his time when he was 17 years old, Ibn Sina said, "***Here is the human being, where is the other sciences?***" saying; When he attempted to deal with the application of music - observing the greatness of the science of music with astonishment- "***Here is science, where is man?***" started to say.

Ibn Sīnā, like Kindi, used music practically as a psychologist. His phrase "***Inter omnia exerciatia sanitatis cantane melius est" (Singing is the best health-preserving exercise)*** has been in the mind for centuries (Shehadi 1993). Nowadays, making music, especially singing; It strengthens the heart, stimulates intestinal activity, regulates blood pressure, reduces stress hormones, keeps memory fit, and strengthens trachea muscles.

The meaningful qualities in music are largely based on the conditions of the sound or the effect the music exerts on the listener: "***If the melody is similar in qualities (shamail), then the soul applies (adapts) to that quality and what it belongs to***". Avicenna returns here as a psychologist to the curative value of what he notices as an aesthetic expert.

In this context, Ibn Sīnā describes music personally as follows: "*Music is a mathematical science that studies sounds in terms of their compatibility with each other and the time periods between these sounds in order to know how a melody is composed.*" Briefly, music is a mathematical science that deals with the study of sounds and related rhythms (Korlaelçi 1984). In this case, the science of music; It also examines whether voices are numb, disaggregated and even duration. There are two main elements in the above recipe. These two elements are directly related to some principles of other branches of science. Some of them are arithmetic, some are with physics; In very few cases it is related to geometry.

Aristotle, Pythagoras, Aristoxenes etc. The ancient Greek philosophers agreed on the harmony and disharmony of sounds in the saying "*harmony in music is what brings a person to peace"*. Some Islamic scholars also followed them. In fact, Safiyyuddin did not content with Ibn Sīnā's description of the note as "*the sound that comes out as a synonym with time in high-pitched and pesty*" and added as follows: ***"It is a sound that is equal to time in a degree of shrillness and pestiness and is pleasant to nature."*** (Yusuf 1962).

## 3. Sound and the Source of Sound

Before Ibn Sīnā entered the theory of music, he focused on the subject of music, the sound and the function of the sound. He stated that his evaluations on this subject are based on some assumptions and mental experiences; explains that the subject is analyzed within the framework of these correct assumptions and philosophical method.

According to Ibn Sīnā, who points out the importance of "sound" by saying "***The first thing we like in music is the heard and felt qualities of the sound***", sound is like other sensible things. So for him the real criterion for sounds is the satisfaction or dissatisfaction of our hearing. For example, ***"some scents, even though they belong to the same type as normal and resemble it, may cause discomfort to the senses due to their excess, density and sharpness."*** he says. It's like the musky smell, which is extremely beautiful, irritates us when it is excessive. Although the sun's rays are beneficial to us, this is the kind of discomfort when excessive. Because in this case, our senses will be tired and uncomfortable. So is the sound: It will be pleasant or unpleasant by itself. When he is strong, our ears will be disturbed by him.

At the same time, according to Ibn Sīnā, ***"when a note is repeated (in the same pitch) at the level of treble and pestiness, this does not produce any musical composition. For composition arises between things (notes) that differ from each other in any way.*** "

The composition actually calls out to our mind power beyond our sense of hearing. In other words, "composition", the position of music related to shape; "Word" can be considered as its position regarding imitation between music-human and natural features. This is what Ibn Sīnā calls this "meaningful sound" of music (Turabi 2004)

According to Avicenna, ***"we like the sound qualities of the sound; more importantly, we like the reflection of the natural world outside music and the familiar qualities of man in sounds***; I mean, there are 3 things we like about sound:

a. The qualities of sound as sound,
b. Similarities between meaningful qualities of music - human - natural actions,
c. Organization of melodies in a musical composition.

To put it briefly, sound is not a sensation; It may seem pleasant or unpleasant to us, compared to our grasp, judging the idea he left in our soul and the role he played in the composition. So it is not our hearing power that makes musical compositions pleasant to us; it is our ability to reason that derives various suggestions from that composition." Hence the harmony between sounds, harmonious melodies and regular rhythm deeply captivate the soul. In short, we can call this "**personal pleasures**". The composition that a person falls in love with in sounds that are in order, is hidden in the strokes that imagine the sounds or in his proximity to the temperaments.

Avicenna asks: "*How should the voice be?*" He answers the question as follows: ***"Music, apart from its need for sound curtains; It should also have a measured (false / clear) sound range that we can apply to the melody-rhythm duo "***. According to him, whatever genre - in terms of the structure of the voice and the qualities of its meaningful character - should at least delight the listener. The "meaningful sound" a person makes can be for love or to dispel loneliness. People naturally compose melodies for various purposes; but a song - whatever its function - is different from a bird cry. In this sense, Ibn Sīnā clearly claims the functional importance of sound in human-animal life.

At the same time, although the natural sound and musical sound are the continuation of the "holy", they are actually part of the same reason, and a meaningful sound plays a different role in the life of living things than music. Composition and lyrics in music are formed on the same ground. But while meaningful sound is used for survival and communication, music is abstracted from this functional role.

Ibn Sīnā, who stated the existence of sound in animals, as the reason for their coming together; He put forward the reproductive order that God created among them. Because reproduction was provided by mating and mating by getting closer to each other. This discontinuous rapprochement includes animals that leave after fencing; to be able to contact when necessary, to call for help, to remember each other, to warn against danger, etc. Allah has given them the voice as a tool for such needs. Ibn Sīnā, here; It stands at a functional point regarding the efficiency of communication through sound in situations where human-animal individuals and species encounter in life. In humans, this function plays a more important role than animals. Because we are guided by the need to share what is inside of us. This type of sharing and communication comes to life-limiting loneliness. According to Ibn Sīnā, when both human and animal are filled with a strong feeling at the moment of relief, they express it by means of "**calling**". It is for this reason that there is always a desire to turn to sound in human beings. People are different; mute, raise, lower, quickness, etc. such as making the sound more functional, making it suitable for many purposes.

In this context, the philosopher, who attributes a different meaning to "**imitation of sounds**", states that imitation is more suitable for human beings and that one enjoys imitation and enjoys finding the things they are looking for in this imitation.

Sound, which is the main subject of the introduction in the music part of Şifa, is mostly limited to the sound used in "**communication**" by human-animal species. Avicenna does not mean by "**natural sound**" the swaying trees, trembling volcanoes, or the sounds emitted by thunder, or their effects on living things. The sound he is talking about here is the sound that Aristotle talked about earlier. His interpretation, simply of the function and natural position of the sound, is also a means to explain the essence of music.

Concerning the origin of music, Ibn Sīnā is completely opposed to the Muslim Pythagoreans who put forward the relationship between music and celestial bodies. He prefers a naturalistic rather than a mystical explanation for the origin of music. On specific points he states that humans and animals instinctively use this - meaningful voice - to express certain things and communicate with each other. Avicenna attributes to this instinctual source a broader function than the ongoing experiences of humans and animals and the expressions of the satisfaction or dissatisfaction they reach as a result of these experiences. In his view, meaningful voice and music - in general - are a reaction to contentment or discontent. He distinguishes with his teacher Farabi at this point: Farabi determines a direct route to music in the form of origin itself rather than this instinctive source. According to Farabi, meaningful results of pleasant or unpleasant life experiences can be seen in the sad-joyful genres of music. According to Ibn Sīnā, the same source; it could be used to explain meaningful sound in general and to explain the source of music in particular.

In summary, in this philosophical preface, Ibn Sīnā emphasizes the communication feature of the sound, especially the meaningful voice, which is functional in animal and human life. At this point, Hıfni considers Avicenna as an authority. Because, Ibn Sīnā regarding this issue; He guides thinkers who interpret music as a functional language, such as Charles Darwin (1809–1882), British thinker Herbert Spencer (1820–1903), and Carl Bücher (1847–1930).

Darwin; He argues that "*music melts into the generality of life*". However, it attributes to music functions such as a beauty that will make males desire females and thus the development of the species. Spencer is of the opinion that "music is a civilized language with a special effect." Bücher, on the other hand, attributes "*music to helping living things.*" In the light of this information, the famous music historian Curt Sachs summarizes the issue as follows: "*Perhaps among these thinkers, Spencer's view that" music was originally an expressive language* "is the closest to the truth. The language he meant is not the language used today among people; They are animal sounds that have certain meanings. In the development stages of humanity, the desire for dialogue, mutual agreement and speech has carried these voices to the level of modern languages they come from today. "

## 4. Music and Astrology

Ibn Sīnā expresses at the beginning of the work that he is completely far from the idea that establishes a connection between music and celestial bodies. Farabi, for whom Ibn Sīnā guided him, is of the opinion that the celestial bodies do not produce any musical or anti-musical sound. This situation does not allow the claim that there is any similarity between heavenly and earthly music. According to Ibn Sīnā, celestial bodies can produce music as a result of their rapid rotation in their orbits; however, the similarity that may exist between these and human musical compositions is a random congruence that at best corresponds to the theory of our music. Those who confuse these extra musical ties are those who, as explained, are surprised by the original and the coincidental. Arithmetic connections can of course be made here; but this is a means to apply to the similarities between music and human nature traits, as will be seen at the end of this chapter. Therefore, while Ibn Sīnā demonstrates the autonomy of the science of music, he declares that such extra-musical connections within their existence and possibilities cannot guide us in understanding the essential nature of music. As far as we can see he speaks of the similarity between music and human nature; But this similarity is neither the focal point of the nature of music nor the source of the taste we get from listening to music (Yusuf 1962).

While explaining his methodology in the introduction of his work - anonymously - some have been the subject of his criticism. With the expression "a group of old philosophies", the Greek philosophers, with the expression "they inherited without sorting them", Kindi, "the helpless persons" and İhvan-ı Safa; By "colleague friends" he means Farabi.

## 5. His Thoughts on Music Therapy

Avicenna recommends occupation, shock, suggestion, music and biomedical methods for the treatment of mental illnesses. In this respect, he can be regarded as the founder of today's modern psychiatry. He says that the most effective way of treatment is to increase the mental and spiritual powers of the patient. For this, he advises him to listen to music and get together with the people he loves. This situation can be considered among the reasons why the philosopher emphasized "**sensation**" in music like Aristoxenes and Farabi. "***Singing is the best health-preserving exercise.***" is remarkable in terms of briefly summarizing the effect of music on the human mind and metabolism.

For now, no information has been available on what types of music the thinker might have used for health protection and treatment purposes other than singing-listening. However, it is seen that he interspersed his assumptions about his psychological effects in his lectures in *Cevamiu İlmi'l-Musiki.*

According to the philosopher, small intervals lose their aesthetic value when they come one after another. Large ranges, on the other hand, are magnificent when used alone, not being mixed with small ones. The person gets more of the pleasure he gets from the moderate intervals from the melodies that are mainly used in large intervals.

The author states that the balanced intervals, translated with the phrase "**large superparticular",** relax the person and the person loses himself between those intervals. He declares that the transition between distant sounds gives a feeling of excessiveness and compulsion, and the transition from one note to the next one evokes laziness and stupidity and leads to stagnation. Based on these views of the philosopher, a theory in the style of "**harmony in sensation**" can be developed and its mental and physical effects can be examined.

Ibn Sina speaks of three types of "genders" which are grouped by music scholars unanimously as **"kavi (strong / diatonic), mu'tedil (mild, medium) and rahve (weak)**. He conveys that noncavid sexes give the impression of weakness, addiction and demoralization. Stating that "Rahve" can be named as "mulevven" (chromatic / colored) or "te'lifiyye" (enharmonic / harmonious), "mild" can be named as "rasima", he declares that these breeds are not used in their own land and their nature does not like them. Here, "**dislike of nature**" can be considered as a psychological concept together with its causes and effects.

Philosopher's thoughts about the cruise in terms of explaining the mental effect of the melodic structure:

"It should be known that the transition to the treble notes evokes angry characters. Transition to pest notes; expresses understanding, humble and balanced characters. Departures based on descent, which are obtained by spinning ascent, give the soul a prominent, wise and noble mood with a glory of sorrow. The contrary of these passages gives a delight inclined to lightness together with a sadness that is inferior to the soul. "

The practical equivalent of these sentences can be concretized by research.

The philosopher examines this concept under two headings in his talk. 1. "muvassal" (continuous), 2. "detailed" (discrete). After making the definition of these, it is stated that all of the classical (Iranian and Hüsrevani) compositions were created with mimassal ka; indicates that this has the ability to improve the state of the soul. Psychological points draw attention in these determinations of the philosopher.

## Conclusion

In the classification of Avicenna's sciences, music is one of the four sciences; these are arithmetic, geometry, astrology-astronomy and music. For, this classification has been accepted by Muslim scholars for a long time, with the translation of the works of Euclid, Ptolemy, Phythagoras and other Greek masters on music into Arabic. In this context, we see that Kindi and Farabi realized this. For this reason, the title of Ibn Sina's work on music is *"Cevamiu İlmi'l-Musika" (Music Science, the Third Branch of Riyazi Sciences)*.

Philosopher Ibn Sina accepts and applies Farabi's briefly expressed thoughts in the field of music; It examines, develops and turns them into assertive theories by expanding them further within its own systematic.

According to Ibn Sīnā, music; *"It is a job based on what is always better"*. Because it expresses personal taste. What he means is beauty, virtue. In other words, the feature in music must include numerical principles and proportions and these must be sound, in other words harmonious.

Avicenna takes the Farabi side against the Muslim Pythagoreans in terms of making music subject to a theory-based study. Like Aristoxenes who lived before him; He reexamined the science of music - the rules and elements of music - as an auditory phenomenon. It really is; It confirms, for example, that intervals and ratios can be thought of in their own time.

According to Ibn Sīnā, who points out the importance of "sound" by saying "*The first thing we like in music is the heard and felt qualities of the sound*", sound is like other sensible things. So in his eyes, the sounds are as far as the satisfaction or dissatisfaction of our hearing.

"Among the living" sound imitated "is neither the jewel of the music, nor its most pleasant situation." This view is a different aspect of Ibn Sīnā who claimed his independence from the Greek masters. Here, Ibn Sīnā explicitly asserts the functional importance of sound in human-animal life. As far as we can see he talks about the similarity between music and human nature; But this similarity is neither the focal point of the nature of music nor the source of the taste we get from listening to music.

Since they can be described, Ibn Sīnā expressed the sound intervals with mathematical proportions and listed them according to their relative degrees in vocal harmony. According to Ibn Sīnā, there are double or half ratios between all sounds. The two compatible voices are always in a numerical ratio. He divides the ranges into harmonious and incompatible.

Ibn Sīnā, who almost did not deviate from the line of Farabi in music theory and philosophy; While this was based on the theory of music, he was not a simple follower of the Greek music theory, he based his works on the music performed in his period. The fact that he used the Pythagoras scale does not show that he followed the theories put forward by the Greeks. Because this pentatonic scale was used in China long before the Hellenistic civilization and was found in West Asia independent of any Greek influence. Even today, it is not possible not to see the theories of Ibn Sīnā in the theory of Turkish, Iranian and Arab music and not to hear the voices based on those times.

## References

Bardakçı, Murat, *Maragalı Abdülkadir*, İstanbul 1986

Çelikkol, Erdinç, *Türk Mûsikîsi Nazariyatı*, Bursa, 1987, s.54; Arel, s.67

Çetin, M. Nihad, "Aruz", *DİA*, İstanbul 1991, III, 424

Dânişpejûh, Muhammed Taki,"Mûsikînâme", *Hüner ü Merdum*, h. 1354, s. 150

Evliyâ Çelebi, *Seyahatnâme*, İstanbul h. 1314/m. 1898–9, I, 622

Farmer, Henry George, "Mûsikî", *İA, İstanbul 1993*, VIII, 680

Farmer, Henry George, "The Lute Scala of Avicenna", *JRAS*, 1939, II, sa. 39, 256

Farmer, Henry George, *Historical Facts for the Arabian an Musical Influence*, New York 1970, s. 331–332

Farmer, Henry George, *Târihu'l-Mûsika'l-Arabiyye*, (Terc: Hüseyin Nassar), Kâhire 1956, s. 259

Farmer, Henry George, *The Sources of Arabian Music*, London 1965, s. 203

Hodgson, Marshall G. S., *İslâm'ın Serüveni* (İz Yay.), İstanbul 1993, I, 422–3

Jenkins-Olsen, Jen and Paul Rowsing, *Music And Musical Instruments In The World Of Islam*, London 1976, s. 40–41

Kaya, Mahmut,"Beytü'l-Hikme", *DİA*, İstanbul 1992, VI, 88

Korlaelçi, Murtaza,"İbn-i Sînâ'da Mûsıkî", *Erciyes Üniversitesi İbn-i Sînâ Sempozyumu*, Kayseri 1984, s. 350

Merâğî, Abdülkadir, *Şerhu'l-Edvar*, Nuruosmâniye Kütüphanesi, nr. 3651

Münzevî, Ahmed, *Fihrist-i Nüshâhâ-yı Hattî-i Fârisî*, Tahran h.1351

Oransay, Gültekin, *Musıkî Tarihi*, Yay-kur, Ankara 1976, s. 16

Picken, Laurence. *Folk Musical Instruments Of Turkey*, New York 1975, s. 586

Sachs, Curt, *The History Of Musical Instruments*, London 1978, s. 242–243

Şa'rânî, Mona Sancakdar, *Târihu'l-Mûsikâ'l-Arabiyye ve Âlâtühâ*, Beyrut 1987, s. 35

Shehadi, Fadlou, *Philosophies of Music In Medieval Islam*, London 1995, s. 68

Turabi, Ahmet Hakkı, *Mûsikî İbn Sînâ*, Litera Yay., İstanbul 2004, s. 3

Wright, Oven, *The Modal System of Arab and Persian Music AD 1250–1300*, London 1978, s. 93

Yekta, Rauf, *Türk Mûsıkîsi*, İstanbul 1985, s. 144

Yusuf, Zekeriya, *Mûsikâ'l-Kindî*, Bağdat 1962, s. 37

## Short Biography of Ahmet Hakkı Turabi

He was born on April 15, 1969 in Amasya. He graduated from Marmara University, Faculty of Theology in 1992. In the same year, he started to work as a research assistant in Turkish Religious Music Department. He studied music at the Turkish Music Conservatory, as well as music lessons at the faculty. In 1993–1994 he studied Arabic at Jordan University and studied Arabic music.

In 1996, "al-Kindi's Music Reseach" received his master's degree with his thesis; In 2002, "Ibn Sînâ 's Kitâbû'ş-Şifâ's Mûsikî" (Ibn Sînâ Mûsikî, Litera Publishing, Istanbul 2004) with his thesis on the thesis; In 2006, "Gevrekzâde Hâfız Hasan Efendi and Musiki Risalesi" (Rağbet Publications, Istanbul 2005) received his associate professorship degree. In 2011 he became Professor.

T.C. In the Itri Turkish Music Awards organized by the Ministry of Culture, it was awarded the "TURKISH MUSIC ACADEMY OF THE YEAR" award.

Marmara, Fatih Sultan Mehmet and the KKTC Near East Universities provide undergraduate and graduate degrees in Religious Music courses.

Prof. Dr. Kadircan H. Keskinbora, M.D., Ph.D.*

# Ibn Sīnā (Avicenna)'s *Canon* and its Influence on Medical Teaching in European Universities

In this chapter, I will attempt to detail the nature, extent, and duration of the influence of Ibn Sīnā's world-renowned work, *The Canon of Medicine,* on the medical education in Europe, and the ways in which it contributed to the overall European cultural development.

## Features of Ibn Sīnā's Canon

Considered as an encyclopedia of medicine, the *Canon* is in many respects distinguished by comprehensiveness and good organization. Praise of Ibn Sīnā's work for these qualities became, indeed, commonplace among Latin commentators. As G. B. Da Monte put it, Ibn Sīnā was moved to write the Canon when he saw that "*neither among the Greeks nor among the Arabs was there any single, complete, continuous book that taught the art of medicine,*" the Hippocratic writings being obscure, Galen extremely lengthy, and Rhazes confusing. Elsewhere, the same author asserted that Ibn Sīnā "*intended to reduce all the monuments of medical art scattered at large in various works of Galen into one, as it were, corpus. Indeed, he collected much dispersed information into appropriate and defined places and arranged it in sequence.*"[1,2]

The most influential of all Arabic medical encyclopedias was *The Canon of Medicine* (*Kitab al-Qanun fi al-tibb*) by Ibn Sīnā (d. 1037), known to Europeans as Avicenna.[3] The compendium consisted of five books: (1) general medical

---

* ORCID ID: 0000-0003-1940-1026; Google Scholar: https://scholar.google.com/scholar?hl=tr&lr=lang_tr&as_sdt=0%2C5&q=%22Kadircan+Keskinbora%22&btnG=

1 Guy Beaujouan, "Fautes et obscurités dans les traductions médicales du Moyen Age," Revue de synthèse, 3rd series, 89 (1968), 143–52.

2 Hakim Abdul Hameed, "Gerard's Latin Translation of lbn Sīnā's Al-Qanun," Studies in Islam 8 (1971), 1–7.

3 Two English translations of the first book only have been published, one made from the Latin version and the other from an Urdu version, but neither adequately represents the Arabic original. See O. C. Gruner, A Treatise on the Canon of Medicine

principles, (2) materia medica, (3) diseases occurring in a particular part of the body, (4) diseases such as fevers that are not specific to one bodily part, and (5) recipes for compound drugs. The first book sometimes circulated separately as *al-Kulliyat* (*General Principles*), or *Colliget* in Latin.[4]

It would be hard to dispute that the *Canon* is a comprehensive work. Few aspects of the traditional Greek and Arabic medicine are left untouched in its five books, which total about a million words in length. At the same time, the *Canon* needs to be seen as a collection of essentially separate and diverse manuals and reference books as well as an architectonic model of medicine. After going through the prefaces Ibn Sīnā wrote for the entire work and for each of his later books, the reader gratefully returns to the analytical table of contents included in the first editions of Gerard's translation.

Book 1 is divided into four main parts, or *fen* (section), to use the term adapted from the Arabic by the Latin translator. It opens with the statement of principles and handbook of physiology. The *second fen of Book 1* classifies varieties, efficient causes, and symptoms of disease. Diseases are divided primarily into those caused by an imbalance of the four elementary qualities of the body, i.e., its state of being hot, wet, cold, and dry, due to faulty composition, or conformation of bodily parts, and due to *solutio contitmitatis* or *continui,* which can be interpreted, more or less, as trauma. The causes of diseases are categorized as related to the environment, regimen, or psychology.[5] They may be due to any of a wide range of individual physical events, some of which (for example, pain and swelling) the modern reader might consider as symptoms rather than causes. The section on symptomology both lists an array of individual signs of imbalance of complexion, of *solutio continuitatis,* of obstruction, and so on, and reviews the standard means of diagnosis by inspecting pulse and urine. The *third fen of Book 1* concerns the conservation of health: separate sections on pediatric, adult, and geriatric regimen are followed by regimes for the delicate and complexionally imbalanced, and those for travelers. The *fourth and final fen of Book 1* deals with principles of therapy and forms of treatment appropriate for different conditions.

---

of Ibn Sina (London: Luzac, 1930); and O. C. Gruner, The General Principles of Ibn Sīnā's Canon of Medicine, trans. Mazhar H. Shah (Karachi: Naveed Clinic, 1966).

4 Muhsin Mahdi et al., "Ibn Sina," in Yarshater, Encyclopedia Iranica, vol. vol. 3, pp. 66–110.

5 Saul Jarcho, "Galen's Six Non-Naturals. A Bibliographic Note and Translation," *Bulletin of the History of Medicine* 44 (1970), 370–77.

*Book 2* is on the subject of simple medicines; most of them are given in a list—arranged more or less in Latin alphabetical order, presumably by the translator—of individual substances, their properties, and the conditions for which they are supposedly remedies.

In his *third book*, Ibn Sīnā provided *twenty-one fens (sections)* on ailments peculiar to each major organ of the body— ordered from head to toe—and their treatment. Most of the sections are preceded by one or two chapters on the anatomy and aspects of the physiology of the organ in question. *Book 4* surveys diseases and injuries that either affect the whole body or may occur in any part of it, as well as their treatment; of its *seven fens*, the most notable is probably the first concerning fevers, which provides a famous and influential account on the subject.

The *remaining fen of Book 4* concerns the following themes: crisis or critical days in illness; tumors and pustules; *solutio continuitatis* in the form of wounds, bruises, sprains, and ulcers; dislocations and fractures; poisons of mineral, vegetable, and animal origin (including animal bites and stings); and skin conditions. The *fifth and final book* of the *Canon* is an *antidotarium*, or manual on the preparation of compound medicines.

The division of the material into separate sections, and the provision of the analytical table of contents, means that anyone who is interested only in one particular topic—lepra, say, or diseases of the eyes—can easily turn to a few chapters on that subject alone. A reader who is primarily interested in diseases can find a sequence of more or less self-contained treatises offering complementary information. He or she can begin with classification, efficient causes, and symptoms of disease in general in *Book 1, Fen 2,* and proceed to the survey arranged by varieties of treatment in *Book 1, Fen 4.* Then, moving from the general to the particular, there is the account of diseases affecting different parts of the body in *Book 3* and of diseases affecting the body as a whole in *Book 4.*

The results are also fairly satisfactory if one considers the material available to a reader primarily interested in therapy. There is a self-contained survey of treatment methods (*1.4*) and a dictionary of medicinal simples (*Book 2*); much discussion of treatments appropriate for disease of particular bodily parts is found in *Book 3*, and of diseases affecting the entire body in *Book 4*; and *Book 5* provides guidance for compounding medicines. The arrangement has the merit of making it possible to approach the subject of therapy from a variety of different standpoints. One can, for example, relatively easily find an answer to any of the following questions: When and in what conditions is bleeding an appropriate treatment? What are the medicinal powers of cinnamon? What treatments are recommended for deafness? Which ones are recommended for various kinds of fevers? How is theriac compounded? However, although no systematic survey has been attempted here, it is clear that in answering these questions, whether they are with respect to therapeutic recommendations or properties attributed to substances, consistency is not always achieved throughout the text. The discussion of anatomy in general and of the physiology of other major organs in particular (brain, lungs, heart, digestive and reproductive organs, for example) are scattered through the opening chapters of *the twenty-one fens of Book 3.* This separation, which is the result both of Ibn Sīnā's division of medicine into theory and practice and of the classification of bodily parts that he adopted, was, as we shall see, further accentuated by the curricula and practices of medieval university faculties of medicine.

## The Nature of Medical Learning according to Ibn Sīnā

In the first volume of the *Canon*, the first section (*doctrina)* of *Fen 1* opens with a definition of medicine: "*Medicine is the science by which we learn the various states of the human body, when in health and when not in health, whereby health is conserved and whereby it is restored, after being lost.*" Medicine is thus presented from the outset as a science in the Aristotelian sense of a body of knowledge derived by demonstrative reasoning from true premises, but a science with a practical purpose.[6]

The second *doctrina* of *Fen 1*, on the elements, is an admirable illustration of this last principle, since it provides a highly compressed account of those, and only those, parts of a mainly Aristotelian theory of elements necessary to establish the human body as an object in the physical world and to provide the foundations for an understanding of two central concepts of the Greco-Arabic medical theory, namely humoral physiology and the idea of *complexio,* temperament, or *krasis* (that is, the balance of the elementary qualities of hot, wet, cold, and dry in living bodies).

The first two *doctrines* (*doctrina*) of *Fen 1* thus constitute an important statement about the nature of medical learning. The definition of medicine is broad enough to include the study of all aspects of physical functioning of the body. The status of medicine as a science is defended. Moreover, the subject is placed in the context of the Aristotelian natural philosophy, through insistence on medicine's scientific character, the application to it of the concept of the four

6 Nancy G Siraisi, Avicenna in Renaissance Italy. New Jersey: Princeton Univ. Press, 1987, pp. 23,24.

causes, and the assertion that the fundamental physical principles on which medicine rests are drawn from natural philosophy.

## Four Causes and Humor Theory

In composing *Fen 1*, Ibn Sīnā superimposed the Aristotelian scheme of the four causes upon the set of seven natural phenomena, redefining them as a sequence that proceeded from the most remote to the most immediate material causes, and ended with the final causes of the human body.

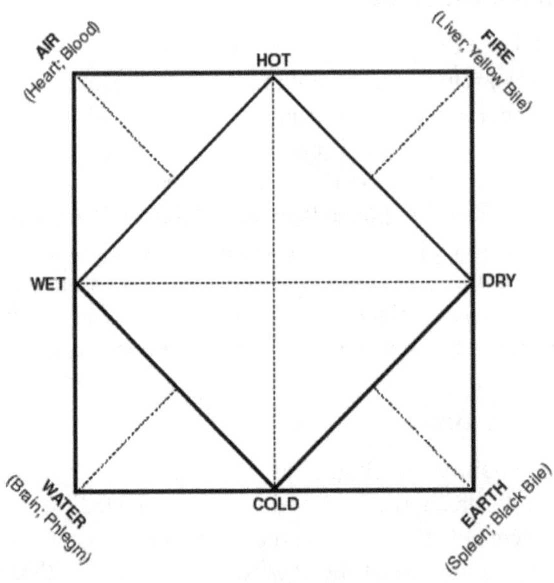


**Figure 1:** The scheme of the four causes and humor theory.

Within this whole scheme, each section leads logically to its successor, and all major bodily functions are neatly fitted into the system. Having learned that the human body, like all other sublunary bodies, is fundamentally composed of the four elements, each with its pair of qualities, the reader proceeds next to *Doctrina* 3 on *complexio.* The balance of the elementary qualities produces, in plant and animal species, as well as in human individuals, in parts of the body, and in medicinal compounds, the *complexio,* which Ibn Sīnā, followed Gerard, defined itself as a quality. Complexion, used in this special sense, is balanced or unbalanced, temperate or intemperate; in reality, however, complexion never achieves perfect balance, although in human beings it can come very close to doing so. A given complexion can only be identified by comparison with one of a series of norms (such as with the ideal for the species or the individual). According to Ibn Sīnā, eight varieties of temperate and eight varieties of distemperate complexion can be identified in this way. Types of medicine, too, can also be described as, temperate, hot, cold, etc. with regard to their effect on a particular body or kind of body.

## The Humors of the Body

*Doctrina* 4 defines bodily humors as liquids into which nutriment is converted. In addition to the four primary humors (blood, phlegm, red bile, and black bile), four secondary humors are identified. All are said to be found in both good and bad varieties. The good varieties of the primary humors are absorbed into and nourish the substance of the body; the bad are "superfluities," which are either excreted or damaging to the body if retained. Thus, discussion of the humors and their role in the body's economy involves attention to digestion, nutrition, and excretion, processes treated in a chapter on the generation of the humors. Topics covered include the stages of digestion and functions of mastication, saliva, stomach, intestines, liver, kidneys, and bladder."[7]

## The Parts of the Body

The topic of the humors is followed in *Doctrina* 5 by that of the *membra*, or parts of the body, which are described here as generated by the humors and sustained by their nutritive activity. The introductory chapter of this section contains generalizations about the *membra* in parallel with those made about the humors and complexions in the two preceding parts of the work. That is followed by five *summae* containing a total of seventy-six chapters on the anatomy of the bones, muscles, nerves, arteries, and veins. Well over half of *Fen 1*, in fact, consists of these chapters on anatomy.[8]

The only part of *Doctrina* 5 regularly taught in European universities was the introductory chapter, and this is all that will be considered here. It is mainly concerned with various ways of classifying bodily parts. The first distinction made is between *membra similia* or *simplicia* (for example, bones, cartilage,

7 Siraisi, ibid, p.27.
8 Siraisi, ibid, p.28.

nerves, ligaments, arteries, and veins) and composite or instrumental members (for example, the hands or the face). It will be observed that this distinction is not quite the same as that between tissues and organs, which it is sometimes said to resemble. Brief definitions of the nature and function of the more important *membra similia* follow. It is only those members that are treated in the subsequent anatomical chapters, and for an account of the chief composite members the reader has to turn to the introductory chapters of each section of *Book 3*.

## Reception of the *Canon* in Europe

The Latin translation of the *Canon* was attributed by his pupils to Gerard of Cremona (d. 1187), and although revisions of the Gerard translation and retranslations of parts of the work began to circulate in the sixteenth century, the twelfth-century Latin text was the original basis of the Western understanding of Ibn Sīnā's book.

The source of inspiration for this endeavor was the reflection of certain ideals of the Renaissance humanism, which appeared around the last quarter of the fifteenth century, in the medical profession. The humanist determination to pay close attention to texts in their original language led to a much closer interest in the relationship of Ibn Sīnā to Galenic sources than ever before. Despite the limited nature of Arabic studies in sixteenth century Europe, there were some efforts to approach the Arabic text in its original. Underlying the several revisions to the text rendered in Latin was the humanist desire for more accurate or, at any rate, more elegant and accessible translations.

Other traces of an influence of the *Canon* outside the universities may be seen in quotations from Avicenna in vernacular medical treatises as well as in the existence of vernacular medical compendia purportedly based on Avicenna's work. For example, a French treatise of which at least two copies survive (both in Italian libraries) claims to be "Avicen en romance." It is a little work on regimen that urges on the reader self-help and self-medication. A complete study might reveal its actual relation, if any, to the *Canon*. Another vernacular treatise compiled in Italian in 1478 also claims to be based on Avicenna.[9]

Finally, the *Canon* played a major role in medieval Jewish medical culture. Nathan ha-Meati translated all five books of the *Canon* into Hebrew in 1279, and Zerahia ben Isaac ben Shealtiel Gracian also independently translated *Books 1 and 2* into Hebrew during the thirteenth century. Nathan's translation

9 Siraisi, ibid, p.47–48.

was subsequently revised by Joseph ben Joshua ha-Lorki in about 1400. One hundred and eleven complete or partial manuscripts of these versions survive, most of them of Spanish or Italian provenance.[10] Thus, the most extensive use of the *Canon* outside the universities in western Europe during the Middle Ages was unquestionably by Jewish physicians (as one might expect, given that Jews were excluded from universities, were possessors of a learned medical culture, and in contact with the Arabic world). Nonetheless, the influence of the *Canon on* Western medical thought was chiefly exercised through the adoption of parts of the work as university textbooks.

Didactic medical poetry was also a popular device, with rhyming quatrains that enabled the student or practitioner to easily remember the basic ideas. Ibn Sina wrote one that was especially popular, judging from the large number of manuscripts and commentaries preserved today.[11]

As mentioned before, Ibn Sīnā's *Canon* was published in the West at around the same time as certain other important encyclopedic medical works of Islamic origin as well as a series of long surveys of note by Galen. At the end of the twelfth century, a carefully and widely designed fundamental curriculum including other short Hippocratic and Galenic works and texts known as *Ars Medicina* and *Articella* was beginning to take shape. But among all the medical works published up to that time, the most systematic and comprehensive was Ibn Sīnā's *Canon.*

## Canon in Italy

In Italy, the study of the *Canon* seems to have been first undertaken by surgeons associated with Bologna and Padua. Several references to Ibn Sīnā's description of and suggested treatments for the condition or conditions termed *cancer* are contained in Rolando da Parma's exposition of twelfth-century surgery by Roger. The *Canon* may, however, have been used in medical, as distinct from surgical, teaching and study in the *studium* of Siena before 1250. The most prolific medical writer associated with a northern or central Italian school in the middle of the thirteenth century was Petrus Hispanus, the future Pope John XXI (d. 1276), who was the author of a widely used medical handbook, the *Thesaurus pauperum,* as well as commentaries on five of the *articella* works,

10 Benjamin Richler, "Manuscripts of Avicenna's Kanon in Hebrew Translation A Revised and Up-to-date List," *Koroth* 8 (1982), 145'-168',

11 Henri Jahier and Abdelkader Noureddine, Avicenne, Po`eme de la medecine, Urguza fi 't-tibb, Cantica Ibn Sinae (Paris: Les Belles Lettres, 1956).

on works of Isaac, and on the Aristotelian books on animals, and a set of celebrated and influential treatises on logic. Petrus most likely acquired his medical training at Paris before he came to Siena, where he was teaching in 1246; he was apparently still in the latter city in 1250 and perhaps remained there longer. In his commentary on the work on diets attributed to Isaac Judeus, Petrus frequently made citations to Ibn Sina.[12]

The *Canon* was frequently copied in its entirety and much studied as a reference work. However, both the commentary tradition as it developed from the late thirteenth century and academic statutes of the fourteenth and fifteenth centuries make it clear that the whole of the *Canon* was never prescribed as a textbook – the work's length alone would make such a requirement impossible. Instead, portions of the work were isolated earlier for use in teaching separate courses in *theoria, practica,* and probably surgery. At Bologna, the *Canon* had certainly entered the curriculum well before the end of the thirteenth century, judging by the fact that Taddeo Alderotti produced commentaries – presumably based on his lectures – on several short sections.[13] The same is probably true of Padua, since the *Tractatus de conservatione sanitatis* of Zambonino da Gaza of Cremona, who was a regent master of medicine at Padua in 1262, contains citations of Avicenna. At Salerno and Naples, however, statutory provisions of the late 1270s gave no place to the *Canon* in the formal curriculum.[14]

After the turn of the century, some commentaries on the *Canon* published in Spain were preoccupied with issues that seemed at least as much metaphysical or even theological as medical. Thus, for example, whatever the situation at Alcalá de Henares in its humanist heyday, before 1611 Dr. Pedro Garcia Carrero was lecturing there on *Canon* 1.1 and before 1628 on *Canon 1.4.* Moreover, at Salamanca, which was at the height of its reputation as a center of medical education during the sixteenth and part of the seventeenth centuries, the *Canon* seems to have been taught actively and seriously throughout the period, if one may judge by the survival of seven lengthy sets of manuscript lectures on

12 On his studies and career as a professor of medicine, see Richard Stapper, *Papst Johannes XXI Eine Monographie* (Münster, 1898), pp. 4–26.

13 Taddeo commented on a chapter on things eaten and drunk from Canon 1.2, a chapter on lepra from Canon 4.2 and on Canon 4.3. A commentary on a few chapters of Canon 1.4 is doubtfully ascribed to him. For incipits and manuscripts (and in the case of the last an early edition), see Siraisi, Alderotti, pp. 416–417, 422, 425, 426.

14 Salvatore de Renzi, Collectio Salernitana ossia Documenti mediti e trattati di medutna appartenenti alla scuola medica salernitana (Naples, 1852), 1:360–62.

different parts of the work, written by Salamanca medical professors between the 1540's and the 1670's.[15]

## Canon in Medical Schools' Curriculum

In the medical curricula of the universities, the first book of the *Canon,* and especially the first section of that book, was adopted early on as a textbook of *theoria,* i.e. the branch of medicine that acquainted the neophyte with the nature of medical science, the position of medicine in the hierarchy of arts and sciences, and the proper relationship of medicine and philosophy, as well as with the basic principles of physiology, pathology, and regimen. Ibn Sina's views may be open to dispute on certain points, but as a whole Canon 1.1 constituted one of the clearest summary expressions available at the time of the principles underlying the system of medical education taught at the universities of Medieval and Renaissance Europe.

Insofar as an overview of physiology was presented to medical students in public lectures at the Renaissance Padua or Bologna, this was accomplished in the course on *theoria* for which *Canon 1.1* provided the text. (Other courses in *theoria* were based on the Hippocratic *Aphorisms* and the Galenic *Ars,* or *Microtechne,* neither of which provided the comprehensive and systematic overview of physiology presented in *Canon 1.1*). Sixteenth-century critics and their modern successors have rightly perceived the division of the study of medicine into *theoria* and *practica* as one of the main weaknesses of the Renaissance university medical curriculum. Nevertheless, the topics discussed in courses on *theoria* were by no means isolated from current debates and scientific interests. For instance, physiological and anatomical debates overlapped in many areas, so that discussions of the implications of sixteenth-century anatomical findings could without incongruity or inappropriateness find their way into commentaries on the *Canon.*[16]

Broadly speaking, medieval medical education was based on a small group of brief texts, the *Articella,* and increasingly upon the *Canon* of Ibn Sīnā. The substance of the teaching of different masters comprised commentary upon these texts. The principal exception to this method of teaching was anatomical demonstration. The essence of dissection was that it was a *practical* affair. It was carefully controlled by regulations within the institutional arrangements of

15 Siraisi, ibid, p.83
16 Siraisi, ibid, p.10

the university and formed a regular, if not frequent element of the curriculum. Probably dissections had been carried out since the Salernitan demonstrations of the insides of pigs in the twelfth century. Human dissection seems to have begun in the late thirteenth century. As a practical affair, dissection and demonstration of the parts did not generate commentary. There was of course the necessary business of glossing anatomical terms as different authors became better known, and this extended to the establishing of sound texts and the correct attribution of works; but anatomical texts of the middle ages that had a direct bearing on dissection did not have the form of a commentary. Nor had there survived from antiquity any suitable text that might form the basis of a commentary. The only commentaries containing anatomical material were those upon book three of the *Canon*, which is much more than an anatomy text. The Venetian presses of Scotus continued through Berengaria's lifetime to publish the commentaries on the *Articella* and the *Canon* that formed the teaching material of the medical schools of Padua and Bologna.[17]

## The Practical Teaching in the Canon

The widest use made of the *Canon* was probably in teaching *practica*. Sections of the work commonly used for this purpose at various times and places included *Part 4 of Book 1, Book 3, and parts of Book 4*. Both the Montpellier statutes of 1340 and the Paduan statutes of 1465 prescribe the whole of Book 1, the latter as part of the instruction to be given by *theorici*. Yet it is clear that *Part 4 of Book 1* (on general therapy) was treated as a text in *practica* by the early fourteenth century, just like it was in later university documents; this is apparent from the title of Dino del Garbo's highly academic commentary on *Canon 1.4*, named *Dilucidatorium totius practice medicine. Canon* 1.4 was regularly the subject of lectures on *practica* at Bologna from 1589 until 1716, and doubtless even before that. It was *Book I* alone, and no other part of the *Canon*, which emerged as a textbook for the teaching of medical *theoria*. It was adapted for this role by selective omission. Of its four parts, or *fen*, it seems likely, as we have just seen, that *Canon 1.4* was moved to the sphere of *practica*. Moreover, in prescribing this book, the Bologna statutes of 1405 indicate omissions from *Fen 1 and 2*, and require only five chapters of *Fen 3*. The portions of the *Canon* used in teaching medical theory were therefore usually drawn from the first two fens

17 French, R.K. 1985. "Berengario da Carpi and the use of commentary in anatomical teaching." A. Wear, R.K. French and I.M. Lonie (eds.), The Medical Renaissance of the Sixteenth Century. New York: Cambridge University Press, pp. 223–245.

of *Book 1*; of these two sections, it was the first that was primarily valued as a compendium of basic principles. The oldest Latin commentary on any part of *Book 1* appears to be a set of lectures taken down by Alberto of Bologna from Antonio da Parma, probably at Bologna between 1310 and 1323; these *recollectiones* are on *Canon 1.1* alone.[18]

Surgical teaching in the Italian universities also drew upon practically oriented portions of the *Canon*. The evidence for the use of parts of *Canon* 4 as a textbook of surgery is provided by the considerable interest shown in Ibn Sīnā by the thirteenth-century north Italian writers on the topic of surgery, and also by Dino del Garbo's *Chirurgia*, which is an academic commentary on *Canon* 4.3–5. The *Canon* was regarded by some as useful for anatomical teaching, as indicated by some disparaging remarks of Berengario da Carpi, writing in 1521.[19]

## Humanism and the Canon

The inspiration for these attempts was derived from the importation of some of the ideals of Renaissance humanism into medicine beginning in about the last quarter of the fifteenth century. The humanist insistence upon attention to original texts in the original languages stimulated a closer attention to Ibn Sīnā's relation to his Greek (especially his Galenic) sources than had hitherto been undertaken; and despite the limitations of Arabic studies in sixteenth-century Europe, some efforts were made to approach the Arabic text directly. The humanist desire for more accurate, or at any rate more elegant and readily understandable, translations lay behind various revisions of the Latin texts.

## The *Canon* in the Medieval Universities and the Humanist Attack on Ibn Sīnā

By the 1520's, i.e., the beginning of the period with which this study is principally concerned, the *Canon* in its twelfth-century Latin translation was both a venerable part of a centuries-old tradition of medical teaching and a book that had been for a generation the object of attacks ranging from reasoned criticism to vitriolic abuse.

18 Siraisi, ibid, 54–56

19 "Berengario da Carpi and the Use of Commentary in Anatomical Teaching," in the Medical Renaissance of the Sixteenth Century, ed. A Wear, R K French, and I M. Lome (Cambridge, 1985), pp 42–74.

Broadly speaking, the history of these developments is well-known. Even though its Latin translation was discovered by 1187, awareness about the *Canon* in the West became unmistakably evident at the beginning of the thirteenth century. In the second half of the century, Ibn Sīnā's work was routinely studied and highly prized at the most prominent centers of medical education, and between the thirteenth and fifteenth centuries a whole corpus of commentary on the work was produced by several of the most famous and learned doctors of the period.

At the same time, the critical commentary already made on the Arab-Latin scholastic medicine by Petrarch in mid-fourteenth century was compounded by those of the humanists in the medical profession and was increasingly concentrated on Ibn Sīnā and his *Canon*. Even so, there is still a lot to be learnt about the reception and employment of the *Canon* in the late Middle Ages. The exact place of the work within the context of the thought and culture of medieval Europe awaits a comprehensive analysis of the Qanun's (Canon) tradition of handwriting and its interpretations and the literature regarding the interpretations.

It seems that the extent to which medicine could be 'humanized' was limited. A 'humanist' physician would be aware of himself as being historically severed from the classical world and certainly to place his authors in a time scale suggested by this would be of value, but he could not historicize his texts in the same way as the legal humanists were doing. Taking the aphorisms of Hippocrates as an example again, however much they were seen to be the products of an alien society, they applied to physical and fixed aspects of human nature, not to a changed set of relationships between people. The same applied *a fortiore* to anatomy: a good anatomical text carried the same message as the body itself for the same reason it was not easy to dismiss the commentators, whether their subject was the anatomy of the *Canon* or the densely aphoristic Hippocratic writings. The ultimate object of enquiry was the truth about the physical human body. Moreover, the *Canon* seemed more complete than any Galenic work available and study of it was indispensable. The 'humanist' physician might do what he could to avoid barbarity of language, but the Ciceronian style that suited rhetoric so admirably was not easily suitable for dissection guides and descriptive anatomy (Vesalius was to lose a number of readers for this reason).[20]

Although the approach of medical humanists to the Arabic writers certainly included its share of purely rhetorical and polemical elements, the grounds on

20 French, ibid, 240-2

which the *Canon* was criticized were for the most part both practical and highly specific. The emphasis was primarily on evaluating the extent of the actual usefulness of the *Canon* for contemporary practitioners. Although the defenders of the *Canon* accused its attackers of excessive concern for literary elegance rather than substance, such in fact seldom seems to have been the case. Moreover, Champier's "suspicion of the taint of Islam" was not echoed by other authors. Instead, Leoniceno, Brissot, Fuchs, and Champier himself, as well as others, expended considerable effort in identifying particular instances in which Ibn Sina's supposed misunderstanding of a text of Greek origin or the obscurities of Gerard of Cremona's Arabo-Latin technical terminology produced confusions and errors that led to an imprecise understanding of Galenic physiology and anatomy and to mistakes in therapy and the identification of pharmacological substances. It was indeed the pharmacological portions of the *Canon* that were the chief focus of critical attention, both because these were the parts where the Latin translation was least comprehensible, and because of the growing general interest among early sixteenth-century physicians in medical botany and pharmacology.[21]

## Criticism and Commentaries of the Canon

The *Canon* was used as a teaching text. More specifically, the teaching of the *Canon* was representative of the Renaissance education that tackled the question of how a scientific subject could be taught by means of commentary on a medieval text and synthesizing ancient sources. Here commentaries must be approached with caution, since they do not necessarily reflect classroom practice directly.[22] Commentaries are unlikely to have the immediacy, for example, of the students' annotations of classical texts from the University of Paris in the second half of the sixteenth century.[23]

Despite Ibn Sīnā's justified reputation as an author belonging to medieval studies, the later period is arguably that in which the most thorough study of the *Canon* was undertaken by scholars in the Latin West. It is also that in which the work aroused the most controversy, and in which the process resulting in the obsolescence of Ibn Sīnā's work for Western medicine began. For about

21 Siraisi, Alderotti, pp. 100–103; for Montpellier, Arnald of Villanova, Opera, 15, 15–37.

22 Anthony Grafton, "Teacher, Text, and Pupil in the Renaissance Class-Room: A Case Study from a Parisian College," History of Universities 1 (1981), 37–70.

23 "Renaissance Commentaries on Ibn Sīnā's Canon, Book 1, Part 1, and the Teaching of Medical Theoria in the Italian Universities," History of Universities (1984), 47–9.

the first two hundred years after its introduction into university curricula in the thirteenth century, the *Canon*, although subjected to occasional criticism, was generally and on the whole rightly esteemed as a sophisticated systematization and summary of almost all available medical learning. By about the mid-seventeenth century, despite the *Canon's* great historical importance, its irrelevance to current developments in European physiology was clearly apparent; its long survival thereafter in various university curricula (at Bologna part of the work retained a nominal position until 1800) must be attributed chiefly to academic inertia, as eighteenth-century educational reformers were not slow to point out.[24]

For the interest of the world of Renaissance in Ibn Sīnā's medical writings the following can be cited as evidence. Between 1500 and 1674, there were published at least sixty editions of the full or partial text of the *Canon* in Latin, along with new interpretations of it. These editions and interpretations of the *Canon* provide us with much information concerning the general trends in the Renaissance medicine and about responses given to these new developments in the academic medical community. Following the effects of and interactions concerning these developments by focusing on the publication history of one single text and its interpretations in a continuous line, provides us with a valuable if limited path of knowledge in a complex and, most of the time, bewildering field of intellectual history and history of science. The *Canon* is certainly just one of a series of texts that can be approached in this manner. The latest studies on the Renaissance interpretations of philosophical texts have begun to reveal the full extent of the diversity and richness of this literature, as well as its significance for the history of philosophy and science and their education.[25]

Although almost all of the Latin medical commentaries in the fourteenth and seventeenth centuries were based on university lectures, only indefinite quantities of the extant body of textual material was subject to later reordering and represented only a small portion of all the lectures given during a period that covered several centuries. One possible reason for this fact is that it resulted from the efforts of more ambitious and energetic professors. Another reason could be that some of the interpretations of the Canon had been written by professors that lived before the texts were taught within the legal university

24 Brendan Dooley, "Science Teaching as a Career at Padua in the Early Eighteenth Century. The Case of Giovanni Polem," History of Universities 4 (1984), 41–51.

25 Charles H. Lohr, "Renaissance Latin Aristotle Commentaries: Authors A-B, "Studies in the Renaissance 21 (1974), 228–89.

curricula or who died prior to their use. Still another reason could be that when the publication of traditional text commentaries lost its ability to polish one's reputation in academic or scientific circles, new commentaries were no longer printed.

If the number of commentaries is any guide, the most highly valued of all the parts of the *Canon* used in teaching *practica* was Book 4, especially its first section on fevers. At least eighteen Latin commentaries on *Canon* 4.I were written before 1500.[26] The earliest known Latin commentary on the *Canon* is, as already noted, on this section. It is also the subject of one of the last publications of any medieval Latin commentary on the work, namely that by Giovanni Arcolano (Arculanus, Herculanus, d. 1458), reissued at Padua in 1685. By contrast, Thorndike and Kibre list only seven commentaries on *Canon* 1.4 written before 1500. Commentaries on the whole of Book 3 are even fewer (perhaps none, since Gentile da Foligno's, which covers most of the book, appears not to be complete); however, the various subdivisions of this part of the *Canon* gave rise to fairly numerous commentaries by different authors in separate short sections. Despite the requirement for the study of *Canones secundi Avicenne* in the Bologna statute of 1405, there appear to be few extant commentaries on *Canon 2, Canon* 5, and the antidotarium, which appear to have been relatively little studied in the schools, and to have attracted commentary only from the indefatigable Gentile da Foligno.[27]

Even though Latin commentaries on sections of the *Canon* appeared toward the end of thirteenth century, its main interpretations were chiefly products of a period between early fourteenth century and mid-fifteenth century. The few commentaries written before 1300, which are mostly short pieces, are seen not to have had much lasting influence, and the composition of important commentaries appears after around 1450. Jacques Despars (d. 1458), began his decade of preparation for his commentaries on Canon 1.3 ve 4.1 after leaving his position as regent master in medicine. Apart from Despars, the most significant Latin commentators of the *Canon* in the fourteenth and fifteenth centuries are Dino del Garbo, Gentile da Foligno, Giacomo da Forli, Ugo Benzi, and Giovanni Arcolano. To these most prominent figures may be added the names of Antonio da Parma, Tommaso del Garbo, Marsiglio di Santa Sofia, Giovanni Matteo Ferrari da Grado and Biagio Astario.

---

26 Charles H. Lohr, ibid.

27 Carl C Schlam, "Graduation Speeches of Gentile da Foligno," Mediaeval Studies 40 (1978), 96–119.

In the fourteenth and fifteenth centuries, the commentary practice on the *Canon* can be deemed to be at its most variegated in the well-developed schools of Northern Italy. This productivity attained local prestige, which explains the high rates of selection of such commentaries by Italian printers for publication, and helped provide a rich supply of manuscripts with widening and continuous influence.

We should stress once more the fact that for the different branches of medical education, it was not only the wide contributions attributed to the different sections of Ibn Sīnā's *Canon*, but the production of commentaries on Ibn Sīnā's works during the fourteenth and fifteenth centuries which served their advancement. The men who were considered the most select masters in the Italian medical schools enjoyed very high reputation among their contemporaries and the following generation of intellectuals. The Latin commentaries of both Ugo and Lockwood went to print multiple times.

We have already noted Roger Bacon's complaints that the *medici* of his day relied too heavily on Ibn Sīnā's classification of diseases and expended too much energy on disputation irrelevant to the task of healing. In the next century, Petrarch grounded his much paraded hostility to medicine in part on a disdain for "Arab lies," for as he explained to his correspondent, the physician Giovanni Dondi, "*I hate the whole race.*"[28]

As one might expect, Petrarch's dislike of Arabic medical advice, like his similar attitude toward scholastic natural philosophy, seems more to have been inspired by religious, moral, and literary than by scientific considerations. Similar views were not necessarily an integral part of various other evaluations of medicine by fourteenth- and fifteenth-century literary humanists. For example, Coluccio Salutati, who was strongly critical of many aspects of the medicine of his day, referred to Ibn Sīnā approvingly as a "*remarkable man who brought great light to medicine.*"[29] Moreover, as already noted, the leading scholastic commentators on the *Canon* were on the whole kindly treated by their humanist contemporaries.

Specific criticism of the *Canon* and its Latin commentators in this period must be understood as part of a broadly based attack on Arabs in general, which aroused controversies in university faculties of medicine throughout Europe

28 Gerhard Baader, "Medizinisches Reformdenken und Arabismus im Deutschland des 16. Jahrhunderts," *Sudhoffs Archiv für Geschichte der Medizin mid der Naturwissenschaften* 63 (1979), 270.

29 Siraisi, Avicenna in Renaissance Italy, 67.

and generated a fairly large literature. Recent studies have charted the progress of these arguments not only in Italian humanist circles, but also in the schools of Montpellier, Paris, Tubingen, Alcalá and some other parts of Germany and Spain. Yet because segments of the *Canon* played a prominent part in university curricula, and because the sections on simples and the composition of remedies in Ibn Sīnā's work were both lengthy and notably problematical, in medical circles criticism of Arabic scholars frequently tended to focus on Ibn Sina. Although controversy over the issue of the Arabic medical writers probably reached its height in the late 1520's and early 1530's in France and Germany, criticism of Ibn Sīnā was already an important ingredient in the medical teaching of Nicolò Leoniceno at the University of Ferrara in the last decade of the fifteenth century.[30]

The criticism of the *Canon* was not always limited to the scorn directed against it by the fourteenth and fifteenth century commentators but was closely related to the emphasis made on the differences that separated medical doctrines from humanist ideas, an emphasis which was highly exaggerated. For the physicians educated at the schools of Northern Italy, the acceptance of Ibn Sīnā's humanist criticism involved the aim of displacement if not a complete rejection of their distinguished predecessors. Especially with respect to pharmacology, the establishment of certain errors or mistranslations in the *Canon* and the diminishing reputation of previous scholastic commentators, would turn into an enduring devotion to Ibn Sīnā. Some of the late fifteenth- and early sixteenth-century critics of the Canon had, as we have seen, supported their arguments by referring to passages which showed how Ibn Sīnā's diverged from Galen, Dioscorides, or other ancient medical authors, but such accounts were incomplete as well as polemical in intent.

The *Canon* survived in the medical curriculum of many a university. It continued to be seriously studied in several universities including some of the foremost centers of medical education, and to be consulted by practitioners. The academic, administrative and professional tradition; the facility of the chapters of the *Canon* for introduction to the teaching of Galenic physiology and pathology; and the faith added by the Arabs to the remedies inherited from the Greeks – all of these factors contributed to this result. More fundamentally, the trust in the power of philosophical eclecticism and humanist philology in reclaiming the essence of ancient wisdom made it difficult or even impossible

30 Luis Garcia Ballester, "The Circulation and Use of Medical Manuscripts in Arabic in Sixteenth-Century Spain" *Journal for the History of Arabic Science* 3 (1979), 183–99.

for the majority of the sixteenth century intellectuals to criticize the works of Ibn Sina.

Thus, in the case of the *Canon,* the introduction of philological humanism into medicine, which engendered the attack on Arabic influence, also served to engender the opinion that the cause of sound medical teaching would be better served if the *Canon,* instead of being scorned, was supplied with an improved Latin text and a modern body of commentary, both of which would clarify Ibn Sīnā's relationship to Galen and confirm or enlarge the practical usefulness of the work.

Until that time, there had been numerous abridgements and explanatory commentaries composed on parts of the *Canon.* Although the earliest abridgement of the *Canon* seems to have been by al-Ilaqi (d. 1068), a pupil of Ibn Sina, it was not until the late twelfth century that a serious need for aids to understanding the work was felt. The Egyptian Jewish physician Ibn Jumay, who died in 1198, composed possibly the earliest commentary on the *Canon.* In the next two centuries, commentaries and epitomes followed in rapid succession, and it was this industry of glossing and condensing the *Canon* that assured the encyclopedic work its preeminent position in medieval medicine.[31] The most widely read of all abridgements of Ibn Sina's *Canon* was the one titled *al-Mujiz* (*The Epitome*), written by the Syrian physician Ibn al-Nafis, mentioned earlier in connection with his own encyclopedia. Al-Nafis also composed a commentary on the *Canon* that became an authoritative work in its own right. Both *The Epitome* and the commentary continued to be copied and read over the following five centuries, often generating further commentaries and supercommentaries.

The medical defenders of the *Canon* in sixteenth-century Europe valued the work essentially for its Galenic doctrines and pharmacological compendia. But the fundamental humanist contention that Galen is best studied from Galen is hard to gainsay. And to arrive at a satisfactory understanding of the possible range of meanings underlying Arabo-Latin botanical and pharmacological terminology would call for an investment of effort likely to be greater than any medical results would justify. What is unquestionable, however, is that the approach adopted by Rinio, Graziolo, and Costeo and his partners was the one most likely to secure the position of the *Canon* in their own milieu. The scholars who edited or revised the Canon accepted the need to find explicit

31 Iskandar, *Catalogue of Arabic Manuscripts on Medicine and Science in the Wellcome Historical Medical Library*, pp. 33–64; E. Savage-Smith, *Islamic Medical Manuscripts at the National Library of Medicine* (http://www.nlm.nih.gov/hmd/arabic).

justification for the continued study of Ibn Sīnā. They, therefore, did much to clarify Ibn Sīnā's relationship to Galen, and used improved editorial techniques to highlight inconsistencies and obscurities within the text. It seems likely that their editions facilitated an evaluation of the merits and defects of the one-time "prince of physicians" in a much more detached manner than before.[32]

In fact, in certain circumstances courses on Canon 1.1 were clearly given for the purpose of teaching philosophy and science as much as for medical instruction.

*In the age of Zabarella and Cremonini the university was still a fairly important center of Aristotelian natural philosophy, a subject of renewed interest to some medical men, among them William Harvey (at Padua 1599–1602). And of course the Venetian and Paduan contacts made by Galileo during his sojourn at Padua (1592–1610) show the presence in those cities of a few intellectuals open to radically innovative scientific approaches.*[81]

Challenges to Galen came from Vesalian anatomists, Paracelsians, modern Aristotelians, followers of Fernel and Argenteno, and various other medical innovators. Nonetheless, the chief effect of the medical humanism of the early sixteenth century had been to reinforce Galen's authority, and that authority was still predominant at the century's end.[33]

By about the 1550s, the victory of Galen over the Arabic medical scholarship was in one sense fairly complete. Few physicians could thereafter have defended Ibn Sīnā as an independent authority against Galen. But a good deal of the evidence that had served to dethrone Ibn Sīnā as a prince of physicians in his own right could also be interpreted as offering reinforcement for the belief that the *Canon,* apart from its pharmacological sections, contained reasonably accurate summaries of Galenic teaching suitably simplified for student use. Furthermore, the attention devoted to the *Canon* by Da Monte, whose commentaries became well known, provided a model for the way in which a Galenist and *modernus* of stature might lecture upon Ibn Sīnā without doing violence to his principles, and in itself constituted an endorsement of the continued usefulness of parts of the *Canon* as introductory textbooks. This intellectual climate, as well as the vagaries of university politics, help to explain not only the survival of a place for Ibn Sīnā in the Paduan curriculum, but also its actual enlargement in the last decade of the sixteenth and first decade of the seventeenth century. Throughout the second half of the century, leading professors at Padua continued to lecture

32 Siraisi, Avicenna in Renaissance Italy, p.173–4.

33 Bylebyl, p.363–4.

on the *Canon* and to preserve their lectures for publication. *Canon* 4.1 was the subject of surviving lectures given by Trincavella as first ordinary professor of *practica* in 1553, by Alessandro Massaria in the same position between 1587 and 1598, and by Capodivacca as the secondary ordinary professor of *practica* in 1579. As well as at least six copies of the complete *Canon* (three of which appear to have been large, and doubtless expensive, folio editions) and four of *Canon* 1.1, the government owned copies of the commentaries on *Canon* 1.1 by Da Monte (three copies), Oddo Oddi (three copies), Paterno, and Santorio of Da Monte on *Canon* 1.2; and as part of larger collections of their works, of Trincavella (two copies) and Capodivacca (nine copies) on *Canon* 4.1.[34]

Monau's comment about Ibn Sīnā's pharmacology therefore belongs to a context of which the most current anatomical findings and controversy were also part. Hence, proposed or actual changes in the amount of time devoted by professors at Padua to public lectures on portions of the *Canon*, of which there were several between 1579 and 1602, were not, in the main, introduced because of controversies over the wisdom of teaching from Ibn Sīnā's work. Instead, the principal issues had to do with the need for coverage of particular kinds of medical subject matter, the proper balance between *theoria* and *practica* and between public and private instruction, scheduling problems, university finances, conflicts between the interests of the various groups affected—professors and the Paduan College of Philosophers and Physicians, students, the university, the Riformatori dello Studio and the Venetian Senate—and competition for jobs between individuals. Nonetheless, these episodes were revealing of the current situation in which the *Canon* was taught.[35]

In 1591 a Dogal decree was issued which re-started a course on Canon 3, stating that "the experience has shown a chair in the Third Book of Ibn Sīnā's Canon is very beneficial and necessary" and thus emphasizing the excellence of the scientific knowledge it contains. In In 1598 came the appointment of a second lecturer on Canon 3. Andrighetto Andrighetti, who gave a lecture on the *Canon*, taught on special subjects relying on certain sections of the *Canon* during the first decade of the seventeenth century, which included skin diseases and eye diseases. To the place of Ibn Sīnā in the curriculum, there was proposed a more significant change in 1600 that went far beyond a restoration of brief courses on Canon 3. That year, Orazio Augenio who was Paterno's successor as the first ordinary professor of "theory" petitioned the Riformatori for

34 Siraisi, Avicenna in Renaissance, 106–8.

35 Siraisi, ibid, 110.

the reinstitution of public lectures on Canon 1.2. According to Augenio, the omission of Canon 1.2 was even more serious than those of Canon 1.3 and 1.4 which were similarly stipulated by the university statutes. Canon 1.3 (which concerned dietary regimes) could be neglected up to a point and the lectures on the Book 3 of the *Ars* covered basically the same material as Canon 1.4. But Canon 1.2 covered much more central and serious topics, the neglect of which was certain to be leave a big gap in medical teaching.[36]

Explicit support for the *Canon* was avowed only by Augenio himself and Annibale Bimbiolo, although Vigonza noted his acceptance of it as a text for use by *theorici*. Augenio's conviction that *Canon 1.2* was a useful textbook treating essential subject matter was not part of any general campaign to enlarge the study of Ibn Sīnā; as we have seen, he found no fault with the practice of passing over other sections of Book 1. However, Bimbiolo, by now first extraordinary professor of *theoria*, submitted an elaborate scheme for interweaving the study of works of Galen and Hippocrates pertaining to diseases, symptoms, pulse and urines with that of portions of the *Canon*, all within the space of three years. The teaching of *Canon* 1 was to be expanded in the first year, that of *Canon* 4 in the third, and *Canon* 5 (compound medicines) was to be introduced in the second. Therefore, Bimbiolo claimed that the entire theoretical and practical medicine explained in in all five books of the *Canon* would be discussed in the *studio* each year. The chair established for Negro, which combined lectures on *Canon* 1.2 with clinical instruction and demonstration in a hospital, lasted only until his death in 1626. Thereafter the lectures on causes and symptoms of diseases were quietly reabsorbed into the regular curriculum, and the hospital instruction on pulse and urine continued separately. The episode of the institution of this chair, like that of the restoration of the lectures on *Canon* 3, testifies primarily to the importance attached to expanding the public curriculum in *practica*.[37]

## After 1620's Teaching the Canon at Padua and Bologna

As the problems Malpighi had with his colleagues in Bologna attest, in seventeenth century there was a powerful resistance against all forms of intellectual change in schools of medicine.[38] What is more, traditionalism was

---

36 Siraisi, ibid, 113.

37 Siraisi, ibid, 118–9.

38 Howard B. Adelmann, *Marcello Malpighi and the Evolution /Embryology (Ithaca, 1966), vol 1, pt 1, "The Life and Works of Marcello Malpighi " Ibid., 1:128–34.*

reinforced thanks to increasing provincialism that left Northern Italian universities behind. Despite the presence of certain advanced scientific circles in the academic medical environment, the overall picture in Bologna and Padua, like elsewhere, suggested a decline in the number of registered students and in the ability to attract foreign students. Leiden's rise as an international center of medical education played a role at the second stage.

Although the courses in the curriculum were generally seen as a formality, in 1640s a professor in Bologna could propose to elucidate the first three doctrines of Canon 1.1 or sometimes skip all. Conditions such as these did provide much excuse for the sluggard as much as the modernist not to spend time for teaching on or listening to lectures about classical books. But some instructors conscientiously persisted on covering the Canon as part of the list of course subjects proposed by the faculty members at Bologna in 1640s and courses taught by Girolamo Santa Sofia at Padua in 1651.[39]

These courses would undoubtedly have been an invigorating intellectual experience, but without much use to a student whose aim was just to get a passing grade on Canon 1.1. G. B. Morgagni, who was a more prominent figure in the world of medicine, decided on the following less than radical solution when invited to Padua to give a public lecture on Canon 1.1 early in his career. At first glance, Morgagni put more emphasis on physiology than Bacchetto and less than on general science. He offered his students a superficial explanation of modern ideas and only mentioned Ibn Sīnā as a historically significant figure.

At Padua, lectures on *Canon 1.1* and on the other books in *theoria* finally gave way to other newly designated courses in the fields of physiology and pathology in 1767. Lectures on *Canon* 1.1 and 1.4 were finally abandoned at Bologna in 1716 (only to be replaced by lectures on Galen's *Methodus medendi*). One can only conclude that Morgagni took for granted that the traditional titles of the chairs had really become simply a designation of subject matter, and a memorial

39 fol 448, lectures on *Canon* 1.1–3 to be given for whole of 19 December 1646, by Franciscus Caelius, fol 450, *explications* of *Canon* 1.4 to be given by Franciscus Caelius for the whole of *20* December *1642* (twenty-six headings), fol 454, Franciscus Caelius on *Canon* 1.4 for the whole of 23 June 1643 (thirty-four headings) Professors were obliged to submit schedules of their forthcoming lectures to the Assunteria, the regulatory magistracy established to oversee the universities, in an effort to oblige them to fulfill their statutory obligations; Giorgio Cencetti, Gli archivi *dello Studio Bolognese* (Bologna, 1938), p 93.

to a text of historical importance. The plea was successful, and *Canon* 1.1 continued to find a nominal place in the official curriculum at Bologna until 1800.

## Ibn Sīnā: Physician and Philosopher

Although Ibn Sīnā made a sharp distinction between the two roles, he was both a physician and a philosopher. Over and over again, he warned the readers of Fen I that the physician should not himself study the natural sciences and instead ought to accept the results provided by the experts in the field. At the same time, the knowledge and ideas derived from philosophy in general and Aristotle's thought in particular actually play a considerable role *in? I.* According to the version attributed to Gerard, Ibn Sīnā informed his readers of the acceptance of the brain as a principle. In certain passages of Doctrina 6 on virtues, Ibn Sīnā returned extensively to the matter of the differences between Aristotle's and Galen's physiologies, and explained that the animal and natural powers were connected, respectively, to the heart, brain, and liver. In one of these passages, while stating that the Aristotelian perspective is correct, he inquired to Medicus whether a particular organ is responsible for any given faculty and whether, as it did not make a difference for purposes of medical treatment, it was his duty to investigate the issue due to his title as a physician.

Ibn Sīnā was not the first or oldest among the writers in the Arabic language who set out with the purpose of making a schematic outline of Greco-Arabic medicine structured around the division of theory and practice. The compilation of brief medical arguments attributed to Joannitius and known as Isagoge, begins with the claim that medicine is divided into theoretical and practical branches, and proceeds to evaluate the natural things, unnatural things, and things against nature (i.e. diseases).

A portion of Ibn Sīnā's materials were shown to have been derived from Rhazes (d. 925) medical encyclopedia. Another forerunner of and possible source of inspiration for the *Canon* was the medical study written by Haly Abbas (d. 994). When compared to these other studies, the *Canon* is more extensive than the much abbreviated Isagoge and offers an intellectually more demanding explanation, and its organization is easier to understand than Rhazes' works. Haly Abbas' study is fully comparable to the *Canon* in terms of scope, complexity and structure. It is divided into ten theoretical and ten practical books. The contents of the first four books on theory are roughly parallel to Canon I.1.

What gave Canon 1.1 its distinctive role was precisely Ibn Sina's philosophical inferences. As in Ibn Sina's philosophical writings, elements originating from a multiple of sources were brought together. Indeed, Ibn Sīnā's well-known readiness to incorporate both Aristotelian and Neoplatonic ingredients to his own philosophical system, seems to have aroused interest in its relationship to Galenic thought that also includes both Aristotelian and Platonic elements.[40]

Such, in barest outline, was the *Canon* as translated by Gerard of Cremona or his associates. The scope and organization of the work, the mass of practical information it contained, the author's summaries of Galenic thought (though sometimes inadequate in detail), and the philosophical context in which Ibn Sīnā succeeded in placing medicine while preserving its independence as a distinct science—all initially secured for the *Canon* a place of honor in medieval western European medicine. Medical works of Arabic origin reached the West through two main channels, namely the translations of Constantinus Africanus of Monte Cassino, and those of the Toledan school of the twelfth century. Of these, only the Constantinian translations penetrated the Salernitan schools in the period in which Salerno was still at its height as a center of medical culture. Hence, the Salernitan teaching of the twelfth and early thirteenth centuries, as reflected, for example, in the collections of Salernitan questions edited by Brian Lawn, shows almost no identifiable use of Ibn Sīnā. The introduction of the *Canon* instead took place as part of the general dissemination of the corpus of scientific and philosophical works translated by the Toledo school. Toledo appears not to have been especially famed as a center of medical learning, but the medical component in the body of scientific texts translated there is considerable.[41]

Although some of his knowledge of Ibn Sīnā's anatomy and physiology may have come via Ibn Sīnā's compendium *De animalibus*, in addition to, or instead of, the *Canon*, Albertus' use of Ibn Sīnā's pharmacology shows that he was definitely familiar with Book 2 of the latter work. Another friar who probably drew on the *Canon* at a relatively early date (although here, too, the simultaneous or alternative use of Ibn Sīnā's *De animalibus* is a possibility) was the Franciscan encyclopedist Bartholomaeus Anglicus; his *De proprietatibus rerum*, probably composed in Paris between 1230 and 1250, contains several citations of Ibn Sīnā in Book 4 on the human body. And around 1250, the canon of Amiens and physician and surgeon Richard de Fournival listed all five books of the *Canon*

40 Philip De Lacey, "Galen's Platonism," American Journal of Philology 93 (1972), 27–39.

41 Heinrich Schipperges, Die Assimilation der arabischen Medizin durch das lateinische Mittelalter. Sudhoffs Archiv für Geschichte der Medizin und der Naturwissenschaften, Beiheft 3 (Wiesbaden, 1964).

in the section of his library devoted to "lucrative sciences," that is, medicine and law. And the *Canon* continued to be used in contexts other than the developing university medical faculties. Thus, it was drawn on by Vincent of Beauvais in the thirteenth century and Henry of Langenstein in the fourteenth.[42]

Furthermore, the presence of the *Canon* in monastic libraries presumably attests to its usefulness both as a general work of reference and for the infirmarian. St. Augustine's Abbey possessed five volumes of parts of the *Canon*, some of which seem to have been acquired in the late thirteenth or early fourteenth century. Taddeo Alderotti himself willed his four-volume copy of the *Canon* to the Franciscan friars of Bologna.[43]

It seems likely that parts of the work (for example, Book 2 on simple medicines, and Book 4, Part 1, on fevers) may have been used as manuals of practice by literate *medici* who were not university graduates. Some of the Latin collections of excerpts, maxims, or *flores* from the *Canon*, which apparently began to be compiled before the end of the thirteenth century, may also have been used outside the schools. Other traces of an influence of the *Canon* outside the universities may be seen in citations of Ibn Sīnā in vernacular medical treatises as well as in the existence of vernacular medical compendia purportedly based on Ibn Sīnā's work. For example, a French treatise of which at least two copies survive (both in Italian libraries) claims to be "*Avicen en romance*." It is a little work on regimen that urges on the reader self- help and self-medication. Hence, the *Canon* was studied alongside, not instead of, translations of Greek medical texts; at both Bologna and Montpellier, for example, in the years around 1300 leading medical masters expounded a rather substantial corpus of Galen's treatises. The high reputation achieved by the author of the *Canon* in the university milieu was doubtless chiefly owing to the suitability of various parts of his work as textbooks for teaching different branches of the medical curriculum, although Ibn Sīnā's status as a philosopher and the attention he gave to differences between Aristotle and Galen must also have served to enhance the value of the *Canon* in the eyes of physicians in the thirteenth-century university environment.

42 Nicholas H. Steneck, Science and Creation in the Middle Ages, Henry of Langenstein (d 1397) on Genesis (Notre Dame and London, 1976), p 144.

43 Mauro Sarti and Mauro Fattorini. De claris Arcchigymnasii Bononiensis professoribus a saeculo XI usque ad saeculum XIV, ed Carlo Albicini and Carlo Malagola, 2 vols. (Bologna, 1888–96), 2 227.

On the basis of manuscript evidence, Danielle Jacquart has established that the study of the *Canon* began at Paris between about 1230 and 1258. The most prominent northern French medical author of the second half of the thirteenth century, Jean de St. Amand (d. before 1307), who may have taught at Paris and whose works were no doubt known there, drew heavily upon the *Canon* for his *Areolae*, a pharmacological compendium. In addition, one of the earliest commentaries on *Canon* 4.1 (fevers) is attributed to this author.[44]

## Latin Biography of Ibn Sīnā

The history of the Latin biography of Ibn Sīnā is a subject that has yet to be fully studied. Prior to the sixteenth century, very little information about his life from Arabic sources appears to have been available in the Latin West. Moreover, several stories circulated that could have no counterpart in the authentic Arabic biographies of Ibn Sīnā. Three different biographies of Ibn Sīnā appear in the various sixteenth-century Latin editions of the *Canon*, biographical information is also contained in a brief note by Andrea Alpago included in the 1527 and various subsequent editions. The short life included in the Venice edition, the 1507 edition, and other early editions may possibly be based on an Arabic source, but contains little specific information other than medical detail about the cause of Ibn Sīnā's death.

However, more extensive as well as authentic information was provided in the well-known life of Ibn Sīnā by Nicoló Massa, which was printed for the first time in Paolo Alpago's second edition of the *Canon* (Venice, 1544). This life was actually a free Latin rendering of the biography written by Ibn Sīnā's pupil Abu Ubayd al-Juzjani, whose name was Latinized as Sorsanus. Massa's work made available for the first time in the West a reasonably full account of Ibn Sīnā from a contemporary Arabic source. A few more items of information about Ibn Sīnā were subsequently added by Plemp, who could draw upon a much wider body of learning about Muslim history and culture than was available to any of the sixteenth-century Italian scholars who worked on the Latin editions of the *Canon:* in the life of Ibn Sīnā prefaced to his own edition of the *Canon*,[45]

---

44 Danielle Jacquart, "La réception du Canon d'Avicenne: Comparaison entre Montpellier et Paris au XIII' et XIV' siècles," Actes du ito Congrès national des sociétés savantes, Montpellier, 1984, section d'histoire des sciences et des techniques II. Histoire de l'école médicale de Montpellier (Paris, 1985), pp. 69–77.

45 The Arabic life in question is edited and translated into English in The Life of lbn Sīnā, ed. and tr. Gohlman Bibliotheca universalis, sive catalogus scriptorum

Plemp announced that his intention was merely to supplement Massa's version of Soranus' biography. This he did by supplying a precise calculation of Ibn Sīnā's dates based on an understanding of the relationship between Muslim and Christian calendars, providing references to later Arabic accounts of Ibn Sina.

## Adoption of Ibn Sina by Christian Saints

At Montpellier, the study of the *Canon* in the medical schools seems to have begun in the middle of the thirteenth century. It has been demonstrated that the first medical author at Montpellier to make extensive use of the work was Cardinalis, who was already a master in the faculty of medicine in 1240 and who died about 1293. Ibn Sīnā is among the authors prescribed for study in the papal bull of 1309 establishing a medical curriculum for Montpellier, but the portions of the *Canon* are not specified, and the substitution of other works is expressly permitted.

Benedetto Rinio called not only upon classical tradition and the modern work of Alpago, but also upon medieval sources in defending Ibn Sīnā. He noted that Ibn Sina's merits as a philosopher had earned the approval of Albertus Magnus, Thomas Aquinas, and Duns Scotus, "*lights of the whole world.*" Moreover, he pointed out that the long tradition of lecturing on the *Canon* in the Italian medical schools had produced the commentaries of "*the great speculator Gentile, the clear expositor Giacomo, and the subtle disputant Dino.*"[46] In the following decade, Costeo and Mongio echoed some of the same themes. They, too, deplored the prevalence of scorn for the Muslims, while pointing out that no one had yet produced a work that surpassed the *Canon* in organization, comprehensiveness, generally accurate presentation of Greek medicine, and range of medicaments. They took the war into the enemy's camp with the assertion that the Muslims were disliked by those who had entered medicine without any study of the dialectic and philosophy and were therefore incapable of appreciating the weighty and recondite statements of Arab authors (by contrast "the Greeks, indeed, with their suavity in words and copious effusion of speech are not difficult to understand"). And in Costeo's preface to Book 4 the argument culminates in a diatribe against the "Galenici," who act "*as if it were a sin to add anything to Galen's writings or as if it were a virtue to know nothing he did not know.*" This, he said, was certainly quite unlike the behavior of any

---

locupletissimus, in tribus linguis, Latina, Graeca, et Hebraica, authore Conrado Gesnero (Zurich, 1545), 1 i ior-i r.

46 Siraisi, Avicenna in, p.168.

men of real distinction in any branch of science, and certainly unlike Galen and Aristotle, who had never hesitated to criticize their predecessors.[47]

Paolino, like Costeo and unlike Rinio and Graziolo, acknowledged that there were contemporaries and also an earlier generation of medical teachers that discouraged their students from studying the *Canon*. Paolino presents a fairly balanced historical perspective how hostility to Ibn Sīnā and the Canon began among the medical humanists. Not able to dismiss earlier critics of Ibn Sīnā, Paolino asserted that these critics did not base their opinions on a close study of the Canon and were instead participating in a polemic regarding a new medical sect that had arisen in their own time. This Galenic sect aimed to unite sound medical teaching with elegance of expression. The Galenic faction stigmatized those who valued the substance of learning alone and were suspicious of rhetorical embellishments as "Ibn Sīnās" or "barbarous" within the context of the division in the medical community. Paolino believed the quarrel was more about translators than about medical content: since Arabic was linguistically much more distant from Latin than Greek, it was scarcely surprising that translators from Arabic had committed "barbarisms" in Latin. In Paolino's view, Ibn Sīnā's critics should have learned Arabic and translated him in good Latin style, instead of casting slurs on a great writer.

## Ibn Sīnā's Canon in the Renaissance

For the Latin Middle Ages and the Renaissance, Ibn Sīnā was of course a leading authority on psychology, although his reputation in this field was chiefly based on his *De anima* rather than the *Canon*.[48] Nonetheless, in the latter work, too, he weighed the validity of such classifications of brain function as *sensus communis, phantasia,* as well as imaginative, cogitative, estimative, and rational powers (the last of these being associated with the rational soul and reserved for humankind alone). *Fen* 1 finally concludes with a chapter in which it is pointed out that many of the body's actual operations require the cooperation of both natural and animal powers.

Ibn Sīnā's Canon played a unique role in the Renaissance era as a topic that attracted the attention of scientists working during the earliest stages of Arabic

47 Siraisi, ibid.

48 Ibn Sīnā's psychology is contained principally in his De anima, also known in Latin as Sextus de naturalibus; see Ibn Sina Latinus. Liber De anima seu Sextus de naturalibus l-ll- III, ed. Simone Van Riet, with introduction by G. Verbeke (Louvain and Leiden, 1972)].

and Eastern studies in the West. The *Canon* continued to be taught and studied in Latin, with somewhat more careful attention paid to revised and partly re-translated versions of the Latin text. In this way, a revised version of a twelfth-century Latin translation of the *Canon* produced by the Padua-educated doctor Andrea Alpago (d. 1522), thanks to his knowledge of Arabic, was widely disseminated and published in Padua. It is doubtful whether some of the Italian scientists who were involved in the later annotated editions of Alpago's text, which was accepted by the College of Philosophers and Physicians, had any knowledge of Arabic. As the *Canon* entered the medical curriculum at Padua and Bologna, the international dominance in medical education moved from Bologna to Padua to other northern institutions as well. For this reason, the history of the Canon assumed significance in the context of a regional medical culture with all its manifest novelty and creativity in the sixteenth and early seventeenth centuries, and its special ties to antiquity as well as to early and middle Renaissance periods.

## Renaissance Translators, Editors, and Commentators of the Canon

As pointed out before, there is still much to learn about the history of the Latin translations of the *Canon*. But it is especially necessary to study the version produced by Gerard of Cremona in the light of the original text. What is more, it seems that apart from Alpago's research, none of the other revisions or partial translations in the sixteenth century, be they in Arabic or Hebrew, have been subject to a detailed study from a textual point of view. But according to what has been previously recorded, it is clear that none of the editions of the *Canon* published in Italy in the sixteenth and early seventeenth centuries included a completely new translation made directly from the Arabic text. Alpago's work on the *Canon* contained a dictionary of technical terms and an explanatory note in addition to the corrections made in the Gerard of Cremona edition. Graziolo's version of Book I is different from that of Gerard, but was similarly not translated directly from the Arabic. Other than Ledesma's studies in Spain, the remaining partial translations published in the sixteenth century – the ones that belonged to Mantino and Cinqarbres in France – were carried out from Hebrew.

The Latin editions of the *Canon* in the sixteenth and seventeenth centuries, and Cremona's re-printing of certain parts of the translations of the Gerard translation, served teachers and students of medicine for generations. On their own, these editions have a lot to tell us about the medical education during the Renaissance and Ibn Sīnā's place in it. The emphasis on the errors of the twelfth century translator by both the detractors and defenders of Ibn Sīnā, fed the belief that a more satisfactory presentation of the text of the *Canon* would once again make Ibn Sīnā's contribution to medicine correctly assessed and appreciated.

In terms of content, the Latin editions of the *Canon* published after 1500 are divided into six categories:

1) The full text produced at the office of Gerard of Cremona before 1187, without comments or "modernization" of the text or instrument;
2) one or more of the books into which the *Canon* was divided, accompanied by the Latin commentary written between the thirteenth and fifteenth centuries;
3) all or most of the *Canon* containing the textual revisions and apparatus contributed to by fifteenth and sixteenth century medical scientists;
4) one or more of the short sections of the work used as a university textbook, comprising stand-alone texts or collections of short pieces like *articella*;
5) compendia or collection of maxims based on the *Canon*;
6) and lastly, re-translations of sections of the work.

These publications can generally be divided into three chronological groups, each marked by the variations in the types of content just mentioned. At the same time, the delineation of these three groups must not be allowed to conceal the extent of the overlaps or continuities between them. Aside from one exception, the first group comprising twenty two editions printed between 1500 and 1525, essentially continue the approaches and presentations originating from the Northern Italian schools as well as Montpellier, Paris and other main Western university centers from thirteenth to fifteenth centuries. Among the twenty nine Latin editions published between 1526 and 1608, an effort to revise the text or its presentation comes to the forefront. Most of the later productions can once again be related to education in Northern Italian universities. Furthermore, this group, which includes the editions that make up the main subject of the present discussion, chronologically coincides with an active phase in the Italian schools of production and publication of commentary on the *Canon*.

Finally, a small group consisting of nine editions was published between 1609 and 1674. These contained the efforts of Northern European Arabists to supply an improved Latin text of the *Canon*, more comprehensive in certain respects than the previous efforts.

No further volumes of Plemp's edition and translation appeared after that, but in the following year, 1659, Pierre Vattier, the physician to the duke of Orleans and the author of treatises and translations, some of them in French, on various aspects of the Middle Eastern or Muslim culture, published in Paris a Latin translation of some excerpts from *Canon* 3.1 having to do with mental disease.[49] Finally, in Augsburg in 1674, Welsch, a practicing physician who had studied at Padua, published his edition and translation of two chapters of *Canon* 4.3 on parasites.[50]

Kirsten, Plemp, Vattier, and Welsch, presented their work as being part of a larger project, but none seems to have produced any more work on the Canon. Certainly, their efforts had little impact upon the practice of lecturing on the Canon in the medical faculties of the Italian universities. Only Plemp chose to translate parts of the Canon still prescribed as textbooks, and as G. B. Morgagni said that Plemp's translation was not better than that of Gerard of Cremona in the Italian schools.

Whether or not Plemp was right that some people in his day thought there had actually been two Ibn Sīnās, in a metaphorical sense, the Renaissance Ibn Sīnās was certainly a split personality. One was the author of systematic summaries of Galenic teaching used as textbooks for formal university instruction. It is now possible to have a fairly good idea of the way his work was used in courses on *theoria* and *practica*. The other Ibn Sīnās was the compiler of remedies and *materia medica*, and a much more elusive character. Pharmacology was an area in which Renaissance physicians often acknowledged that the Muslims had added to the knowledge produced by the Greeks. Trust in *Canon 2* and 5 seems to have been widespread among working physicians; it certainly extended well beyond the Iberian and Italian academic circles in which the "academic" Ibn Sīnās found his chief Renaissance home. Expressions of praise for Ibn Sīnās's usefulness for the practitioner almost all relate to his *materia medica*. Moreover, Ibn Sīnās's reputation in this regard seems to have survived a number of specific criticisms of misleading or incomprehensible items in his pharmacology. Yet both the pharmacological and the linguistic capabilities of the sixteenth century must surely have limited the actual usefulness of *Canon*

49 Moritz Steinschneider, Die europäischen Übersetzungen aus dem Arabischen bis Mitte des 17. Jahrhunderts, Sitzungsberichten der Kais Akademie der Wissenschaften in Wien, Philosophisch-Historische Klasse, 149 (Vienna, 1904), p. 79, no. 117.

50 Welsch (1624–77) was the author of a number of other medical works, all of which appear from their titles to be on practical aspects of medicine; see Biogr Lex., 6:236–37.

*2* and *5*. Among the many remaining ambiguities about the place of Ibn Sīnā in the larger picture of Renaissance medicine is that of the extent to which his pharmacology found any real use or understanding.[51]

In the broader context of Renaissance learning, the *Canon* provides instructive examples of techniques of text editing, of the extent and limitations of language studies, of the impact of printing on a scientific discipline, and of the development and varieties of commentary. Ironically, the history of the Arabo-Latin *Canon* provides powerful confirmation of the central importance of Greek studies in sixteenth-century learning. As far as attempts to purify the Latin text of the *Canon* were concerned, Greek medicine played a more important role than Arabic or Hebrew linguistic studies. The Renaissance editors of the work learned their trade in the school of Greek medical humanism. To the degree that their enterprise involved an attempt to demonstrate Ibn Sina's dependence on Galen, it was directly parasitical upon Renaissance Galenism, which provided the tools in the shape of the Renaissance editions of Galen and their apparatus.

## The Canon and Boerhaave's Studies

Da Monte's endeavor to use *Canon* 1 as a unified introductory medical textbook may be related to the revival of the ancient five-fold division of medicine into physiology, pathology, semiotics, hygiene, and therapy. This scheme (which does, in fact, outline the content of *Canon* 1) was available through various texts translated into Latin during the Middle Ages, but apparently seldom used by fourteenth- and fifteenth- century scholastic physicians, who preferred the division into *theoria* and *practica*. The replacement of the division into *theoria* and *practica* by the fivefold scheme and of teaching by commentary through direct exposition of the subject led ultimately to the production of textbooks of the variety known as "the institutes of medicine," of which Boerhaave's is the best known. Perhaps Da Monte's set of commentaries may be regarded as representing a very early stage in this process.

Herman Boerhaave's *Institutiones mediate* (Leiden, 1707), is divided into sections on physiology, pathology, symptomology, hygiene, and therapy. According to G. A. Lindeboom, Boerhaave explained the phrase "*institutiones medicae*" to mean "*the general aspects of theoretical medicine as well as the general precepts of practical medicine. On the basis of physiology the Institutes give*

51 Siraisi, Avicenna in, p.356.

*general points of view on pathology, symptomology and therapy, which are to apply later to individual cases. So the term theoretical medicine, sometimes used for the Institutes, is less exact. Apparently, the Institutes consisted of a course that formed an introduction to clinical medicine.*"[52] There is little doubt that Da Monte thought of his commentaries on *Canon I* as a set. He lectured on *Canon 1.2* immediately after *Canon 1.1.* He had already expounded *Canon 1.2*, when he wrote on *Canon 1.4.*

At Padua, however, Da Monte's approach to the problem of unifying medical teaching left no lasting impression on the curriculum. Later commentators explicitly stated, as Da Monte had not, that *Canon* I as a whole encompassed the five parts of medicine, but *Canon* 1.1 alone continued to be the subject of lectures on Ibn Sīnā in the course on *theoria. Canon* 1.2 again fell into disuse after Da Monte's death, although, it was briefly reintroduced early in the next century. By the time the traditional statutory division between *theoria and practica* was finally abandoned at Padua in the 1760s, the age in which *Canon* 1 could be perceived as a viable textbook was long over.

## Use of Canon in Medical Education at European Universities after Sixteenth Century

In northern Europe, not only did the *Canon* retain at least a formal place in many university curricula, but statutes or directives specifically mandating its continued use were issued: for example, at Jena in 1591 (where *Canon* 1.1 and 4.1 were to be read alongside a range of Hippocratic and Galenic texts), in Wurzburg in 1610, in Ingolstadt in 1611, and at Louvain in 1617.[53] Furthermore, although few actual sets of lectures based on the *Canon* written after 1520 in universities north of the Alps appear to have survived, evidence of continued use of Ibn Sīnā by physicians is easy to find.

The University of Paris had the largest medical faculty in the sixteenth-century Europe. One might suppose that, despite the survival of highly traditional curricular arrangements until the French Revolution,[54] the *Canon*

52 Herman Boerhaave The Man and His Work (London, [1968]), p 58.

53 Heinz Goerke, "Die medizinische Fakultät von 1472 bis zur Gegenwart " in Ludwig-Maximilians Universitat in ihren Fakultäten (Berlin, 1972), 1 191 (re Ingoldstadt); Ernst Giese and Benno von Hagen, Geschichte der medizinischen Fakultat der Friedrich-Schiller- Universitat Jena (Jena, 1958), pp. 17–20.

54 Charles Coury, "The Teaching of Medicine in France from the Beginning of the Seventeenth Century," in The History of Medical Education, ed C. D O'Malley (UCLA Forum in Medical Sciences, no. 12, Los Angeles, 1970), pp. 121–72.

would be effectively ignored by the sixteenth-century Parisian Hippocratics and Galenists. This was probably the case as far as the use of portions of the *Canon* as textbooks for the systematic presentation of Galenic medicine was concerned.

Lyon was another major center of medical learning and activity in sixteenth-century France; there, the absence of a university was perhaps more than compensated for by the surgical education available at the Hôtel-Dieu, and the presence of an active college of physicians, and a flourishing medical publishing industry. In Lyon, Jacques Dalechamps produced his important work *Chirurgie Françoise,* a translation of Book 6 of Paulus Aegineta's work, accompanied by his own commentary. And writing the latter he drew frequently upon Abulcasis, and occasionally upon Ibn Sīnā; furthermore, he drew attention to his use of these authors on his title page. As soon as one begins to look closely, one sees many signs that the *Canon* was still read and used, and to some extent still openly acknowledged and appreciated.

Lange, like many other sixteenth-century German physicians, had been trained and had his professional and scientific ideas formed in Italy.[55] And in Italy, Ibn Sīnā continued to play a prominent role in the curriculum of the most celebrated schools. Moreover, in the Low Countries and the German lands, manifestations of interest in the *Canon* continued well after 1600. In the seventeenth century, this interest took the form of several attempts, to retranslate the text directly from the Arabic.

Doubtless many more examples could be added to the enduring use of Ibn Sīnā in northern Europe in the first half of the sixteenth century. The use of Ibn Sīnā is unlikely to have been less, and may in fact have been more, widespread in the years around 1600. The overall impression left by various scattered references to Ibn Sīnā by northern medical authors, and from the way some of them used his work, is that the *Canon* was valued chiefly as a reference work for the practicing physician, and for its pharmacological and therapeutic recommendations. For a much more active tradition of university teaching based on the *Canon* after about the 1520's, one must turn to southern Europe, that is, to the Iberian peninsula and to Italy. From these regions, too, there are expressions of appreciation for the *Canon* considered as a storehouse of Islamic *materia medica,* or a handy guide to treatment. The *Canon* as a text on which to base university lectures on medicine were regarded in the sixteenth and seventeenth centuries highly enough to give rise to numerous Latin editions for the use of

55 Nutton, "Humanist Surgery," pp. 92–93.

professors and students and to engender the continued production of new lectures and commentaries especially on specific parts of Ibn Sīnā's work.

The major Italian centers of medical education, and particularly the University of Padua, attracted large numbers of foreign students (especially Germans), as a result of which the influence of the form of medical education offered at Padua was very widely felt.[56] At the same time, the output from Italy of editions of the *Canon* and of new commentaries on it was a good deal larger than that produced in all the rest of Europe put together. Hence, the Italian schools offer both the largest body of material for a study of the influence of the *Canon* on the Renaissance and early modern medical education, and of the most striking examples of the interaction in the medical ideas of the period of humanist Galenism, scientific innovation, Aristotelian and eclectic natural philosophy, and Galenism in its medieval Arabo-Latin form.

In Pisa, the only lectures on *Canon 1.1* appear to have been given by poorly paid *extraordinarii* in the early stages of their generally undistinguished teaching careers that seldom produced of written works of any kind. Hence it comes as no surprise to learn that apparently the only surviving commentary on *Canon* 1.1 by a professor at Pisa is a highly abbreviated and wholly unoriginal exposition. This was written, probably early in his career, by Giuseppe della Papa (1649–1735), who achieved modest success later in life as a grand-ducal physician and the author of a few minor medical works.[57] For other portions of the *Canon* we seem to have no commentaries from Pisa, unless Argenterio's own work on fevers is to be considered as one.

The concentration at Padua, Pavia, and Bologna—the three major Italian universities of the period—of the active pursuit, and indeed renewal, of the practice of writing commentaries on the *Canon* in the sixteenth and early seventeenth centuries was clearly not due to any more vitality in those institutions as a whole. However, local conditions that fostered special attention to the *Canon* at Padua certainly existed. Attention has, for example, been drawn to manifestations of interest in Ibn Sīnā as a philosopher in late fifteenth-century Paduan circles. In a more practical vein, it was of course the Venetian presence in the Middle East that made possible the textual work of Ramusio and Alpago, and the Venetian printing industry that disseminated Alpago's revised edition of the *Canon*.

---

56 Bylebyl, "School of Padua", p.335.

57 Venice, Biblioteca Marciana, MS lat VII.23 (3491) A brief notice of Del Papa's career is included in Nouvelle Biographie Générale (Paris, 1862), 29:155.

In Bologna in the late sixteenth and seventeenth centuries three ordinary professors and three or four extraordinary professors of *theoria* normally expounded *Canon 1.1* as part of a three-year cycle of texts; a similar number of professors of *practica* taught *Canon 1.4*, and apparently *Canon 4.1*, as two parts of a three-year cycle. At Padua, an essentially similar arrangement prevailed as regards *Canon 1.1* and *4.1*; *Canon 1.4* seems not to have formed a regular part of the Paduan curriculum in this period.

Nonetheless, among earlier teachers whose lectures do not survive, sets of lectures on the *Canon* from the sixteenth and early seventeenth centuries do not appear notably truncated or cursory. A full academic year's course was usually supposed to amount to about eighty or ninety lectures.[58] To take a few rather randomly chosen examples from manuscripts, Matteo Corti left 63 lectures on *Canon 1.1*; Girolamo Capodivacca 77 lectures on *Canon 4.1*; and Bernardino Paterno's lectures on *Canon 1.4* fill a volume of 277 leaves. Furthermore, while it was rather common for a lecturer not to get through the whole of *Canon* 1.1, the treatment of individual topics and the length of individual lectures were usually quite expansive. For example, Giambatista Da Monte's exposition of *Canon* 1.1 in the printed version amounts to about 80 percent of the length accorded to the same portion of the work by that extremely prolix scholastic Gentile da Foligno.[59] It seems fair to assume from these surviving examples that during the sixteenth century a significant number of the prescribed lectures on Ibn Sīnā at Padua, Bologna, and Pavia were actually delivered and were not pro forma treatments.

## Conclusion

*'Medicine is a science from which one learns the conditions of the human body with regard to health and the absence of health, the aim being to protect health when it exists and restore it when absent.'*[60]

58 Administrative reforms at the University of Siena m 1589 included the stipulation that each professor must give at least ninety lectures in the academic year; see Damlo Marrara, Lo studio di Siena nelle riforme del Granduca Herdmando I (1589 e 1591) (Milan, 1970), p. 22.

59 Based on a very rough estimate and comparison of the number of words in Da Monte, comm Canon 1.1 (Venice, 1557), and Gentile da Foligno, comm Canon 1 1 (Pavia, 1510—for this edition see Appendix 1).

60 Mona Nasser, Aida Tibi, Emilie Savage-Smith. Ibn Sina's Canon of Medicine: 11th century rules for assessing the effects of drugs. J R Soc Med 2009;102:78–80. DOI 10.1258/jrsm.2008.08k040

After this famous opening sentence, Ibn Sīnā continues:

*'Someone might say to us that medicine is divided into theoretical and practical parts and that, by calling it a science, we have considered it as being all theoretical. To this we respond by saying that some arts and philosophy have theoretical and practical parts, and medicine, too, has its theoretical and practical parts. The division into theoretical and practical parts differs from case to case, but we need not discuss these divisions in disciplines other than medicine. If it is said that some parts of medicine are theoretical and other parts are practical, this does not mean that one part teaches medicine and the other puts it into practice – as many researchers in this subject believe. One should be aware that the intention is something else: it is that both parts of medicine are science, but one part is the science dealing with the principles of medicine, and the other with how to put those principles into practice.'*[61]

Ibn Sīnā begins the second book (on simple drugs, or *materia medica*) with a discussion on the nature and quality of drugs (they were each assigned a pair of qualities, cold or warm, dry or moist), and the way that mixing them influences their effectiveness. The second chapter (*maqalah*) of Book 2 is 'On knowledge of the potency of drugs through experimentation (*tajribah*)'. "*You can tell the potency of drugs in two ways, by analogy* (qiyas) *and by experiment* (tajribah). *We say experimenting leads to knowledge of the potency of a medicine with certainty after taking into consideration certain conditions.*"[62]

However, Ibn Sīnā's *Canon* was not greeted everywhere with praise. In Spain, for instance, when Abu al-Ala Zuhr (d. 1131) was presented with a copy, he so disliked it that he refused to put it in his library, preferring to cut off its margins for use in writing prescriptions for patients. He also composed a treatise criticizing the materia medica in the *Canon*. This hostile reaction on the part of the progenitor of a five-generation family of prominent Andalusian physicians raises the question of whether medicine in Islamic Spain developed with less dependence upon the ideas of Ibn Sina than it did elsewhere. Abu al-Ala Zuhr's son, Abu Marwan ibn Zuhr (Latin. Avenzoar), wrote several important works, including *The Easy Guide to Therapy and Dietetics*, translated into Latin as *Thaisir*, while his compatriot Ibn Rushd (Averroes; d. 1198) wrote the widely read *Book of General Principles* (*Kitab al-Kulliyat*), known in Europe as *Colliget* (the same name by which the first book of the *Canon* was known).[63]

---

61 Mona Nasser, ibid.

62 Mona Nasser, ibid.

63 Roger Arnaldez, "Ibn Zuhr," in Gibbs et al., Encyclopaedia of Islam, vol. 3, pp. 976–9. For the anecdote regarding the copy of the Canon, see A. Z. Iskandar, A Catalogue of Arabic Manuscripts.

Other criticism has been that the sheer size of Ibn Sīnā's chapters, reinforced by titles such as *The Canon*, gave them an aura of authority that was to prove stultifying rather than invigorating. Furthermore, the medical historian Michael McVaugh noted: "*however much [such treatises] might emphasize the importance of practical knowledge, or the nature of medicine as 'art', the effect of their very structure was to favor the logical element over the clinical.*"[64]

Physical subjects were closely related to medicine and were generally taught by men of medicine. Aristotelian philosophy of nature could be done in a way that provided the basis of medicine as a whole, but only after the solution of certain problems. The first of these concerned the fact that Ibn Sina made partial citations to these works of Aristotle; moreover, he was not always in agreement with the medical knowledge derived from Galen. The second was the fact that the greatest single authority in medical education fast became Ibn Sina and his *Canon*, which had to be reconciled with Aristotle and Galen.

When Ibn Sīnā examined the general principles of anatomy especially in the first book, he scattered the topographical details to the sections in the third book dealing with organic diseases. The commentator on anatomy was left to bring them together himself. Berengario adds that despite his citations to Rhazes, Ibn Sīnā was the first to be recognized in the West and that due to the lucidity of its content and design, the *Canon* had a wide reception.[65]

A significant portion of the techniques for constructing solid texts consisted of the forty-page anatomical "catalogue" given throughout the discussion and especially in the early sections of the study as well as the research on historical terminology included within the lexicon.

The remark by Berengario that the goal of correctly listing anatomical terms is to construct their meaning in accordance with the way in which they were historically used by past authors, cannot be much improved upon as a "humanist" program. The bulk of Berengario's philological research, however, was directed toward significant authors writing in Arabic.

In particular, the third book of the *Canon*, which presented a comprehensive medical perspective from anatomy to treatment, became the path followed by the men of medicine. This was exemplified by Gentile la Foligno who was

64 Michael McVaugh in Edward Grant, ed., A Source Book of Medieval Science (Cambridge, Mass.: Harvard University Press, 1974), p. 715 n. 1.

65 French, R.K. 1985. "Berengario da Carpi and the use of commentary in anatomical teaching." A. Wear, R.K. French and I.M. Lonie (eds.), The Medical Renaissance of the Sixteenth Century. New York: Cambridge University Press, pp. 223–245.

one of the old commentators Berengario quoted extensively. The first section of the commentary on the third book of the *Canon* is the common exercise concerning the wisdom and goodness on God. God the Creator is presented to us as *artifex istius mundi:* God the "practical craftsman". God's hand is never so evident as in the microcosm that is the human body and the special interest of the physician.[66]

According to Berengario, in order to understand the author's mind, the reader ought to make utmost effort ("ultimo conatu") to discover which author uses a particular term and what that term can mean in different contexts. Then, the terminology can be simplified in two ways. The first is having a good Latin word taken from an approved writer replace all its synonyms, for "tail fat" means "fatty" in a way that makes all its other synonyms redundant. The second is to avoid all barbarism and corruption in translation.[67]

After the mid-eleventh century, multiple copies of the *Canon* were made particularly to render the ideas more accessible; commentaries were written to clarify the contents and open diverging opinions to debate; and the number of theses on a single topic was multiplied.

When discussing anatomical knowledge and its acquisition, Berengario makes use of the tradition of commentary on the third book of the *Canon* involving anatomic material. Generally speaking, the *Canon* became the biggest single authority of the period covering the two centuries before Berengario. As in other fields, while Aristotle's works on logic and physics supplied the basic instruments for academic studies in medicine, the essence of the matter was provided by Ibn Sīnā's non-Aristotelian *Canon*.

Aristotelian natural science can principally extend to cover medicine and the rest of the natural phenomena. However, on the subject of medicine there was no Aristotelian study, and men of medicine gathered the essential elements of this discipline from elsewhere. This subject did not extend to other areas of the natural world and, as a consequence, the medical commentators of the *Canon* regarded medicine as a field with clearly delineated boundaries not to be crossed over in either direction.

The third book of the *Canon* was vocational and practical; it was the only text mentioned in the 1405 Bologna curriculum for practical courses. Gentile's commentary advances the theme of a skilled doctor who achieves medical virtuosity by covering and never straying from the path that extends from the

66 French, R.K. 1985 ibid.
67 French, R.K. 1985 ibid.

subject of practical anatomy to that of application of medication in equal degrees. Gentile's explanatory remarks refer to the training of the doctor with an emphasis on the fact that even though philosophers may possess satisfactory explanations for the causes of parts of the body or types of effect of medications, experience, like the one involving the form of a certain medication and its actions, is the only source of attaining knowledge.

The output of the editions of the *Canon* after 1608 reflects both the fact that works in Arabic came too late to make an impact on medical education and that old works in Latin were durable. These were a series of publications starting with the first print in 1522 and covering the entirety or a large portion of the *Canon*, and quite different in character from other translations of classics of medicine, reflecting the awareness about Ibn Sīnā's humanist criticism. The majority of the scientists involved in the production of this series of editions were interested in the *Canon* not directly but only as a means of transmission of Galenic medical education and Greco-Arabic pharmacology.

On the other hand, the Renaissance education based on the *Canon* was still a component of mainstream contemporary medicine. The editions and commentaries of Ibn Sīnā's work that are the products of the Renaissance era and at the fact that it was still being used at the beginning of the seventeenth century must be examined more closely.

## Bibliography

Adelmann H. B. (1966). Marcello Malpighi and the Evolution /Embryology (vol 1, pt 1). The Life and Works of Marcello Malpighi Ibid. Ithaca. 1, 128–34.

Arnaldez R. Ibn Zuhr, in Gibbs et al., Encyclopaedia of Islam, (vol. 3). 976–9.

Baader G. (1979). Medizinisches Reformdenken und Arabismus im Deutschland des 16. Jahrhunderts, Sudhoffs Archiv für Geschichte der Medizin mid der Naturwissenschaften. 63, 270.

Ballester L. G. (1979). The Circulation and Use of Medical Manuscripts in Arabic in Sixteenth-Century Spain. Journal for the History of Arabic Science. 3, 183–999.

Canon 1.1 (Venice, 1557), and Gentile da Foligno, comm Canon 1 1 (Pavia, 1510).

Beaujouan G., (1968). Fautes et obscurités dans les traductions médicales du Moyen Age (Revue de synthèse, 3rd series). 89, 143–52.

Biblioteca Marciana. (1862). MS lat VII.23 (3491) A brief notice of Del Papa's career is included in Nouvelle Biographie Générale. Venice. 29–155.

Boerhaave H. (1968). The Man and His Work. London. 58.

Cencetti G. (1938). Cli archwi dello Studio Bolognese. Bologna. 93.

Coury C. (1970). The Teaching of Medicine in France from the Beginning of the Seventeenth Century. The History of Medical Education. (Ed.) O'Malley C. D. (UCLA Forum in Medical Sciences, no. 12). Los Angeles. 121–72.

De Lacey P. (1972). Galen's Platonism. American Journal of Philology. 93, 27–39.

De Renzi S. (1852). Collectio Salernitana ossia Documenti mediti e trattati di medutna appartenenti alla scuola medica salernitana. Naples. 1, 360–62.

Dooley B. (1984). Science Teaching as a Career at Padua in the Early Eighteenth Century. The Case of Giovanni Polem. History of Universities. 4, 11–51.

French and Lonie I.M. (eds.). The Medical Renaissance of the Sixteenth Century. New York: Cambridge University Press. 223–245.

French, R.K. Wear A. (1985). Berengario da Carpi and the use of commentary in anatomical teaching. French, R.K. Wear A. Lonie I. M. (ed.). (1985). Berengario da Carpi and the use of commentary in anatomical teaching. The Medical Renaissance of the Sixteenth Century. New York: Cambridge University Press. 223–245.

Gesnero C. (1545). Bibliotheca universalis, sive catalogus scriptorum locupletissimus, in tribus linguis, Latina, Graeca, et Hebraica. Zurich, $110^r$-$111^r$.

Giese E. and Von Hagen B. (1958). Geschichte der medizinischen Fakultat der Friedrich-Schiller- Universitat. Jena. 17–20.

Goerke H. (1972). Die medizinische Fakultät von 1472 bis zur Gegenwart. Die Ludwig-Maximilians Universitat in ihren Fakultäten. Berlin. 1, 191.

Grafton A. (1981). Teacher, Text, and Pupil in the Renaissance Class-Room: A Case Study from a Parisian College. History of Universities. 1, 37– 70.

Gruner O. C. (1930). A Treatise on the Canon of Medicine of Ibn Sina. London: Luzac.

Gruner O. C. (1966). The General Principles of Ibn Sina's Canon of Medicine. (Translate: Shah M. H.). Karachi: Naveed Clinic.

Hameed H. A. (1971). Gerard's Latin Translation of Ibn Sīnā's Al-Qanun. Studies in Islam. 8, 1–7.

Ibn Sina Latinus. Liber De anima seu Sextus de naturalibus l-ll- III, ed. Simone Van Riet, with introduction by G. Verbeke. Louvain and Leiden, 1972.

Iskandar. Catalogue of Arabic Manuscripts on Medicine and Science in the Wellcome Historical Medical Library. 33–64.

Jacquart D, "La réception du Canon d'Avicenne: Comparaison entre Montpellier et Paris au XIII' et XIV' siècles," Actes du ito Congrès national des sociétés savantes, Montpellier, 1984, section d'histoire des sciences et des techniques II. Histoire de l'école médicale de Montpellier (Paris, 1985), pp. 69–77.

Jahier H. and Noureddine A. (1956). Avicenne, Poème de la medecine, Urguza fi 't-tibb, Cantica Ibn Sinae. Les Belles Lettres. Paris.

Jarcho S. (1970) Galen's Six Non-Naturals: A Bibliographic Note and Translation. Bulletin of the History of Medicine. 44, 370–77.

Lohr C. H. (1974). Renaissance Latin Aristotle Commentaries: Authors A-B. Studies in the Renaissance. 21, 228–89.

Mahdi M. et al. Ibn Sina, in Yarshater. Encyclopedia Iranica. (vol. 3). 66–110.

Marrara D. (1970). Lo studio di Siena nelle riforme del Granduca Herdmando I (1589 e 1591). Milan. 22.

McVaugh M. Grant, E. (ed.). (1974). A Source Book of Medieval Science. Cambridge, Mass.: Harvard University Press. 715, 1.

Nasser M, Tibi A, and Savage-Smith E (2009). Ibn Sina's Canon of Medicine: 11th century rules for assessing the effects of drugs. J R Soc. 102, 78–80. DOI 10.1258/jrsm.2008.08k040.

Richard Stapper, Papst Johannes XXI Eine Monographie (Münster, 1898), pp. 4–26.

Renaissance Commentaries on Ibn Sina's Canon. (Book 1). (1984). Part 1 and Teaching of Medical Theoria in the Italian Universities. History of Universities. 47–49.

Richler B. (1982). Manuscripts of Avicenna's Kanon in Hebrew Translation A Revised and Up-to-date List (Koroth 8). I45–I68.

Sarti M. and Fattorini M. (1988–96). De claris Archigymnasii Bononiensis professoribus a saeculo XI usque ad saeculum XIV. (Ed.) Albicini C. and Malagola C. (2 vols.). Bologna. 2, 227.

Savage-Smith E. Islamic Medical Manuscripts at the National Library of Medicine. Access Address http://www.nlm.nih.gov/hmd/arabic

Schipperges H. (1964). Die Assimilation der arabischen Medizin durch das lateinisch Mittelalter. Sudhoffs Archiv für Geschichte der Medizin und der Naturwissenschaften, Beiheft. Wiesbaden. 3.

Schlam C. C. (1978). Graduation Speeches of Gentile da Foligno. Mediaeval Studies, 40: 96–119.

Siraisi, Nancy G. (1987). Avicenna in Renaissance Italy - The Canon and Medical Teaching in Italian Universities after 1500. Princeton: Princeton University Press.

Siraisi, Nancy G. (1990). Medieval & Early Renaissance Medicine: An Introduction to Knowledge and Practice. Chicago: The University of Chicago Press.

Siraisi, Nancy G. (1981). Taddeo Alderotti and His Pupils: Two Generations of Italian Medical Learning. Princeton: Princeton University Press.

Steinschneider M. (1904). Die europäischen Übersetzungen aus dem Arabischen bis Mitte des 17. Jahrhunderts. Sitzungsberichten der Kais Akademie der Wissenschaften in Wien. (Philosophisch-Historische Klasse, 149). Vienna. 79, 117.

Steneck N. H. (1976). Science and Creation in the Middle Ages' Henry of Langenstein (d 1397) on Genesis. Notre Dame and London. 144.

Wear A. French R. K. and Lome I. M. (Ed.). (1985). Berengario da Carpi and the Use of Commentary in Anatomical Teaching. The Medical Renaissance of the Sixteenth Century. Cambridge. 42–74.

## Short Biography of Kadircan H. Keskinbora

He has studied medicine at Hacettepe University, Faculty of Medicine (Ankara/Turkey). He became an Ophthalmologist in 1987, an associate professor in 1999 and a professor in 2007. He concluded his second Ph.D. in "Deontology, History of Medicine and Medical Ethics" in 2006. He still is a professor at Istanbul Bahcesehir University, School of Medicine, Head of Dept. History of Medicine and Ethics. He is a member of various national and international scientific or non-governmental organizations. His Published Books:

**Ophthalmology:** Oftalmolojide Sorularla Eğitim (Education in Ophthalmology with Questions), Oftalmolojide Sınava Doğru (Towards Exam in Ophthalmology), Oftalmoloji İle Kesişen Bilim Dalları (Scientific Areas that Intersect with Ophthalmology)

**History of Medicine:** Göz Nurunun Anahtarı ve Sevinç Hazineleri (Key to Eye Light and Treasures of Joy), Esat Işık: Bilimde, Siyasette, Milli Mücadelede Bir Işık (Esat Isik: A Light in Science, in Politics, in National Struggle), Kanûn-u Sagir of Ibn Sina (The Little Canon of Avicenna), The Little Qanun of Ibn Sina (Peter Lang Publish.).

**Literature:** Düşünen Beyinlerin İnsanlığa Mirası: Özdeyişler (Inheritance of Thinking Minds to Humanity: Aphorisms), Yaban Gülü (Brier Rose - poem book), Mardin Düşünceleri (Thoughts on Mardin - poem book), Ben Suyum (I am water - poem book), İddia (Claim - poem book).

Because of his studies on Avicenna (Ibn Sina), he was awarded the **"International Avicenne Prize"** in Paris/France in 2016.

e-mail: kadircan.keskinbora@gmail.com
hidirkadircan.keskinbora@med.bau.edu.tr

Prof. Dr. Roida Rzayeva Oktay

# Ibn Sina and His Philosophical Legacy

Although philosophy has always been nourished by many sources, it has been significantly influenced by a particular culture, civilization or thinkers in this or that historical period. As a matter of fact, the influence of the Western or the Eastern thinkers on philosophical thought was felt more effectively from time to time. It is often noted that, unlike the philosophy of the West, the philosophy of the East focused on the problem of man, and considers the problem of man from the point of view of practice. At the same time, it should be noted that the natural philosophical, ontological, epistemological, logical foundations of this practical human being cover a huge layer of philosophical problems.

The interaction between Eastern and Western philosophies is a social historical phenomenon. Philosophically, the West has always attracted the attention of the East and the East has always attracted the attention of the West. Both constitute the future philosophical thought at the universal level as a whole (*Современная философия. Восточная философия*). Many world-famous philosophers grew up in the East and influenced the philosophical thought of both the Islamic world and Europe with their discovery and inventions. Therefore, we can say that the Islamic civilization has significantly influenced the course of history.

Although Islamic thinkers have contributed significantly to many areas of science (*Электронная библиотека по философии*, p. 252), it is known that the main influence lies in the field of ideas.

Most of the Greek philosophical and scientific legacy in the West was lost in the period between the collapse of the Roman Empire and the cultural Renaissance of the XIII-XIV centuries. However, many experts point out that in the "Dark Ages" Greek philosophy and science was transferred to another culture (*Электронная библиотека по философии*, p. 250). Although philosophy, science and art in medieval Europe went through a period of stagnation for a certain period of time, cultural development was observed in the East. Muslim thinkers have developed by preserving their own philosophy as well as Greek philosophical thought. Thus, thanks to the Islamic philosophy, Plato and Aristotle in Europe, as well as Neoplatonism, Stoics, Epicureans, Siseron and others started to be understood from different angles again. The philosophy of those mentioned above has begun to be considered historically (Бобоев, 2002).

It is often said that Western philosophy and science was "preserved" in Islamic culture. Some explanations and clear statements are needed here. As mentioned above, Islamic culture was not the passive guardian of Greek culture and science, but they developed the Hellenistic heritage creatively, actively embracing it. Thus, in the intellectual culture of most of the world, until the scientific revolution of the XVI-XVII centuries, the foundation of the new prevailing scientific tradition was laid (*Электронная библиотека по философии*, p. 250). The science of the Muslim East has given an impulse to the development of scientific thought in Western Europe.

In the Middle Ages there were three intellectual centers that were sufficiently independent from each other. But they were all based on ancient heritage. These were Byzantine, Latin monasteries and Islamic culture.

Hence, as historical experience shows, different civilizations have never been separate, the dialogue between civilizations has always continued. Ibn Sina assumed one of the most important tasks in this interaction process and contributed greatly to the universal culture.

In some sources: a) finding the full text of the Organon; b) many translations from Arabic to Latin, recognition of Al-Farabi and Ibn Sînâ are shown as two important cases between 1125 and 1150. (Ülken, 1967, p. 313).

The philosophical and scientific creativity of Ibn Sina has been an important connecting element of the common cultural tradition of humanity. At a time when Oriental science was less developed than Western science, Ibn Sina significantly influenced European science and promoted the subsequent development of not only Eastern but also Western culture and science. Ibn Sînâ's theoretical text and the encyclopedic work of clinical medicine consisting of five books titled "El-Kânûn fî't-Tıb (The Canon of Medicine), which includes the approaches and experiences of Greek, Roman, Indian and Central Asian doctors and "is a broad synthesis of the best in Greek and Arab medicine" (Siraisi, 1987) has influenced universal science for centuries, transcended regional boundaries between East and West, and provided the scientific interaction of East and West. The best indicator of the popularity of this work in both the East and the West is that it has been read as a textbook for centuries in Europe, where it is perceived as a kind of medical Gospel (Holy Book) and is published approximately 30 Latin editions. In addition, this book enabled Ibn Sina to be recognized as the greatest doctor in the West after the Hippocrates in the Middle Ages.

There is no doubt that Ibn Sînâ, who, besides his own philosophy, transferred and introduced classical philosophical inheritance to modern Europe and who is known as "al-Shaykh al-Ra'is" in the Islamic world, among the world-class geniuses raised by the Islamic civilization, has gained an important place in the history of philosophy. While Roger Bacon refers to Ibn Sina as "the greatest philosopher after Aristotle", Maimonides stated that he preferred Ibn Sînâ to Aristotle in his book "The Guide for the Perplexed" (Delil ul-hairin) (*Tarih ve Edebiyat Mecmuası*, 1982, p. 105).

The philosophers who lived in Islamic culture have views in metaphysics, epistemology, logic, morality and many other fields.

Islamic philosophy developed in parallel with early scholastic thought. But this development happened in a different way. At first, Aristotle's thoughts gained attention and his works (especially those on metaphysics, logic and physics) were carefully studied and interpreted. Meanwhile, weight was given to metaphysical and formal logic. Aristotelianism was not sought as it was, but as it was intertwined with elements of Neoplatonism (Бобоев, 2002).

"The biggest representative of Islamic neoplatonism in the Orient was the philosopher whose name was identified with this philosophy by later writers in the East and Europe . . . Abu Ali al-Hussein Ibn Sînâ" (Fahri, 1997, p. 119).

The parallel development of Muslim and Christian philosophies also shows the comprehension of the universal concepts. Ibn Sina reaches conclusions similar to those of the French Scholastic thinker and theologian Petrus Abelardus, but earlier in time (*Электронная библиотека по философии*).

The main philosophical work of Ibn Sina was an encyclopedic book of Kitabü'ş-Şifa (The Book of Healing), which contained the foundations of logic, physics, and metaphysics. He also wrote Aristotle's commentaries and many other books. In these comments he criticized Aristotle's understanding of movement, and his term "violent inclination" (called "mayl qasri") was met with the term "impetus" in the West. Therefore, this study is a manifestation of Ibn Sina's approach to Modern Age Mechanics.

Ibn Sina has developed a unique approach in the field of aesthetics. Ibn Sina seems to have examined the beauty and made the philosophy of the beautiful among the aesthetic values. Although he did not examine the term beautiful as a guiding concept, Ibn Sina seems to have made explanations to make the content of this concept clear. The beautiful was first conceived as an entity and identified with goodness and truth. The beauty of natural beings has been seen in Ibn Sina in proportion to their proximity to balance and harmony. He placed "human beauty" in a different category in the realm of natural being and has laid the groundwork for human spiritual ascension and maturity.

Professor Macit Fahri writes in his book "History of Islamic Philosophy": "The written corpus of Ibn Sina was really voluminous and his works were more sophisticated than those written by earlier philosophers such as Kindi and Razi. In addition, he surpasses all his predecessors, even the great Fârâbî, in the smoothness of his style and his careful handling the issues superficially considered by his predecessors . . . " (Fahri, 1997, p.120–121).

Since Greek was later forgotten, the opportunity to benefit from the roots and morphological principles of Greek science was lost. Europe, which uses Latin since the main antiquities were translated into Arabic early enough, met them much later, when it came face to face with Islamic culture in the 10th century. Usually Kindi, Ibn Sina, and Ibn Rushd were famous figures of the medieval university tradition (*Электронная библиотека по философии*, p. 245). Therefore, the influence of Islamic thought in the West began to manifest as a result of the translations made from Arabic and Greek to Latin since the 11th century.

"The effect of these translations should be divided into two groups: 1) The effect originating from Farabi and Ibn Sînâ and opening the avicennisme; 2) Ongoing influence due to the summaries made by Ghazali from Farabi and Ibn Sina. Farabi and Ibn Sina translations served Augustinisme's settlement or revival. He brought new evidence to support him. Hippone began to make this composition in his work called Doctrina Sacra. This draft played a big role in the 13th century. Avicenna became the Thinker who had a primary influence on Medieval Christian thought because he was useful both directly and to annotate Augustine. . ." (Ülken, 1967, p. 314).

The most famous scientist in Toledo, Gerard of Cremona (1114–1187), to whom are attributed translations of at least seventy separate works, refers both to the most important works of Aristotle, Plotinus, Proclus, Euclid, Galen and to Ibn Sînâ's Canon, which is said to have replaced Galen's writings in the West in that time period (*Ibn Sina*).

Ahmet Gürkan, referring to this subject in his book "Acculturation of the West by Islamic Culture", writes that "Islamic philosophy quickly entered Jewish and Christian schools and occupied the idea of man in the West for four centuries" (Gürkan, 1965, p. 248).

Studying at the medieval university meant first of all to acquire book knowledge. There is a description of the four-year course on medicine at the University of Bologna. Conferences were held every day. The first year was devoted to Ibn Sînâ and his el-Kânûn fi't-Tıb (The Canon of Medicine) textbook. In the second and third years, Galen, Hippocrates and Ibn Rushd were taught. There was repeat in the fourth year. (*Электронная библиотека по философии*, p. 248).

The science of medicine significantly influenced by Ibn Sina, and he was mentioned as the greatest physician of the world history who ruled Islam and Christian medicine for six centuries (*Yeni Türk Ansiklopedisi*, 1985, p. 1365), and was named "the father of doctors" in Latin dictionaries.

The works of Ibn Sînâ, known as Avicenna in the West, genius scientist-encyclopedist, physician and philosopher, naturalist and thinker, poet and literary who have achieved excellence in many his works and actions, are among the outstanding works enriching the world cultural treasure. Dante Alighieri, the Italian poet and politician, mentioned Avicenna's name among the greatest thinkers of all time and tribes. He was interested in medicine, physics, astronomy, philosophy, theology, music and other fields and created valuable works.

"...Ibn-i Sinâ, who is considered the father of medicine, had his greatest influence on Western philosophy" (*Tarih ve Edebiyat Mecmuası*, 1982). They call Ibn Sina the "philosopher of being" because the original part of his philosophy is his teaching about being. Many Christian philosophers adopted Ibn Sina's theory of knowledge instead of Aristotle's theory of knowledge, which led to Avicennism. As we can observe the brightest manifestations of this trend in Roger Bacon's illuminisme, it will develop further in augustinism. Therefore, there was the birth of an Ibn Sina Augustinizm in the West. The terms "Meşrikî" and "Israkî", which became more prominent in the Israkî movement of Suhreverdî, were also used starting from Ibn Sînâ (Ülken, 1967, p. 108–110, 314).

He was influenced by the thinkers before him, especially by Western philosophers, and guided others like Ibn Rushd. Ibn Rushd got his understanding of general rankings and hierarchy between God and man from Ibn Sînâ (*Электронная библиотека по философии*).

It is known that Ibn Rushd in the West and Ibn Sînâ in the East is regarded as genius of Islamic philosophical thought (*Электронная библиотека по философии*), (Бобоев, 2002).

Many famous figures are included in the Ibn Sina School. Some of these were directly affected by him, while others were indirectly affected. Among them Maimonides b. Necib-al-Vasıti, poet Ömer Hayyâm and others are mentioned (Ülken, 1967, p. 114).

Of course, those who comment or criticize their works were inspired by their thoughts in one way or another. Among them are the historian of sects (doxographer) Al-Shahrastani (died: 1153), the theologian Fakhr al-Din al-Razi (died: 1209) and the encyclopedist Nasir al-Din al-Tusi (d. 1273). It is known that many of the famous authors of the XII-XIII centuries have devoted themselves to explaining or annotating the works of Ibn Sînâ (Fahri, 1997, p. 119).

Although Fakhr al-Din al-Razi criticized Ibn Sina in his commentaries to two important works of Ibn Sina, Al-isharat and Uyun al-Hikma, the influence of Ibn Sînâ is also evident on Razi's thought. Professor Macit Fahri writes on this subject: "A careful reading of El-Mebâhis is enough to convince the reader that Râzî owes to Ibn Sînâ" (Fahri, 1997, p. 288 -289).

As Ibn Sînâ had an important influence on Ibn Arabi, it is said that Ghazali was significantly influenced by Ibn Snâ especially in psychology, because he joined skepticism after reading Kitab al-Shifa (Book of the Remedy) and was said to him as "Shifa made Ghazali sick" (Ülken, 1967, p. 105–106).

Ibn Sina had an influence on the philosophy of Albertus Magnus (1206–1280), Bonaventura, Saint Thomas and also Spinoza in the West.

Of course, the above-mentioned thinkers were influenced by Ibn Sina, and some philosophers who were influenced by these thinkers also felt the reflections of Ibn Sina's views. For example, through Albertus Magnus, Ibn Sînâ's classifications of the soul were transferred to many Western Medieval philosophers.

Hilmi Ziya Ülken writes in his book "Sources and Influences of Islamic Philosophy" on this subject: "There is no doubt that the translation of a large part of Ibn Sînâ's works into Latin has made significant changes in Western intellectual life. Et. Gilson explains his influence on Duns Scot in his article. Moreover, the area of influence of his thoughts on the definition and classification of the soul was very wide" (Ülken, 1967, p. 315).

Of course, while the above-mentioned persons agree with some of Ibn Sina's thoughts, they criticize some of them, which is natural.

His students are Al-Juzjani, who wrote the life of the philosopher, the closest to the master was Behmanyar, born in Azerbaijan, Abu Mansur b. Zayla (Ibn Zayla), his favorite student, El-Ma'sumi who writes about him "According to Plato, he is in the same position in my eyes as Aristotle" (death: 1029) (Ülken, 1967, p. 106; *IBN sına*).

Stating that the schematic separation between East and West is relative, we can say that the East and West relations have penetrated each other in the course of historical development as they have been in the past, and contemporary civilization is formed from this fusion. Scientists who nurture and develop science have been trained by acquiring qualities specific to the intellectual life of both. Therefore, it is the cultures that enrich, create and nurture the universal culture.

Intelligence is always in the world of the multitude (*Современная философия. Восточная философия*). The knowledge and thoughts of humanity have been and will be in constant interaction, because science is universal.

Usually, Ibn Sinâ's Canon (book), Al-Farghani's Summary of Astronomy together with Ibn Razi's Al-Kitab al-Hawi and Ibn Rushd's Kulliyat ("Generalities", i.e. general medicine, known in its Latin translation as Colliget) were described as great medical works written in the tradition of encyclopedia. According to Ernest Renan and Georges Sarton, although the above-mentioned works were the most comprehensive works of the period written inspired by Aristotle, they deeply affected Paris scholastic philosophy, but the Islamic world remained unaware of them (*İslam Biliminin Yükselişi*).

In response to the above view, we can say that the name of Ibn Sina has never been forgotten and the tradition of researching his works has always continued.

The works of Ibn Sina still preserve their scientific value and actuality today. Some of his observations and predictions anticipated a series of future discoveries and shed light on universal science.

It is one of our duties to research thoroughly, preserve and develop the rich cultural heritage we have. In this regard, it should be noted that the legacy of Ibn Sina occupies one of the most important places in our great scientific and cultural treasure.

Philosophy in both the West and the East is emerging as a form of social consciousness. The philosophy of the West and the East is directed towards universal human values. The role of Ibn Sina's worldview guidelines in the formation of universal human philosophy can not be reduced.

## References:

1. Бобоев, Ш.М. (2002). *Роль арабо-мусульманской культуры в сохранении и возрождении античной философии.* (22.10.2003) В.В.Ванчугов Российский университет дружбы народов, Факультет гуманитарных и социальных наук, Москва, 18 февраля 2002 года: научная конференция студентов, аспирантов и преподавателей «Диалог цивилизаций: история, современность и перспективы». Секция философии.
2. Cihan, A.K. (2009). *İbni Sina ve Estetik*. Ankara: Beyaz Kule. 1. Baskı.
3. *Электронная библиотека по философии* (Felsefe üzerine elektronik kütüphane). http://filosof.historic.ru Accessed 2 January 2020.
4. Fahri, M. (1997). *İslâm Felsefesi Tarihi*. Çev. Yrd. Doç. Dr. Kasım Turhan. İstanbul: İklim Yayınları.

5. Gürkan, A. (1965). *İslam Kültürünün Garbı Medenileştirmesi*. İstanbul.
6. *IBN sına*. Philosoff.Ru. Accessed 11 February 2010.
7. *İslam Biliminin Yükselişi*. Hazırlayan Ramazan Karakale. http://www.atominsan.com/bilimin_yukselisi.php Accessed 2 June 2011.
8. “Книга спасения” *Избранные произведения мыслителей стран Ближнего и Среднего Востока*. (1961). М.
9. Siraisi, N. (1987). *Avicenna in Renaissance Italy: The Canon and Medical Teaching in Italian Universities after 1500*. Princeton.
10. *Современная философия. Восточная философия*. www.modernphil.pp.ru. Accessed 3 August 2009.
11. *Tarih ve Edebiyat Mecmuası*. (1982). Ocak 1982 Sayısı.
12. Ülken, H. Z. (1967). *İslâm Felsefesi Kaynakları ve Tesirleri. Eski Yunandan Çağdaş Düşünceye Doğru*. Türkiye İş Bankası Kültür Yayınları.
13. *Yeni Türk Ansiklopedisi* (1985). 4. C., Ötüken Yay.


## Short Biography of Roida Rzayeva Oktay

She is the head of Department of Theory and History of Oriental Studies, Institute of Oriental Studies named after Academican Z.Bunyadov, Azerbaijan National Academy of Science. From 2011 until 2017, Rzayeva worked as deputy director at the Institute of Philosophy and Law of ANAS. She has authored five books ***(The Challenges of Contemporaneity: Postmodernity and Multiculturalism*** (Springer), etc.), and authored of over one hundred and thirty publications. Rzayeva gave talks in many countries (South Korea, Great Britain, France, Italy, Greece, Denmark, Russia, Turkey, Cyprus, Lithuania, Belarus, Georgia, Kazakhstan, etc.). She was awarded the Diploma in the field of Humanitarian and Social Sciences at the International competition of the young scientists of CIS, the diploma and the award “Young Scientist of the Year” for the scientific achievements in 2007 (2008), the honorary diploma of Department of Social Studies, ANAS on the occasion of 70-year-old anniversary of ANAS for long and fruitful scientific activity (2015), honorary Diploma of Youth Intellectual Development Centre for distinguishing herself in pursue youth policy (2007), the Diploma of the Ministry of Education of Azerbaijan Republic for the best report at the section of Oriental Studies (2002). She has been officially thanked for organizational, pedagogical and research activity by Turkish Academy of Sciences (2014), the Ministry of Family and Social Policy of the Republic of Turkey (2013), the Ministry of Culture and Tourism of the Republic of Azerbaijan (2011), Ege University of the Republic of Turkey (2010), the Ministry of National Education of the Republic of Turkey (2003-2008).
e-mail: rzayeva2020@inbox.ru

Prof. Dr. Esin Kâhya

# Two Distinguished Physicians, Ibn Sina and Galen

In general, when looking at the history of science, some common features of scientists draw attention. Some of are common features of almost all scientists. For instance, scientists pay attention to details; they have a critical mindset, they are patient; do not accept almost anything without scrutinization; they have an inquisitive spirit, what matters most for them are the research the subjects of which they work on or the problems they try to solve; generally, for scientists, the subjects they work on are of paramount importance; their researches and scientific studies they are interested in are indispensable for them.

All these features of them are also very important in terms of the history of science, because as we follow the course of scientific activities in the historical process, we observe similar behaviors with almost all scientists. The people they were influenced by and guided them in their childhood are similar in terms of their upbringing, basic education, the basic disciplines they have been interested in since childhood, as well as their lifestyles, the continuation of their works in certain cultural centers, their relations with political authorities and their interest in philosophy and mathematics.

In addition to their contributions to science, two of the scientists who will set an example especially in terms of methodology studies are Galen and Ibn Sina. Galen is one of the distinguished physicians who lived in the Hellenistic period. Galen's life can be traced back easily from various sources, except for his last years when mysterious events occurred. He was born in 129 in Bergama where was a settlement that was a cultural center at that time. Galen's father is one of the city's notable rich men, and he has an intense influence on his son Galen. Her mother, on the other hand, did not have a positive effect on Galen. Galen is said to have reported about his mother: "My mother was very angry; she always shouted, like Xantippe (Socrates' wife). I wanted to be like my father; I followed his movements."[1]

His father sent Galen to the city's Asclepion for training. There, Galen learned the basic principles of mathematics, logic, and architecture, and at the

1 De propriorum anim cauius libeli affectum dicnotione et curatione V, 40–41K.

age of fourteen he learned the teachings of almost all philosophical schools. Gaius, one of his teachers, had adopted the Plato philosophy. In this respect, he greatly influenced Galen.

It is recorded that the course of Galen's life changed when he was seventeen. With the influence of his teachers, he concluded that he should receive medical education as well as philosophy education. However, Galen's interest in philosophy never disappeared; He was interested in philosophy throughout his life. In fact, it is understood from his explanations in his work named The Method of Medicine that he discussed with the members of the philosophy schools of the period.

He shows his interest in the subject by saying that the Peripatetics, Stoics, and Platonists differ in logic theory. Indeed, we know that among his teachers there were representatives of Stoic philosophy, Plato philosophy, and Epicurean philosophy.

Regarding medicine education, Galen says: "*At that period they convinced me that a person receiving medicine education should also have philosophy education*".[2] As inferred, Galen's interest in philosophy continued as long as he lived without any decreasing.

Concerning medicine Galen says: "*I studied logic in my youth, and then I started to study medicine; first of all, I did not mind worldly matters. Latterly I tried to divert my worldly time to medicine implementations; I focused on this respect and ignored worldly matters.*" It is interesting that the importance of medicine was not conferred on plentily, however the place of philosophy is already known.

About nine centuries after Galen, the scientist and philosopher Ibn Sina, who lived and who, like Galen, continued to be active not only in his period but also in the following centuries, is also referred to as the 'Physician Ibn Sina'. He is considered to be the second most important philosopher after Farabi in Islamic philosophy. Ibn Sina was born in Bukhara in 980. His father is from the city of Balkh and because of his father's duty, the family lives in Bukhara. Interestingly, Ibn Sina, like Galen, is under his father's influence and his first teacher is his father. In the following years, Natili taught him philosophy. As a Muslim, he first had a religious education and then, like Galen, he took primarily mathematics and logic lessons. Ibn Sina (Avicenna) took a keen interest in logic as well as Aristotle philosophy (Aristotelian logic).

2 De ordine librorum suorum ad Eugeniarıun, xix, 59K.

Like Galen, Avicenna (Ibn Sina) also became famous in young age. He also has a high self-confidence since his young age like Galen; he never accepts any idea easily; he also scrutinizes to perfect his works. He narrates such a story in his work so-called İbn Hallikan, Vefeyat ü'l-âyân: "*One day he reads a poem which he had written at an assembly of distinguished people where the sultan also is present, and ideological arguments are exercised, however he is criticized by one of the people in the assembly; but at the next meeting, before everybody, he goes and leaves a poem he had recently written at the seat of that criticizing person. When that person comes he takes up that left poem, reads it and says. That's it, a poem must be like this*".

Galen received medicine education in Alexandria which was considered as a center of scientific studies at that era. He was interested in medicine however the importance of philosophy in his life continued, but medicine became effective in his travels. He improved his medicine related knowledges in Alexandria. Like physicians Herphilos and Erasistratos he implemented dissections on animals over there. From explanations conferred anatomy, especially regarding muscles skeletal system it is inferred that he implemented dissections mostly on monkeys.[3]

Galen returned from Alexandria to his hometown Bergama at 28 years old. Later he went to Rome, Italy but not stayed long, where was in charge of being a doctor for gladiators. He treated all the fractures and dislocations of the injured in Rome. Galen's works here helped him improve knowledges in classification of diseases and continuities of cases as well as his knowledges of anatomy and surgery.

After some time, Galen returned to his hometown Bergama. But it is known that he went to Rome again and worked with Boetius and executed dissections together with him. However, he did not stay long over there. An epidemic which broke out in Rome at that era caused him to return from Rome to Bergama compulsorily. Galen spent the rest of his life in Bergama. He died at age 87. We do not have plenty of information about his last years of his life as well as about his cause of death. Galen continued to write mostly on medicine until the last years of his life.[4]

---

3 Galen, De Ossibus ad Tirones (On Bones for Beginners, translator: Charles Singer), London: 1952. Galen, De Anatomicus Administrationibus (On Anatomical Procedurs, translator: Charles Singer), London: 1965.

4 Method of Medicine for Glaucon, s. xxii-xxxi

Ibn Sina became famous in young age like Galen. He went to cities such as Jurjan, Kazvin and Hamadan which were cultural centers of Islamic world in that period; As a physician he executed as private physician for several administrators of the period and received their supports.

Ibn Sina's first teacher was his father as Galen's first teacher was his father. Later, he received lessons of philosophy, logic, Islamic jurisprudence from Ismail üz'zahid al-Natılî. In addition, he is also known having taken lessons of nature and religious knowledges. Ibn Sina was also interested in philosophy like Galen. He is known having had a special sympathy to Farabi. A story of him is narrated such as he went to book sellers and notices a book of Farabi on metaphysics when touring old books market; bought the book and after reading said that *"I understood what Aristotle meant now"*.

Ibn Sina treated the Samanid ruler Nuh bin Mansur in Bukhara; thus, he was allowed to make use of his rich library, but unfortunately that library which was full of rare books was burned and he was charged burning it and therefore he was obliged to leave the city.

Ibn Sina first moved from there to Jurjan where he was taken under protection by rulers of the city so that he wrote down some of his works. He could never return to his hometown Bukhara due to fear of the ruler Mahmud The Ghaznavid to have him caught and jailed.

Ibn Sina moved respectively first to Kazvin and then to Hamadan; he started to write down a part of his famous work *al-Qanun fi't Tıbb* which contains works of physics and mathematics as much as his philosophical views in his *Shifa* book. In the meantime, an attempt to catch and jail him by Ghaznavid Mahmud failed, the ruler Şemsu'd Davlah took him under protection and assigned him as vizier (minister).

Ibn Sina treated the sultan in Hamadan and was assigned as vizier. Upon the sultan's death, he left the city, but he was caught and jailed at *Fardajan Fortress*. Ibn Sina continued to read and write during his imprisonment where he is said to have written down a part of *Shifa* and *Qanun* works.

After some time Alau'd Davlah had him released. Under protection of Alau'd Davlah, Ibn Sina dealt mostly with astronomy and mathematics in Hamadan. Over there upon request of Alau'd Davlah, he shaped the first calendar in Hamadan which is still in use in Iran.

Alau'd Davlah respected him a lot. However, Ibn Sina's very active and simultaneously scientific and philosophical life expired here in Hamadan. He was given overdose poison and murdered by his slave in his 57 years of age. Ibn

Sina understood he would die and donated his goods to his slaves, prayed and prepared himself for death. His grave is in Hamadan.[5]

It is known that Ibn Sina exchanged ideas like Galen and sometimes entered arguments concerning scientific methods especially.

Galen who has a critical mindset is known to be under Plato's influence; as a physician he admires Hippocrates. A major part of Galen's manuscripts have been reserved for remarks of texts of Hippocrates; in other words, Galen has adopted views of Hippocrates as basis for his works. Regarding this matter Lloyd says: *"Galen always expressed his admiration to him"*.[6]

Galen admires especially Plato among philosophers. A lot of researchers said that Galed owed his success in philosophy and medicine to Plato. It can be inferred from his works that Galen adopted Plato's method of argument and wrote down the Method of Medicine. When Galen discusses basic principles of medicine he also mentions and discusses other asserted views beside his views.[7]

Ibn Sina is mostly a follower of Aristotle because according to him, logical principles should be taken as basis for the way to truth. By his system of thought we can say that he implemented basic principles of classical logic. It has also determined that he sometimes exchanged views with his colleagues and sometimes argues with them; It can also be said that Galen's discussions are on methods more than scientific data like Ibn Sina's; he replies the thinkers by mentioning names especially in his "' Method of Medicine". Among them Thessalus's name is frequently mentioned.[8]

Ibn Sina as a scientist and a philosopher adopted it as a principle to behave objectively; it is clearly seen that he never accepted anything that he did not observe. He opposes astrology and alchemy. For instance, he rejected transformation theory while working on chemistry. According to him, metals have certain characteristics therefore precious metals such as gold and silver cannot be generated because of chemical processes. He discussed this matter in his Chemistry Article and proved that was impossible with experimental works.[9]

---

5 Günaltay, Şemseddin, İbn Sina'nın Milliyeti, Hayatı, Kültürü, Büyük Türk Filozofu ve Tıp Üstadı, İbn Sina, TTK, Ankara 1937. s. 25

6 Galen, Method of Medicine, Book 1–14, ed. and translate lan Johnston ve G.H. Horsley, Harvard University Press, 2011. p. IX.

7 Galen, Method of Medicine, Book 1–14, ed. and translate lan Johnston ve G.H. Horsley, Harvard University Press, 2011. P.X.

8 Ibid., p.29.

9 Kâhya, İbn Sina'da Kimya, İbn Sina Sempozyumu, Ankara 1984, s. 175–177.

It is known that Ibn Sina sometimes communicated with scientists in scientific matters. He exchanged letters with Ebu'l-Vefa Buzjani and as a result of astronomical research both of them designated that the inclination of ecliptic plane is 23° 31'. Also, he exchanged views with Biruni about the same subject.[10]

Regarding optics, Ibn Sina exchanged ideas with Ibn Haitham as well. Both exercised dark room experiments. As a result of these experiments, he explained that sight of eye is with functions of lens; and added that through the lens, the image falls to a certain point at the back of the eye, so that it is possible to see, but for this fact to occur, there must be a light source in the environment. According to him, image is real, not imaginary.[11] Sight is possible with light rays coming from outside.

Ibn Sina examined how an object moved and rejected Aristotle's remarks and claim that a force applied to an object passes into the air and that the object is transported by the air. According to him, the force moving the object is that the force which gives the object the ability to move.

Ibn Sina has never agreed with Biruni about scientific method. There exist 12 letters on the method subject which they debated. As understood from these, Biruni attached importance to the facts designated by observations one by one, however Ibn Sina attached importance to observations and experiments and focused on generally valid results. Doubtlessly the reason why he thought like this and concluded by paying more importance to logical inferences.[12]

If to compare Ibn Sina with Galen in terms of scientific behavior, both scientists had great interest in learning especially mathematics and philosophy since their childhoods. As a physician Galen gave importance to dissection, but his practice on animals like other scientists of his time such as Erasistratos and Herophilus, and especially on monkeys, which he saw as the closest to human beings, caused him to make some mistakes in the anatomical structure of man, for example, this is clearly seen in the statements he gave about the extremity muscles.

We infer from Ibn Sina's remarks regarding viscera that he exercised dissections to find out the causes of diseases. We know that when he sometimes fails to treat a patient, he wonders why the patient has not made use of the treatment and in order to find out the real findings of the disease he has exercised some dissections. In this respect he clearly mentions in miscellaneous parts of his

10 Sayılı, Aydın, İbn Sina'nın Astronomisi ve Astrolojisi, İbn Sina, Ankara 1986, s. 163.
11 Sayılı, Aydın. Ibn Sinâ'da Işık, Görme ve Gökkuşağı, İbn Sina, Ankara 1986, s.209.
12 Garrison, Fielding H. An Introduction to the History of Medicine, New York 1929, s.261.

work so-called Kanun's third volume that he dissected the corpse and examined the body to find the cause of death of the patient. Doubtlessly, this exercise helped him learn human body better especially in the subject of anatomy and more clearly and specifically compared to his colleagues.[13]

Another prof that how healthy information Ibn Sina has about human anatomy and probably he exercised dissection on human body is the detailed information when he described anatomic structures and locations of organs. For example, regarding kidneys he said that; they were located both on right and left nearby the liver. The left kidney is in solidarity with spleen. Kidneys are nearby spleen and liver.[14]

Another characteristic discerning Ibn Sina from Galen is his close interest in mathematics and music as well as medicine and philosophy. In fact, according to him there are two disciplines in the foundation of music, mathematics, and astronomy. As astronomy provides music with eternity concept and mathematics provides measuring concept.

As a result we can say that even if Ibn Sina and Galen lived in different eras, they look like each other a lot as thinkers and scientists in several aspects very interestingly. As mentioned above in terms of their orientation, scientific formations, interests in science, especially medicine and philosophy, they are two distinguished representatives as well as in terms of their orientation, scientific formation, and their interest in science, especially medicine and philosophy, in the period we can only call the beginning of their life, as well as two successful historical periods. Galen, for the Hellenistic Period and Ibn Sina for the eleventh century which we can name as the golden period.

13 Kahya, Esin ve A.D. Erdemir, Osmanlı'dan Cumhuriyete Tıp ve Sağlık Kurumları, TDK, Ankara 2000, s.51–52.

14 Ibn Sina, el-Kanun fı 't-Tıbb, çev. Esin Kâhya, III. Kitap, 2. Kısım, Ankara 2018, s. 413.

## Short Biography of Esin Kahya

She received the title of Ph.D. of literature in 1971. She was on a scholarship in England between 1973–74 and during this time she conducted research at the Wellcome Institute and British Library. She conducted research on her subject at the Department of Philosophy at Cambridge University and at the Bibliotheque Nationale in Paris. She became associate professor in 1977 and professor in 1982.

She continued her studies as a faculty member and head of the Department of Philosophy. Republic of Turkey Ministry of Culture has served as a consultant in the publishing Condominium.

She is a member of Atatürk Cultural Center, International Medical History Institute, Turkish Medical History Institute, International Science History Institute, Turkish Science History Institute, and Turkish Philosophy Association. She participated in various national and international meetings.

Eighteen books and more than seventy articles have been published. Her articles took place in Belleten, OTAM, Erdem, Bilge, DTCF Magazine, Avicenna, Tanzimat, Felsefe Dünyası, Research (Philosophy), as well as in various common books in Turkish and foreign languages. Some of her prominent publications are as follows: Shemseddin Itaki's The Illustrated Treatise on the Anatomy of the Human Body, Turkey and Turkish People From The Beginning of the Ancient Ages to Today, Medicine in the Ottoman Empire, Science of Medicine in the Ottoman Empire.

Prof. Dr. Michael Such, OMD CM L.A.TCM

# Anthology of Selected Writing of Ibn Sina

This anthology is a translation of the selected writings of the leading, and most influencing philosopher of the Muslim world, Abu Ali Al-Hussein Ibn Sina, also known as Avicenna (980–1037) into the modern Hebrew. It contains Hebrew translations for his entire work, such as: Avicenna's autobiography; About the Essence of Prayer; Treatise on Love; Treatise of the Birds. It also contains long sections of other books, such as the chapter on the soul from the book of Salvation; latest book on the politics and religion of healing; Great Encyclopedia of Avicenna; the last three volumes of the book of Hints and Notes (1). We also added shorter passages, many of which are from the sphere of healing, representing the most typical teachings of Avicenna, such as: the difference between reality and essence; the difference between reality and possible in reality; knowledge of God; preservation of the individual soul.

The Avicenna writings anthology is the second book in a series of modern Hebrew translations of the greatest Muslim writings, published by the Tel Aviv University Press. The first book consisted of the Doctrine of the exemplary city-state of Al-Farabi, which was released in 2007 (2).

Abu Ali Al-Hussein Ibn Sina (980–1037), known in the West under the name Avicenna, was the leading physician of his time, and the most famous and influential philosopher of the Islamic world. Ibn Sina was part of the Islamic philosophy tradition created by Abu Naser Al-Farabi (870–950). His roots go back to the organized study of Aristotle logic, physics, and metaphysics, and he was also influenced by Aplaton in everything related to political philosophy. Al-Farabi Kazakh National University has created that tradition, and it was called the "Second Teacher, second only to Aristotle, but the place is a leading philosopher of Islam soon took Ibn Sina. He was honored, and his writings were studied in many centuries after the influence of Al-Farabi on Islamic thinking died away. Recently, Robert Wisnowski said: "In the intellectual history of post-classical Islam there is nothing like the influence of Ibn Sina [. . .] his innovations in metaphysics are his most significant contribution to philosophy, were discussed before the rise of Islamic Modernism in the late 19th century." Al-Farabi and Ibn Sina were the most prominent philosophers in the Muslim East (3).

The explanation of the influence of Ibn Sina in the next generation of Islamic thinkers, even after studying the scriptures (philosophers from the tradition established by Al-Farabi) was rude and even dangerous is the fact that his writings are more consistent with traditional beliefs of Islam than the writings of the great Falasif like Al Badzh (1085–1138) and Ibn Rushd (1126–1198). The influence of Ibn Sina on the philosophy of the Christian West, especially in the thirteenth century, when Aristotle philosophy leaked into Christian Europe, and Latin Aristotelianism grew, was significant, but smaller than Ibn Rushd, since Ibn Sina was sometimes perceived as departing from statements of Aristotle. This retreat is especially emphasized in the critical position that Ibn Rushd adopted regarding Ibn Sina (4).

We know a lot about the life of Ibn Sina, among other things because he left behind an autobiography completed by his student Al Juzdani (see: Chapter 1) (5). Ibn Sina was born in a small village called Afshana, near Bukhara in modern Uzbekistan, and grew up in Bukhara. Reading an autobiography shows that he was exalted and excelled in his studies under the supervision of private teachers, and then on his own. According to him, upon reaching the age of eighteen, he completed his studies in the science of philosophy and: "In those days, the training material was stored in my memory as it should, better than now, but today it is more mature in me. Since then, nothing has been updated to me since then, and the knowledge that I have is that same knowledge". A few years later, his father passed away, and Ibn Sina left Bukhara and wandered among the cities of Persia.

Ibn Sina was a prolific author who wrote more than a hundred works. The greatest and most famous of them is the extensive essay on medicine Konstitu qi I Medicine, or Canon (Al Kanun fi Altab) and Healing (Alshifaa). Book Canon of Medicine was translated into Latin Gerardosom Kermony of the twelfth century (1150–1178) and became the main textbook of medicine in Europe for five hundred years. This five-volume book was also popular in translation into Hebrew. This conclusion is drawn from the existence of dozens of manuscripts containing partial translations into Hebrew, and the availability of a complete translation into Hebrew of a shortened version. Another proof of the great popularity of the book among medieval Jews is the presence of more canonical manuscripts in Arabic-Jewish than any other Muslim-written book. According to Langermann, there is no doubt that the book of Ibn Sina was the most important text used by Jewish doctors in the Middle Ages and during the Renaissance" (6).

The second book is Healing, the greatest philosophical work of Ibn Sina, an extensive, multi-volume encyclopedia of science and philosophy. There are four parts in Healing: (A) Logic (in the order of the Organon, nine books of Aristotle on logic, including rhetoric and poetics). (B) Physics. (C) Mathematics (quadrivium) is the highest division of the liberal sciences of the Middle Ages: geometry, astronomy, arithmetic and music. (D) Metaphysics. The mathematics of Ibn Sina are based on Nicomachus (arithmetic), Euclid (geometry) and Ptolameus (astronomy), while his natural sciences and metaphysics are based on Aristotle (7).

The philosophical doctrine of Ibn Sina was originally pure Aristotelian, but throughout the years adopted a self-yours form, settled in the tradition of Aristotle. The development of his teachings is described in the book of "Ibn Sina and the tradition of Aristotle" (1). Ibn Sina wrote Healing in the late period of his life (approximately 1020–1027), and it is considered an independent creation, not content with the interpretation of the scientific teachings of Aristotle (see: Chapter 3). Thanks to Ibn Sina, healing took place Aristotle's books as the best source of knowledge and truth gates. This work is a find for most of the teachings and opinions typical of his philosophy.

Ibn Sina is known mainly for his psychological and metaphysical treatises. For example: the perception of the soul and the knowledge of humanity (see: Chapter 5); the perception of essence and reality, distinguishing the essence that tells us what a thing is, from the reality that tells us whether a thing exists at all (see: Chapter 6); metaphysical proof of the existence of God (see: Chapter 7); the distinction of the obligation of reality from the possible in reality (see: Chapter 7); worldview about the divine knowledge of details (see: Chapter 8); perception of prophecy (see: Chapter 9); preservation of the soul (see: Chapter 13); human integrity (see: Chapter 14). (1) A discussion of the views of Ibn Sina on these topics and others is given in the introductions to each chapter of this book.

The philosophical doctrine of Ibn Sina is undoubtedly influenced by religious considerations, mainly Islam, and there are studies discussing this influence, but do not overestimate the size of the phenomenon. Ibn Sina was an original philosopher, confident of himself and his teachings, and avoided submitting to religious orders. So, for example, one of his famous treatises concerns the dualism of the soul and body, and expresses the belief that the soul is a separate object, independent of the body. This treatise perfectly combines the religious faith in preserving the individual soul of a person, but at the same time, in fact, denies the rebellion of the dead, which is the basis of Islamic theology. Ibn Sina discusses the dualism of body and soul through a mental test, given in various forms in several of his writings. The most famous version is given in the first article from "About the Soul", from Healing (8).

Each of us should imagine that he had just been created in the prime of life, but that vision was preventing him from seeing things in the outside world, and that he had been created by falling in the air or emptiness, so that there is no air friction in the fall to the extent obligating to feel it, and the organs are separated so that they do not meet and do not touch each other. Then let him think whether he can confirm his very existence. He will not doubt that he would confirm his existence, despite the fact that he would not confirm the edges of his limbs, neither the cavities of his insides, nor his heart as such, nor his brain, nor anything outside.

Ibn Sina suggests that a person's self-awareness does not necessarily depend on the body or feelings. The perception of the "fluttering person" presented by him teaches that in his opinion we have the ability to acknowledge our existence and confirm it without acquaintance with the body, and without any knowledge of it. This paragraph is reminiscent of Descartes' principle of Cogito ("I think, therefore I exist"), and is perhaps one of Descartes's sources. At the same time, the perception presented here is not going to serve as an evidence but is content with a representation of the reality of the soul, ethereal and not associated with the body. (8) Still, according to Ibn Sina, our awareness of existence (or that which is) can be direct knowledge.

Recently, Peter Adamson investigated the relationship between soul and body in the treatment of Ibn Sina Aristotle's Theology (in short: Theology) in order to assess the neo-Platonic influence of this scripture. One of the most important issues in Islamic and Jewish philosophy in the Middle Ages, was the degree of influence of Neoplatonism on Aristotle philosophers. The researcher was divided on the answer to this question, at least on the most important philosophers like Al Farabi, Ibn Sina and Maimonides. The work of Theology is attributed to Aristotle, but in fact we are talking about the Arabic rephrasing of the chapters of Anad for Plotinus, articles four through six, which became the main text of Arab Neoplatonism. Researchers also disagree on the issue of whether Islamic philosophers recognized that Aristotle was not the author of the Neoplatonic book attributed to him. Ibn Sina himself had a doubt whether Aristotle was the author of the work. As it links to the essays that were deep, he even found a spot treatment. According to Adamson (9), the interpretation of Theology by Ibn Sina gives us "an incomparable opportunity to verify the position of Ibn Sina in relation to the Neoplatonic tradition". Adamson concluded that, at least in the matter of the connection between soul and body, Ibn Sina did not hesitate to criticize and correct the neo-Platonic opinions in Theology in order to reconcile them with his philosophy. That is, Ibn Sina perceived himself as an innocent innkeeper whose role was to judge the teachings of the text. So, for example, according to Theology, the soul is completely separate, and it does not have any need for bodily form in order to achieve perfection. On the contrary, the body actually threatens her. Ibn Sina follows the path of Aristotle and argues that the body and feelings complement the powers of the mind and allow the integrity of the soul. He explains that the rational soul needs feelings in order to extract forms from particular weights, and thus comprehend awareness. To this epistemological need of a rational soul in the body, Ibn Sina added a metaphysical need: the soul needs a source of individuality (individuation), the essence of the body (see: Chapter 5). Therefore, the soul cannot exist before the body, according to Plotinus and the Neoplatonic thinkers.

The personal opinion of Ibn Sina is also not clear enough. His philosophy is very difficult to fully understand, and there are immediacy and obscure terms. An aspiring reader should assume that this philosophy is not known in all its details. There are ideas in the treatises of Ibn Sina, about which even leading researchers disagree. So, for example, there is no agreement about the measure in which the Neoplatonic worldview influenced him, and what his attitude towards mysticism was (see: Chapter 14). While researchers agree about his main opinions - for example, a god who knows everything, it is very generalized, these opinions are not always clear (see: Chapter 8). (10)(11). Even when his main opinions are known, sometimes even their details are vague. I will give two examples: The first example is the teaching of Ibn Sina on inheritance. According to this teaching, the world is inherited from God, obligated by reality, in the light of his knowledge of himself (see: Chapter 8) (11). First, he was created, the first mind that knows three things:

(A) God is necessarily within himself.
(B) His reality obligates in the light of the obligated reality, which is its cause
(B) His reality is possible from the point of view of himself.

Three factors flow from these thinking actions:

(A) Second Mind
(B) The soul is the outermost celestial sphere
(B) The body of this sphere.

In a similar way, from the mental action of the second mind, a third mind is generated, another soul of the sphere of planets, and another body, which is the body of this sphere. So, the teaching of the inheritance of Ibn Sina continues until the inheritance of the last heavenly mind, which is the active mind, from which the world of current and loss is inherited. The first substance and all forms (primarily the forms of the four elements) are inherited from the real mind, "giving the form", and of them all that is under the sky. So explains Ibn Sina in the beginning of his treatise on the soul (see: Chapter 5.):

"When the elements merge in a more balanced merger, that is, a merger closer to equilibrium than the one mentioned above, new entities are formed from these elements, also thanks to the forces of celestial bodies. The first entities are plants." (8)

The theory of inheritance of Ibn Sina combines Neoplatonic and Aristotle influences, and is similar in its foundations to Al Farabi. Did Ibn Sina really believe in this strange theory (strange, at least for the modern reader)? Did he not know Aristotle metaphysics, and did not understand that it does not correspond to the theory of inheritance, for example, described by the author of Theology? Mahsan Mahdi, a leading scholar of the philosophy of Al Farabi, negatively answers these questions in all that relates to Al Farabi. Therefore, according to him, gently at the reader should "distinguish Theorem call metaphysics of political metaphysics oh and theoretical psychology of political psychology." In other words, according to Mahdi (as opposed to looking at his powerful arguments, not every researcher agrees with him), the aim of the Neo-Platonic metaphysics and cosmology, represented by Al Farabi in his popular writings, is to create an alternative metaphysics, the Islamic faith, that is, not real metaphysics, but "political" metaphysics. It is difficult to define a political goal in the theory of inheritance of Ibn Sina, and Mahdi's important arguments about Al Farabi are not valid in the question of Ibn Sina. It is more logical to consider the theory of inheritance of Ibn Sina as one component in its central synthesis between Aristotelianism and Neoplatonism, which is the main goal of his metaphysical project. A study based on various terms for the inheritance and renewal of the world of Ibn Sina, discovered that Ibn Sina believed in both inheriting and updating the world from nothing (12). His intention was to combine the metaphysics of the forced with metaphysics, that is, inheritance with the renewal of the world. Inasnas noted in Ibn Sina "a clear tendency to translate the data of the Islamic religion into real philosophical theory." According to it sees this as an explanation of the popularity of Ibn Sina among Muslims in the west and in the east. He emphasizes the difference between the Neoplatonism of Ibn Sina and the non- Platonist tradition, and explains this by the fact that Ibn Sina saw himself as part of the Aristotle tradition, even in Islamic conditions. Yet, as Inasnas mentioned, the description of the theory of inheritance of Ibn Sina suffers from inconsistency and uncertainty reigns in it about its details.

Another example of vague teachings of Ibn Sina is his attitude to the renewal of RATIONAL soul in time. Eating is an agreement that according to Ibn Sina, immediately after the creation of the human body in real is the relation between the body and soul. But still, it is not clear how the process is going. Most likely, he has in mind mainly the working mind, the last of the heavenly minds. Marmura (13), one of the leading researchers of the philosophy of Ibn Sina, has recently published an article, allowing to understand that even this famous writing has questions without an answer. For example, what is the designated role of the celestial soul (or souls) in renewing the rational individual soul? Why is the human individual soul doesn't inherit from the working mind the way the working mind inherits from the separate mind predating it? What is the effect of the celestial bodies on the bodies in our, lower world? What is the effect of souls of the celestial bodies on the souls of this world? What is the relation between all this and the prophetical impression? What is the difference between the terms "Common sense" (Sekhel Al-Khul) and the "Common mind" (Al-Aqal al-Khuli)? Also, between the "Soul of All" (Naps Al-Khul) and the "Shared Soul" (Al-Naps Al-Khuli)? Did Ibn Sina use those terms consistently? Marmora offers answers to all these questions, and underlines that, despite the uncertainty s about the details of the theory of renovation rational individual and soul in time, the general theory of well-known researchers of Ibn Sina.

Did the thinkers of Islam in the Middle Ages Ibn Sin understand well? It is difficult to answer s to this question in the absence of a general agreement among modern scholars on some issues. For example, did Ibn Sina believe in God's knowledge of private affairs? Did he believe, according to Inasnas, in the renewal of the world from nothing? Abu Hamad Al- Ghazali (1058–1111), the greatest Mutakalim (theologist), a Sufi mystic, and arguably the most famous and respected philosopher and sage of the medieval age, has assumed that he knew Ibn Sina, and even expressed his respect for him as a philosopher. Al-Ghazali accused Ibn Sina, al-Farabi and other Islamic philosophers of heresy, for three reasons: they do not believe in the renewal of the world (out of nothing); did not believe that God knows the details (as opposed to generalizations); they denied the rebellion of the dead. (8)

Al-Ghazali in his autobiographical book "Salvation is of Errors" said he studied philosophy independently, at the age of 30, in order to properly understand the perceptions, he meant to refute:

"And I know exactly what people will not resist s front vices science of sciences, if it is to not delved into its study before its knowledge of its fundamentals compared with the knowledge of the most knowledgeable of the study it, and even surpass him in knowledge, and rise above its rank until it penetrates into the depths and secrets that the one who knew did not know. And then perhaps it peer's error science has a share of the truth . . . understand (i) that the fighter with the school, do not understand it and did not grasp the essence of it, like a shot." (14)

Al-Ghazali believed al-Farabi and Ibn Sina were the best philosophers of Islam, and worthy successors of the Greek philosophy and science. Most of his criticism is directed to Ibn Sina. (14) The accusation that Falasifah do not believe that God knows the details of our world, it was a particularly severe. From this there's a possible conclusion that God can't sent a prophet and to provide him with the divine law: He can't know who abides the law and lives a righteous life, and who doesn't, He can't punish and reward; in addition, He can't follow His creations and can't hear the prayer of the believer. As said, Al-Ghazali assumed that Ibn Sina renounces the divine knowledge of details. Was there truth in his accusations? The view of Ibn Sina on his question is unclear. A proper reading of his essay on the essence of prayer (15) (see: Chapter 10) is worth reading in order to argue whether his words shed light on his personal opinion on God's knowledge.

The charges announced by al-Ghazali threatens the future of philosophy among Muslims, and eventually killed the Aristotle tradition founded by al-Farabi. After the death of Ibn Rushd, who tried in vain neutralize accusations al-Ghazali, the Muslim world almost did not read his writings, as well as the writings of al-Farabi and Ibn Baja. (8) Their fear of references to these wise men is especially noticeable. Nevertheless, the doctrine of Ibn Sina, affected so many thinkers of Islam, and they continued to teach his writings, most likely because of its religious and mystical treatises.

Ibn Khaldun, the great historian of the fourteenth century, was one of the late thinkers of Islam, who appreciated Ibn Sina as a rationalist philosopher and representative of Islamic Aristotelianism (16). He honored him "among the [four] great scholars in the sciences of philosophy among Islam" and among the "heads of the sages of Islam", and mentioned his contribution to logic, mathematics, geometry, astronomy, physics and metaphysics. He called the medical treatise Ibn Sina the "most extensive composition" of physics. But this estimate is expressed by Ibn Sina as a rationalist philosopher, was unusual and reflected the personal philosophical inclinations of the Ibn Khaldun, while at that time the only philosophy that existed among the Islamic community, based on a combination of Kalam (theology), mystery and philosophy.

## The influence of Ibn Sina on the medieval Jew with some thinking

The theme of the influence of Ibn Sina on Jewish thinking in the Middle Ages consists of two questions. First, to what extent did his scriptures in Arabic influence Jewish thinkers? Second- to what extent did his writings, translated to Hebrew, affect the same thinkers? The first question concerns thinkers up to Maimonides, Maimonides himself (1138–1204), and some thinkers who came after him; the second concerns thinkers only after Maimonides.

Surprisingly, from the period of Ibn Sina to the second half of the twelfth century, only a few Jewish philosophers and theologians were interested in Ibn Sina, or any other Islamic philosopher, who could be recognized as referring to the followers of the al-Farabi school of Falasifah. One of the few acquaintances with Ibn Sina was Rabbi Judah Ha-Levi. His book Kuzri (The Khazar) (17) partially criticizes the Aristotle philosophy of Islamic philosophers. Shlomo Pines pointed out that the description of the philosophical world in "Kuzri" based on think Ibn Sina and Ibn Baja, but we almost did not hear it in the period of Jewish philosophy Ha-Levi who would have been under the influence of Islamic philosophy. The young friend of Ha-Levi, Abraham Ibn Ezra (1089–1067) was influenced by some of the writings of Ibn Sina, for example, in his mention of the knowledge of God about the details, and the distinction of the obligation of reality from the possible in reality (18). But we are talking about an exception to the rule, and in any case, it is almost impossible to classify Ibn Ezra as a philosopher in the format of Falasif. Joseph Ibn Tzadik was also aware of the reality of differences liable possible in reality, Ibn Sina, but also it is even less than the Ibn Ezra, it may not be so s described as a philosopher of a series Falasifah. According to Pines, Ha-Levi was deeply impressed by him [Ibn Sina], and perhaps tried, despite criticism of philosophy to combine his own ideas, at least to some extent, with the framework of Ibn Sina. (6) There is no doubt that Ha-Levi was familiar with the writings of Ibn Sina, and sometimes quoted them, but they also were not a follower of this school.

Despite that, we can clearly state that Ibn Sina was known among the thinkers of the Spanish Jews, and had them comment and criticism, at the latest, from 1130's, a period in which he influenced the Ha-Levi and Ibn Ezra. Some scholars believed that Ibn Sina influenced earlier Spanish-Jewish thinkers who lived in the eleventh century, such as Ichak Ibn Giat, Shlomo Ibn Gvirol and Bahya Ibn Pakudu. But there is no unequivocal evidence of the influence of Ibn Sina on Jewish thinking until the period of Ha-Levi and Ibn Ezra (6).

The first Jewish thinker who can be called a follower of Ibn Sina is Abraham Ibn Daud (1110–1180), the author of the book Great Faith (Emuna Raba), the first Jewish Aristotle composition. Despite the fact that the name of Ibn Sina is not explicitly mentioned, there is no doubt that it was he who served as the main philosophical source for the book of Ibn Daud, and it was from him that Ibn Daud draws knowledge in his research on basic topics, for example, God and the human soul. Soon after the publication of the book of Ibn Daud, it was overshadowed by another book, which touched upon Aristotle's philosophy and science, the Guidebook of Maimonides, Confused (More Nevohim). (19) The issue of the influence of Ibn Sina on Maimonides is very confusing. It is well known that Maimonides appreciated Al-Farabi more than Ibn Sina. In a famous letter written by him to the end of his life to Shmuel Ibn Tivon, the one who translated "The Guide for the Perplexed" to Hebrew, he recommended some philosophers worthy of being read and which are not worthy of it. He greatly praised Al Farabi, Ibn Badzhu and Ibn Rushd. The praise to Ibn Sina comes with a condition "And the book of Ibn Sina, despite the fact that they possess great accuracy and subtle reading, are unlike like a book by Abu Nasser al- Farabi, but his books are helpful, and he himself a man worthy of this session words and contemplation of his works." (20) This assessment Ibn Sina's not standing next to lavishly praise unto others Falasifah, but is at the very end of the nuc s ma, like "remembered in the end." At the same time, the fact that this litter cautiously praises of a sage, or even does not mention it at all does not mean that this thinker s not influenced by Maimonides, but it is possible that Maimonides did not want to pay attention to those things or encourage reader interest in his writings.

Today it deemed accepted - thanks largely to Pines- that the influence of Ibn Sina on Maimonides in the guide was more than reflected in the cautious praise to Ibn Tivon, and from the fact that it is not mentioned explicitly in the guide. It seems that Maimonides, like Ibn Rushd, who heavily criticized Ibn Sina, believed that one should not study real sciences - that is, Aristotelian ones – based on Ibn Sina (20). Such a science should be studied by means of the works of Aristotle, interpreted by and explanations of Ibn Rushd and the great Greek - Alexander of Aphrodisias and Temisiem- on par with the works of the great philosophers, al Farabi and Ibn Baja. How, then, does Ibn Sina fit into the works of Maimonides? And how are his writings useful?

Pines pointed out that Ibn Sina influenced Maimonides in the following aspects: Description of God as obliged by reality, the truth of which is similar to his essence; Maimonides negative theology, some aspects of the theory of prophecy; perhaps also in his perception in the matter of the rational work of God. Zeev Harevi showed that Maimonides believed that metaphysical proof that Ibn Sina gave to the existence of God depends on unprovable assumptions eternity of the world. (21) Therefore, Maimonides did not find Ibn Sina's metaphysical proof a full one. Yet Harevi believes that due it is the lack of demonstrative metaphysical proof according to Maimonides, the later found appeal in the metaphysical assumptions of Ibn Sina, whose "metaphysical representation of the most intelligent and sublime." In all that concerns Maimonides asserts Harevi, "there is no point in trying to Execute tough philosophical methodology during discussions of metaphysics." The topics in metaphysics or theology, in which the Aristotelian science loses its advantage, the words of Ibn Sina can be applied. Harevi agree that Maimonides turned to the metaphysics of Ibn Sina, as it is "direct thought s in the most effective way to cognition of the unknown." This statement perfectly matches Pines said that the method of Ibn Sina's "more in line with the religious approach . . . and no doubt the religion itself be what it perceived in the Middle Ages, when compared with orthodox Aristotelian teachings." (21)

Many years ago, it was argued that Ibn Sina is likely to serve as a direct source for nonstandard s motions Maimonides Arabic term Ishq (desire) to the god of love (19, part 3, p. 51). An article soon to be published by the author of those lines agrees with Pines- who asserts that the discussion of Ibn Sina external prayer (meaning ritualized) and inner manner- that day for it's true service influenced the discussion of Maimonides prayers and questions mental labor. Influences of this type are not surprising. These differences thus increasing the assertion that, although Maimonides small version of Ibn Sina and physics of Aristotle, the legends of Ibn Sina on god measurement and the relationship between man and God, play a roll helpful hints and instructions for it in places where it is not it was possible to move on solid ground demonstrative proof a God.

Jewish followers of Aristotle appeared after Maimonides, definitely inspired by Maimonides and Ibn Rushd- expressed little interest in Ibn Sina and with a few of his works have been translated into Hebrew. For them, Ibn Sina hot s and was Aristotle s skim wise, but it was not considered credible. The greatest translator of scientific texts from Arabic into Hebrew Kalona, the son of Kalomi, separated from Ibn Sina " the most important philosophers" - Alexander of Aphrodisias, al- Farabi, Ibn Baja and Ibn Rushd. Ibn Sina sometimes "strayed too much from the path of Aristotle," and apparently, he could not serve as a worthy guide for those wishing to delve into the words of the Greek. In this criticism he had many supporters among Aristotelian thinkers, such as Rabbi Gershom ben Levi and Joseph Ibn Kaspi, and they also do not care for the scientific writings of Ibn Sina (22).

When Aristotelian philosophers like Itzhak Al-Balagha, Moshe Narvoni and Moshe Ben Yehuda mentioned philosophy of Ibn Sina, in the representation of Al - Ghazali in the intention of the Philosophers, they did used it as a starting point for the teaching of Aristotelian science, Ibn Rushda. And yet, gradually it was discovered that the philosophy and science of Ibn Sina influenced the train of thought in the post-Maimonid period. In the thirteenth century, Jewish scholars such as Shmuel Ibn Tivon and Shem Tov Falkira studied the treatises of Ibn Sina and quoted excerpts from his Arabic writings in their Hebrew writings. Hillel ben Samuel of has cited the Latin translations. (6) Of those Hebrew writers who wrote in Arabic, Ibn Sina definitely influenced Moshe Halawi in the thirteenth century, and Joseph Ibn Vikar in the fourteenth century. Some Jewish thinkers who studied the writings of Ibn Sina during this period suggested that his statements fit well with religion, compared with the statements of other Falasif. There were also those who preferred the philosophy of Ibn Rushd (such as Shem Tov Falkir), but recognized the value of Ibn Sina. As already mentioned, only a few of his works were translated into Hebrew, with the exception of the Canon of Medicine, other medical writings and some paragraphs cited by Ibn Tivon, Falkir and some others. The main translator of Ibn Sina was Todor Todorasi, in whose anthology of translations of philosophical works (dated 1343), he contained paragraphs on physics and metaphysics from the book of Salvation, and several chapters and paragraphs from other books of Ibn Sina. Maoro Zonte argues that Todora's interest in Ibn Sina, as well as the other sages mentioned above, was caused by the inability to combine Jewry with the rigid Aristoteles of Ibn Rushd, as well as from the feeling that the philosophy of Ibn Sina is better aligned with traditional Judaism.

Apparently, the translation "Salvation" by Todros was not popular and did not have much influence. He has survived in only two manuscripts. Dov Schwartz demonstrated that the philosophical circle of interpreters of Abraham Inz Ezra, operating in Christian Spain in the second half of the fourteenth century, accepted some of the conclusions of Ibn Sina, but there is limited evidence that members of the circle were familiar with the writings of Ibn Sina in the original source. (23) Perhaps some of them did not even know that the decisions adopted by him were formulated by Ibn Sina. It is possible, nevertheless, to assume that they knew a short synopsis of the philosophy of Ibn Sina, for example in Al Ghazali's "Intentions of Philosophers," but there is no clear evidence that they studied this text. In fact, Al-Ghazali's processing of the writings of science and logic by Ibn Sina was popular in Hebrew translation only in the fifteenth and sixteenth century, when they were studied as an alternative to the Aristotle science of Ibn Rushd.

Hasdai Kreskas (1410–1340), (24) who wrote revolutionary criticism at the end of the fourteenth century to Aristotle's Physics, was perhaps the only Jew to thoroughly study the work of Al Ghazali, "The intentions of philosophers," translated into Hebrew, as an alternative to the physics of Al Rushd. Kreskas appreciated Ibn Sina and those who were influenced by his ideas, such as Al Ghazali and Ibn Daud. He usually preferred the original version of Al-Ghazali's writings of Ibn Sina, possibly because the text of Al-Ghazali was more accessible and understandable to him than the texts of Ibn Sina, although, perhaps, because of more simple and understandable wording of Al-Ghazali. After Crescas, in the fifteenth century, the Intentions of the Philosophers became the most popular philosophical text in Hebrew. It was through this essay, and with the help of sharp criticism of Al Ghazali to the philosophy and theology of Ibn Sina in refuting philosophers, and not through it numerous translations of the works of Ibn Sina in Hebrew, the Jews fully learned the teachings of Ibn Sina.

This is a brief description of the influence of Ibn Sina on post-Maimonid Jewish thinking refers to influence in the West. In the east, in Egypt, Yemen and other countries, interest in the philosophical tradition of Falasiph was small, from the thirteenth to sixteenth century. Their philosophy deviated greatly from Aristotle's perception, and was mixed with mysticism and esotericism. If there was a Muslim philosopher who influenced Jewish thinkers in the east during this period, then it was Ibn Sina. Paul Penton noted that some of the "observational writings" of Ibn Sina were rewritten in Hebrew letters at that time. They were attracted not so much by the science of Ibn Sina, as by his more mystical teachings.

## Avicenna's Influence on Scholastic Thinking

The most famous and most often translated into Latin philosopher of Islam among the scholars was, of course, Ibn Rushd. As already mentioned, he was the most important interpreter in the West, the key to understanding the writings of Aristotle. After Ibn Rushd, Ibn Sina had the greatest influence on Islamic scholars. His significant influence was in the field of psychology and metaphysics, through the translation of Healing into Latin (called Sufficientia), although the parts relating to the logic and science of nature in Healing were translated into Latin and were widely known. The science and philosophy of Ibn Sina was known thanks to the Latin translations of his other writings, as well as through the hints and references of philosophers to Al-Ghazali. That is, the greatest work of Ibn Sina in medicine, The Canon of Medicine was very popular in Europe, thanks to the translation of Garardos of Kremona, (6) quickly became the main text in the universities taught medicine.

The thinking of Ibn Sina began to influence scholars at an early stage - already at the end of the twelfth century - and continued to influence in full force throughout most of the thirteenth century, during which she gained influence among significant Latin scholars, such as Dominic Gundisalvi (the first to use material from Psychology Ibn Sina), John Blend, Guyem from Avenra, Jean Mile Rochelle, Albert Magn, Roger Bacon, Thomas Aquitaine, Henry Magnet, Sijar of Barbant and Johannes Dones Scotus. (25) Therefore, the direct influence of Ibn Sina on these philosophers concentrated on philology and metaphysics, but also extended to logic, physics and theology. New studies have been able to significantly determine and clarify the essence and exact scope of this influence. To understand Aristotle, the scholars consulted with the writings of Al Rushd. Ibn Sina is particularly interested in them because of his intellectual freedom. Sometimes, he intentionally left Aristotle and presented his personal philosophy — psychological, metaphysical, and theological opinions, which could, carefully and prudently, be combined with the foundations of the Christian faith. (26)

## The Importance of Ibn Sina Today

We described the great influence of Ibn Sina on Islamic, Jewish, and Christian philosophy during the Middle Ages. What is its importance to us today? We see that sometimes his teachings are difficult to understand, and sometimes suffer from inconstancy. Definitely, there are things that are still incomprehensible even to the best researchers. And yet, despite the difficulty of his teachings, and despite the criticism directed at them, Ibn Sina was the most respected, most important and most famous philosopher of the Islamic world. He had original and charming ideas that influenced thinkers not only in Islam, but also in Jewish and Western philosophy. This wisdom is worth learning today.

## Reference

(1) Gutas, D. (2014). *Avicenna and the Aristotelian tradition: Introduction to reading Avicenna's philosophical works. Including an inventory of Avicenna's authentic works*. Brill.

(2) Al-Farabi, A. N. (2007). Directing attention to the way to happiness. In *Classical Arabic philosophy: An anthology of sources*. (J. McGinnis & D. C. Reisman, Trans). USA: Hackett Publishing Company, Inc.

(3) Wisnowski, R. (2015, November 3). *Avicenna and Avicennism* [Video file]. Retrieved from https://cmes.fas.harvard.edu/news/avicenna-and-avicennism
(4) Ceylan, Y. (1993). A critical approach to the Avicennian distinction of essence and existence. *Islamic studies*, *32*(3), 329–337.
(5) Avicenna, Goldman, W. E. & Al-Juzajani (1974). *The Life of Ibn Sina.* Albany, NY: State University of New York Press.
(6) Harvey, S. (2009). *Antologiya lekitvey Ibn Sina* [Anthology of the writings of Ibn Sina]. Tel-Aviv: Taupress.
(7) Guitas, D. (2016, September 15). Ibn Sina. In: E. N. Zalta (ed.) *The Stanford Encyclopedia of Philosophy* (Fall 2016 Edition). https://plato.stanford.edu/entries/ibn-sina/
(8) Avicenna (2009). *The physics of the healing* (J. McGinnis, Trans.) Provo, Utah: Brigham Young University Press.
(9) Adamson, P. (2001). Aristotelianism and the Soul in the Arabic Plotinus. *Journal of the History of Ideas*, *62*(2), 211–232.
(10) Zarkasyi, H. F. (2011). Ibn Sina's Concept of Wajib al-Wujud. *TSAQAFAH*, *7*(2), 375–388.
(11) Ahmed, S. (2017). *The Disagreement between Avicenna and al-Ghazali on the Issue of the Pre-eternity of the Universe, how their Arguments Originated from Greek Philosophers and their Effect on Muslim Philosophers* (Doctoral dissertation, University of Wales Trinity Saint David).
(12) Inasnas, n.a.
(13) Marmura, M. E. (1965) "al-Ghazali and Demonstrative Science", Journal of the History of Philosophy, 3,183–204
(14) Al-Ghazali (2008). *The confessions of Al-Ghazali: Rescuer from error* (C. Field, Trans.). Dodo Press.
(15) Ibn Sina (1960). *Al-Shifa': Illahiyyat,* (M. Y. Musa & S. Z. Dunya, eds.) Cairo: n.d.
(16) Mihirig, A. (2017, November 27). The myth of intellectual decline: a response to Shaykh Hamza Yusuf. *Maydan.* Accessed February 19, 2021 at https://themaydan.com/2017/11/myth-intellectual-decline-response-shaykh-hamza-yusuf/
(17) Ha-Levi, J. (2012). *The Kuzari–The Book of Refutation and Proof on the Despised Faith* (N. Bashir, Trans.). Freiburg an Niedersachsen: Al-Kamel Verlag, 2012.
(18) Langermann, T. (2018, October 22). Abraham Ibn Ezra. In: E. N. Zalta (ed.) *The Stanford Encyclopedia of Philosophy* (*Winter 2018 Edition*). https://plato.stanford.edu/entries/ibn-ezra/

(19) Maimonides, M. (1904). *Guide for the perplexed* (N. Friedlander, Trans.) (4th ed.). New York:

(20) Maimonides, M. (n.d.). *Igeret aRambam ZaL to R. Shmuel Ibn Tabon Zal im tshuvot al sheelotav* [A letter from Maimonides RIP to R. Shmuel Ibn Tavon RIP with answers to his questions]. Retrieved from http://www.daat.ac.il/daat/vl/rambamuvno/rambamuvno18.pdf

(21) Harevi, Z. (1988). *Sefer hayovel leShlomo Pines bimlot lo shmonim shana* [Shlomo Pines jubilee volume on the occasion of his eightieth birthday]. Jerusalem: Mandel Institute for Jewish studies.

(22) Freudenthal, G., & Zonta, M. (2012). Avicenna among medieval Jews the reception of Avicenna's philosophical, scientific and medical writings in Jewish cultures, east and west. *Arabic Sciences and Philosophy, 22*(2), 217.

(23) Schwartz, D. (2000). Avicenna and Maimonides on immortality: A comparative study. In: R. Nettler (ed.) *Medieval and modern perspectives on Muslim-Jewish relations* (pp. 185–197). Hardwood Academic Publishers.

(24) Zadik, S. (2018). *Bikoret amada aaristoteli shel R. Hasdai Kreshkash vesifro aavud shel Avner miborgos* [Rabbi Ḥasdai Crescas' critique of Aristotelian science and the lost book of Abňer of Burgos]. *Tarbiz, 77*(a), 133–155. Retrieved from http://www.jstor.org/stable/23607180

(25) Zaimeche, S. (2017). The impact of Islamic science and learning on England. *Muslim Heritage.* Accessed February 20, 2021 at https://muslimheritage.com/islamic-science-learning-england/

(26) Leuprecht, P. (2012). Second Stage–Faith and Reason. In *Reason, Justice and Dignity* (pp. 31–73). Brill Nijhoff.

## Short Biography of Michael Such

The President of the Israeli Avicenna association who has written many medical articles and researchers in the fields of Oriental and Chinese medicine that have been published in country's such as the republic of Uzbekistan, Israel and in the Russian federation.

For his medical and research work, he has been given recognition and awards from the republic of Uzbekistan many times. An honored professor from the Ibn Sina Bukhara state medical university of Bukhara.

A lecture Professor at the "East West" college Israel. Dental DS, Senior degree. A member of the European Traditional Chinese Medicine Association (ETCMA) and a member of the Israeli Chinese fellowship and in the US fellowship AAAOM. Former Chief department of dermatology psoriasis. Chinese endocrinology and gynecology.

Ferdi Koç, Assoc. Prof.

# Comparison of the "Cevâmi-u 'İlmi'l-Mûsikā" Section in Ibn Sīnā's Kitabu's-Shifa with Abdulkādir Meragi's Câmiu'l-Elhan in Terms of Musical Theory[1]

## 1. Introduction

Although studies on the theory of music in the Turkish-Islamic world began to appear at the end of the 8th century, 11th centuries appear to be the period in which extensive and valuable works were written. For the first time in the Turkish-Islamic world, the physical and mathematical principles of music have been emphasized by the translation of the works on Greek music theory into Arabic. The works of the Greeks on the music theory serve as the basis for the relationships of the music theory in the Islamic world, especially in the relations of music-mathematics and music-physics. This issue is clearly understood in the works of music theory written by Kindî (d. 874), Fârâbî (d. 950), İhvân-ı Safâ (X. cent.) and Ibn Sīnā (980/1037).

Our research is based on the comparative analysis of the "*Cevâmiu İlmi'l-Mûsikā*" section in Ibn Sīnā's *Kitâbü'ş-Şifâ* and Abdülkādir-i Merâgî's *Câmiu'l-Elhân* in terms of musical theory. In our study, both the Greek music theory, which Ibn Sīnā benefited from in her musical theory, and the contributions of later period music scholars such as Kindî and Fârâbî to theoretical studies, her own musical thought and theory will be discussed.

However, Safiyüddîn-i Urmevî, which is the basis of modern music theory, has given its final form with his additions to the seventeen interval system revealed in his works of music theory, the thought of the theology of Abdükādir-i Merâgî, which provides its intelligibility, system, the first and most important of the five works of music theory brought into existence through his contributions will be examined the system of theory in *Câmiu'l-Elhân*.

---

1 Assoc. Prof. Dr. Ferdi Koç, Sakarya. Üniv. State Conservatory. E-mail: fkoc@sakarya.edu.tr

The essence of our study consists of the comparative examination of the *Cevâmiu İlmi'l-Mûsikā* section written by Ibn Sīnā and *Câmiu'l-Elhân* written by Merâgî on his musical theory. In this comparative study; a comparative analysis of Ibn Sīnā and Merâgî's musical understanding will be made under the headings such as description of music, formation of sound, reasons of treble and pestiness, compatibility/incompatibility of intervals, intervals, sound sequences, transition (seyir), ikā and instruments.

In this study, it is aimed to reveal the differences in subjects such as change, progress, sound physics, and intervals on the subjects of music of the music scholar's Ibn Sīnā and Merâgî, who have a period of about four hundred years between them.

## 1.1. Ibn Sīnā and Works of Musical Theory

Ibn Sīnā was born in 980 in the village of Efşene near Bukhara. In order to express his extraordinary position in the world of science and philosophy, Islamic thinkers named him "Şeyhü'r-Reis", and medieval scholars and thinkers "prince of philosophers" and "avicenna" (Alper 1999:319). He trained himself very well in mathematics, geometry, philosophy, medicine, astronomy and religious sciences. He has also produced valuable works in the field of music, especially in medicine, philosophy, religious sciences. In the field of music, Ibn Sīnā has devoted chapters to music in three encyclopedic works and has opened titles in some of his treatises. Encyclopedia sections and treatises include:

1. "*Cevâmiu İlmi'l-Mûsikā*" section in *Kitâbü'ş-Şifâ*
2. "Muhtasar fî İlmi'l-Mûsikā"section in *Kitâbü'n-Necât*
3. Department of music at *Dâniş-nâme-i 'Âlâî*

Along with these chapters, there are valuable information about music in the treatises called Risâle fi'l-Hurûf, Risâle fi'n-Nefs, Risâle fi Beyâni Aksâmi'l-Ulûm li Hikemiyye ve'l-Akliyye, el-Kânûn fi't-Tıbb (Turabi 2004: IV).

Ibn Sīnā used the mûsikî works of Kindî, İhvân-ı Safâ and especially Fârâbî as a source in his music writings along with the famous Greek scholars such as Aristo, Themistius, Öklid (Can 2001:11). He accepted Fârâbî's musical system, applied it and turned it into a theory. He made valuable studies on sound, the source of sound, the treatment aspect of music, and astrology.

### 1.2. Abdülkādir Merâgî and Works of Musical Theory

Abdülkādir-i Merâgî's the date of his birth is not certain and it is shown in the sources between years 1340–1350. He was born in Meraga, Southern Azerbaijan, within the borders of present-day Iran. He first learned many sciences and music from his father. He left Meraga at a young age and went to Tabriz, where he became famous for musical knowledge and performance. It was protected by Sultan Şeyh Üveys (1356–1374), Sultan Celâleddin Hüseyin (1374–1382), Sultan Ahmed Bahâdır (1382–1410), the rulers of Celayir the period. In 1398 he was sent to Samarkand with the engagement given by Timur. After Timur's death, he was attracted by Sultan Halil (1405–1409). Due to the defeat of Sultan Halil to his brother Şahrûh (1405–1447) in the struggle for power, he migrated to Herat, the center of Science and art of the period. Merâgî, who became more famous for composing Nevbet-i Müretteb during his time, organized makam and ikā cycles on musical theory and invented instruments. However, the following six musical writing works have been produced:

1. *Câmiü'l-Elhân*
2. *Makāsidü'l-Elhân*
3. *Kenzü'l-Elhân*
4. *Risâle-i Fevâid-i Aşere*
5. *Şerh-i Kitabü'l-Edvâr*
6. *Zübdetü'l-Edvâr*

Merâgî died in a plague epidemic in Herat in 1435.

## 2. Comparison of the "Cevâmiu İlmi'l-Mûsikā" Section in İbn Sīnā's Kitâbü'ş-Shifâ With Abdülkādir Merâgî's Câmi u'l- Elhân in Terms of Musical Theory

### 2.1. Definition of Music

Ibn Sīnā music, "It is a mathematical science that investigates sounds in terms of whether they are compatible with each other and the time periods between these sounds in order to know how a melody is composed. This description of music implies that it covers two areas of research. The first of these is the study of the states of sounds, this part is called composition. The second area of research is the time periods between sounds. This part is called rhythm (ikā)." identifies with his statement (Turabi 2004: 6)

Merâgî, in his work, firstly describes the definition of Fârâbî: "the meaning of music is tunes. The tune is called a variety of sound groups, sorted in a specific format. The same way (but) certain style of sound groups are also given this name. Through these arranged and composed sound groups, the letters that form poetic words that are poured into a particular form of poetry and mediate a number of general topics are connected together." his statement, later Safiyüddîn-i Urmevî's definition: "It is a limited and appropriately arranged form of various, limited tunes." he has stated. Merâgî also referring to the description of Ibn Sīnā in his work "Some of the scholars also said that the science of music consists of the science of mathematics, which talks about harmony within itself or how the irregular gaps seen between times are harmonized, and some said that this science consists of instrumental and human arts that improve (correct) harmonies and harmonies." wrote his description (Sezikli 2007:88). When the definitions of music of Ibn Sīnā and Merâgî were examined, Ibn Sīnā made a technical definition in the form of mathematical expression of the compatibility of sounds and periods between sounds, and Merâgî, in particular, took Fârâbî and Safiyuddin-I Urmevi as sources and defined music as a collection of harmonious sounds of poems, provided that the periods between sounds (ikā) remained the same.

## 2.2. The Reasons of Sound Hıghness and Lowness

In Ibn Sīnā's work, it is stated that the reasons for the shrillness of sound are the tension of the wire, the strength, the smoothness of the surface, the frequency of wave particles in the air, and the reasons for pestiness are the exact opposite. However, the shortness, hardness, tension and smoothness of the wire, the narrowness of the air outlet in the wind instruments, its proximity to the blowing place are the reasons for its highness; The looseness, length, roughnÃÅess of the wire, its flexibility, the width of the void volume in which the air circulates in blown instruments, the distance from the blowing place to the point where the air comes out are the reasons for sound lowness (Turabi 2004:7).

Merâgî mentions in works that the shortness, thinness and tension of the strings are the reason for sound highness, and the length, thickness and looseness are the reasons for sound lowness. In blown instruments, the hardness of the breath blown, the location of the sound being blown close to the place, the narrowness of the hole blown and the space of air circulating in the instrument are recorded as the reason for the highness, the reverse has been noted as the cause of lowness. Merâgî also added that moisture in the string will cause lowness in strings (Sezikli 2007:98).

When the expressions of Ibn Sīnā and Merâgî on highness and lowness are compared, they are similar and complementary to each other. Merâgî explained this issue at length and the fact that the moisture in the stringed instrument causes lowness is not found in Ibn Sīnā's work.

## 2.3. Congruence and Incompatible Intervals

Ibn Sīnā has long described the state of congruence and incompatıble of sound intervals in his work. That is to say, two voices at the same high and low pitch do not create (notes) intervals. Interval occurs between two voices with different highness and lowness levels. If this occurring sound range leaves a nice effect on the ear, it is congruence; if it leaves an ugly effect, it is incompatible. The compatibility between the two sounds can be explained as follows: "Each of the two voices has a mathematical equivalent. If the value of the range between two sounds corresponds to an integer, the sounds are compatible, and if the range does not correspond to an integer, the sounds are incompatible." The reason for congruence is arithmetic in the form of integer multiples of the ratio of one sound to another sound, but providing the arithmetic ratio without having to be integer is the first reason for congruence. Ibn Sīnā, on the other hand, referred to Pythagoras as saying that he could establish compatibility in alternative (without integer) ratios. Here, Ibn Sīnā explains that the reason for congruence is mainly due to the fact that the ratio of two sound ranges is certain (Turabi 2004:11). Merâgî made similar remarks with Ibn Sīnā on the issue of congruence and incompatible. In addition to Ibn Sīnā's views, Fârâbî and Safiyüddîn-i Urmevî's views were included. Merâgî used the expressions interval quantity and relation instead of the merital interval ratio (Sezikli 2007:94).

## 2.4. Types of Compatible Intervals (Bakiye, Mücennep, Tanini, Quaternary, Quintet, Octave)

Ibn Sīnā divided the compatible intervals into three classes. These are: large, medium, and small ranges. Large intervals are intervals in which each of the notes is more than the other. These octave intervals are called as (ellezi bi'l-küll).

The middle intervals are the intervals with the greatest difference in fractional value between the two notes. Between these two notes there are ratios such as ½, 1/3, ¼, 1/6. The most used in this interval type is the quintet ratio of 2/3 and the quadrant interval ratio of ¾.

Small intervals are small intervals from the quadruple interval. These are called as lahni interval. These are called such as: tanini, mücennep, bakiye (Turabi 2004:15).

Merâgî examined the issue of compatible intervals in more detail in three classes, major, medium and minor, such as Ibn Sīnā. The smallest unit of this is called the bakiye range, two bakiye ranges with mücennep, three bakiye ranges with tanini range obtained. Ibn Sīnā's 2/3 quintet and ¾ quintet range has given more detailed explanation. Merâgî, referring to Safiyüddîn, combined two tanini of the full quadruple range and one tanini of one bakiye or two tanini together in different combinations, gave a frequency value of 498 cents, and revealed a range of three tanini and one bakiye range and two tanini with a frequency value of 702 cents in a full quintuple compatible range of 2/3. From here, Merâgî revealed a range of 7 full quads and 13 full quintets (Sezikli 2007:67).

It is understood from this that Ibn Sīnā actually described the foursome and the five revealed by Merâgî in a more closed expression.

Ibn Sīnā and Merâgî explained the octave interval in two different ways, starting with the small intervals and explaining the four and five intervals. Ibn Sīnā in his work completely tanini and bakiye intervals, combining different combinations of four and fives intervals to create an octave interval here refers to Pythagoras (Turabi 2004:54). Merâgî combined the quartets and quintets in a way of creating a richer interval using the bakiye and the mücennep and tanini intervals, creating melodically richer octave intervals (Sezikli 2007:68), he has taken Safiyüddîn Urmevî system to further. Merâgî combined the full quadruple and quintet intervals to form the fully congruent twelve sequences, which were later called the twelve maqams, while Ibn Sīnā here created six fully congruent sequences, as he used only the bakiye and tanini intervals. Ibn Sīnā named the intervals of four and five as genus, and Merâgî called the interval of four-five "buud".

## 2.5. İntikāl (Melodic Progression)

Ibn Sīnā explained the subject of c as follows: "the sequencing of the notes in the octave range" (Turabi 2004:57). Ibn Sīnā define intikāl as moving from low to high in melodic progression descending intikāl, from high to low in melodic progression ascendant intikal. Starting from the middle voices, high and low sounds are called as descending - ascendant intikāl. Descending and ascendant avengāl Ibn Sīnā said that it was done in two forms of direct and rotational transition. If the return is one time, it is called "single spinner intikāl", and if it happens many times, it is called "consecutive spinner intikāl" (Turabi 2004:57).

Merâgî described the subject of avengāl as similar, referring to Fârâbî, Ibn Sīnā and Safiyüddîn-i Urmevî (Sezikli 2007:214).

## 2.6. Îkā

Ibn Sīnā describes the subject of Îkā in his work as follows: "Îkā is an appreciated measure for the time of the innings in nature. Îkā is melodic if voiced, if the letters are laid out poetry." In other words, short or long times are entered between equal times. Every repetition of these in a given period has been considered as an ikā period. In ikā, the palpable time interval between two beats is considered unit time. When the second strike is struck, the feeling of the first strike is lost, and the multiples of this unit time interval become the multiples of the times that fall between the strike intervals. When the syllables in the beats are closed, the sound is turned off but when it remains open it is connected to the other beat. The syllable being open as closed sâkin is named with hareke. Sâkin letters are nun, be, te, cim, dal, tı, kaf, kef, lam, mim. Hareke extension letters are elif, vav, ye. For example, if ten is a sâkin stroke, then ten is also a moving stroke. Also there is no single time for tâ and ten hits. Sâkin's time from nu to ten, with hareke te time's 1.5 times becomes. After making these technical diagnoses, Ibn Sīnā named the time of te as light, the time of ten as heavy light, the time of tâ as light heavy, and the time of târen as heavy. Ibn Sīnā considered the time of heavy as a unit time, and stated that this time would not change in an ikā cycle, and that the execution of an ikā cycle with a different version was called tad'if. Ibn Sīnā here also expressed the patterns of aruz through the periods of ikā (Turabi 2004:62).

Ibn Sīnā explained the types of ikā used during his period after giving the basic information about ikā. The types of ikā are divided into muvassal and mufassal. Muvassal ones are hafif, sakil hafif, hafif sakil and sakil. Hafif is folded by sakil, sakil are the solid power of hafif. So they are interchangeably. Mufassal is the strokes made by entering times at different times between units of time in an ikā cycle. Examples of these beats such as tenen tenen, ten ten ten ten, tân tân tân tân were diversified by Ibn Sīnā (Turabi 2004:81).

Merâgî, in his work on the subject of ikā, said of Fârâbî, "Îkā is to appreciate the times of strokes. The amount and proportion at certain times is to go to certain tunes" and Safiyüddîn Urmevî's "Îkā is the whole of the beats, and there are certain –equal Times - of the amount between them. This time and times, the accuracy and equality of a right tab'ı selim (talent from creation) with the balance you can notice the "he described in the form of (Sezikli 2007:225). He has not made any original identification. Merâgî explained that ikā was related to the poetry measure, using aruz patterns of beats, as Ibn Sīnā did. He explained that the strike times consisted of three elements: sebep, fasila and veted. On the basis of the Ikā elements "reason is two: sebeb-i sakîl, sebeb-i hafif. Sebeb-i sâkil, as in the word tene consists of two movements. Because, in here both of the two strokes are hareke. In sebeb-i hafif, as seen in the following example, the first letter is hareke, the second is sâkin: ten. Veted also has two types: veted-i mecmû, veted-i mefrûk. The first two letters of Veted-i mecmû are hareke, the last letter is sâkin. They say veted-i mecmû because the hareke of this is somewhere. The first letter of the Veted-i mefrûk is hareke and the middle letter is sâkin. Like tân. The reason it is called reserved is that the letter sâkin is located between the two harake. There are in fâsıla two parts: the first is fâsıla-yı suğrâ as in the following example, the first three of the four letters of the last letter of hareke is sâkin: tenenen. Fâsıla-yı kübrâ, as in the following example, the first four of the five letters of hareke and the last one is sâkin: tenenenen" told with sentences (Sezikli 2007:226). Merâgî also explained the subject of muvassal and mufassal ikā in more detail, as in the work of Ibn Sīnā. The cycles of the ikā named sakîl-i evvel, sakîl-i sânî, sakîl hafif, remel, hafîfü'r-remel and hezec were described as described in the books before him. Later ikā cycles used in his own period sakîl, hafîf, çıhâr-darb, türkî-i asıl, muhammes-i râh kerd, remel ve hezec çenber strokes are shown. In addition, Merâgî also described the strokes of îkā cycles Darbü'l-feth, devr-i şâhî, devr-i kumriye, darbü'l-cedîd ve devr-i mieteyn, which is his invention (Sezikli 2007:229).

We should say that the subject of ikā in the works of Ibn Sīnā and Merâgî is essentially the same when compared. A closed explanation is made due to the use of ikā cycles in execution in the process during the period of Ibn Sīnā's recipes. In Merâgî's work, Merâgî style is more understandable since it was understood during the period of ikā cycles and found its value in execution. Later uses on the six basic strokes described by Ibn Sīnā, Merâgî also demonstrated the ikā cycles and the strokes of his own found ikā cycles.

## 2.7. Instruments

Ibn Sīnā has opened a valuable chapter in his work under the title music instruments. He described instruments as follows: "instruments are divided into different parts. Some of them have strings and fret that are played, such as" tanbur "and" barbat" (oud). Some of them have strings and no frets. These varieties "şahrud", "zü'l-ankâ" and "feceste" at strings like grows on the surface of the instrument; and "sanc" ve "silyak" like strings of the instrument the gap grows between the two sides, and the third part is have the strings and frets as "rebap" they played like a drawn bow, those with no strings but blown from one end like "mizmar", hand-blown instruments such as "mizmârü'l-cerâb" (torbalı mizmâr, gayda, tulum), known as "surnay", which are blown through the hole, such as "yerâ'a". Sometimes it is made by integrating into one another, as in the

Greek instrument known as "ergûn". It is possible to invent instruments such as "Sanc" struck with sticks" he describes the subject of instrument with his sentences. On the other hand, he mentions that the most famous instrument since the past is the oud. In his work he talks about the performance of the oud instrument and how it is used in music theory (Turabi 2004:108).

Merâgî has also opened a department under the name of music instruments. In this section, especially after the human larynx, the most perfect instrument is the Ud-ı Cedîd, where ten wires are connected. There is no doubt that the use of oud as an instrument of musical theory for centuries has an important effect. On the other hand, he divided the instruments into three classes: stringed, blown and percussion. He gives technical information about how these instruments are made and how they are played, which he has divided into three classes in his work (Sezikli 2007:217). When this is taken into account, Merâgî examined the instruments in great detail according to Ibn Sīnā. The development of music performance and the passing of at least four centuries has an important role in the formation of the instruments here.

Merâgî instruments are divided into three classes:

Stringed instruments: Ûd-ı kâmil, ûd-ı kadîm, tarabu'l-feth, şeştây, tarabrûd, tanbur-ı şirveniyân, tanbûre-i Mogolî, rûh-efzây, kopuz-ı Rûmî, Evzân, nây-ı tanbûr, rebâb, muğnî, çeng, egri, kânun, kemânçe, gijek, yektây, terentây, sâz-ı dolab, sâz-ı gâibî-i murassâ, tuhfetü'l-ûd, şidirgû, pipa, yatugan, şahrûd, rûd-ı hânî.

Blown instruments: Nây-ı sefîd, zemr-i siyeh nây, surnây, nây-ı balabân, nây-ı çâver, nefîr, burgu, mûsikār, çıpçık, organon, nây-ı enbân.

Percussion instruments: Sâz-ı kâsât, sâz-ı tâsât, sâz-ı elvâh-ı fülâd.

## 3. Conclusion

As a result of the research, the "*Cevâmiu İlmi'l-Mûsikā*" section in Ibn Sīnā's *Kitâbü'ş-Şifâ* and Abdülkādir-i Merâgî's *Câmiu'l-Elhân* were compared in terms of musical theory. It was understood that Ibn Sīnā benefited from the works of previous music scholars such as El-Kindî and Fârâbî along with Grek philosophers like Pisagor while writing his work.

Abdülkādir-i Merâgî was writing his in work, it is obvious that he benefited from the works of music scholars such as Kindî, Fârabî, Safiyüddîn-i Urmevî ve Kutbuddîn-i Şirâzî, and therefore his research area was wider. This is because Ibn Sīnā wrote the work about four centuries later.

In comparing the two works in terms of musical theory, it was revealed that Ibn Sīnā's statements had to be explained because the development of musical performance had just begun. In Merâgî's statements, however, it was observed that the subjects of fret, ikā, cycle, were transferred more to musical performance, as it was more understandable and reciprocated during the period of musical theory and playing system.

In terms of musical terminology and system of expressions in Ibn Sīnā's work as a last word, it can be said that it was the second work after Fârâbî in the beginning as a contribution to the establishment of music theory into a certain system.

## References

Alper, Ömer Mahir (1999). İbn Sînâ. Encylopedia of Islam. İstanbul: Turkey Religious Foundation, vol. 20, p. 319.

Can, Cihat (2001). XV. Yüzyıl Türk Mûsikîsi Nazariyatı (Ses Sistemi) [Unpublished Doctoral Dissertation]. İstanbul: Marmara Univ. Social Sciences Institue, p. 11.

Sezikli, Ubeydullah (2007). Abdülkadir Merâgî ve Câmiu'l-Elhân'ı. [Unpublished Doctoral Dissertation]. İstanbul: Marmara Univ. Social Sciences Institue, pp. 20–238.

Turabi, Ahmet Hakkı (2004). Mûsikî-İbn Sinâ (Translation). İstanbul: Litera Publication, pp. IV-108.

## Short Biography of Ferdi Koç

He was born in Adapazarı,1977, TURKEY. He began Turkish music education in Sakarya Music Association in 1992. He took oud lessons from Necati Çelik in İstanbul. He graduated the Electronic and Computer Education Department of Sakarya University in 1999. Between the years of 1999 and 2012,in Bakırköy Music Conservatory Foundation, he benefited from Nevzat Atlığ, Fatih Salgar, Faruk Salgar ve Cengizhan Sönmez. He became research assistant in Conservatory Department of Sakarya University in 2000. In 2003,he completed his higher education thesis, headed "Musical Analysis of the Sultan III.(3rd)'s Compositions";in Marmara University Turkish Religious Music Department and in 2010, his doctoral thesis,headed `the role and importance of Abdulaziz b. Abdulkadir Meragi and his Nekavetu'l-Edvar music book in Turkish Music Theory. In 2012, he became assistant professor in Sakarya University State Conservatory Turkish Music Department. In 2015, He became an associate professor of music / performance (oud). He participated in lots of concerts in our country and abroad. Ferdi Koç, married Selma Füsun Koç, is a academic staff in Sakarya University State Conservatory Turkish Music Department and he has been doing academic researches on Turkish music.

Peter Starr, Ph.D.

# Alchemical Texts Ascribed to Ibn Sīnā and the Role of Alchemy in Science

**Abstract:** Although Ibn Sīnā's *Kitāb aš-Šifā'* (Book of the Healing) contains a clear refutation of alchemical transmutation, it presents some ideas which were beloved of alchemists. There is also one treatise, strongly influenced by Abū Bakr ar-Rāzī's alchemy, which is ascribed to Ibn Sīnā from an early date. Perhaps, at least during one period of the great philosopher's life, he believed in and studied alchemy? A good question, to which I give the good answer that we do not know, at least not with certainty. A reading of the treatise, called *Fī al-Amr al-mastūr*, leads to the question of how much we believe ar-Rāzī could have been formative in the development of Ibn Sīnā's thought, and to the recognition that the treatise contrasts with known works of our author. On the other hand, open admiration for ar-Rāzī as theologian and alchemist was forbidden in polite society, so a hidden dimension of Ibn Sīnā's life is not impossible. In general I will argue that, illicit though it often was, alchemy was more widespread and influential than many people recognize.

**Keywords:** Ibn Sīnā, Avicenna, Alchemy, *Kitāb aš-Šifā'*, Book of the Healing, *Fī al-Amr al-mastūr.*

## Introduction

Ibn Sīnā (Avicenna) is occasionally referred to in the books of Georg Agricola (m. AD 1555), who is known as 'the father of mineralogy'. For example, in a book on the causes of rocks and minerals, Georg Agricola disputes Ibn Sīnā's statement that stones can form through a 'power' in water:

> Then Avicenna states that there is some kind of power (virtue), which makes stones from waters poured into its vessel, and from its motives and sources. But he never properly explains what this power is.[1]

1 Deinde Avicenna afferit vim quandam esse, quae ex aquis propter suum alveum effusis, et ex animantibus atque stirpibus efficiat lapides. Sed que sit ea vis nequaquam satis explicit. (*De ortu et causis subterraneorum*, 1546, IV, p. 55, lines 12–15.)

Ibn Sīnā mentions this theory of 'vis' (power, virtue) in *Kitāb aš-Šifā'* (Book of the Healing) in these words: "We know therefore that in that ground there must be a congealing, petrifying virtue which converts the liquid to the solid." A little later Ibn Sīnā continues: "[like salt, it is] transformed by heat, and in that the advent of heat coagulates them. Or it may be that the virtue is yet another, unknown to us."[2] This is the uncertainly about the theory which the German expert on mines and minerals noted.

Naturally, Georg Agricola knew only the works of Avicenna found in Latin translation. He has in mind a concise treatise, which in the Latin West had been detached from Ibn Sīnā's great *Book of the Healing*, and shortened under the name *De congelatione et conglutinatione lapidum*.[3] It is in fact two chapters from *Kitāb aš-Šifā'*.[4] To be precise, this treatise is two chapters from the Natural Sciences section, Subject (*Fann*) 5, Discourse (*Maqāla*) 1, Chapters (*Faṣl*) 1 and 5. Chapter 1 gives an account of the congelation and conglutination of stones (from which the Latin treatise as a whole gets its name), and on the cause of mountains, while Chapter 5 lists the four species of mineral, followed by a

---

2 فعلمنا أيضًا أنّ لتلك الأرض قوّة معدنيّة تحيل السيال إلى الجمود . . . تتقلّب بمعاونة الحرارة فلمّا يصيبه الحرّ يعقّده أو قوّة أخرى مجهولة عندنا

Madkūr (ed.), *Kitāb aš-Šifā'*, Nat. Sciences 5.1.1, p. 4:6–7, 12–13. In the Holmyard/Mandeville ed., p. 72.12–73.1, 6–7.

3 In the West, *Kitāb aš-Šifā'* was circulated as different books. Best known were parts of the Logic, the first parts of the Natural Sciences (called *Suffientia*), the Psychology (*De anima*), and the Metaphysics. The transmission of Ibn Sīnā's mineralogy is further complicated by the fact that it was often placed after Aristotle's *Meteorologica*, and this book, called *Mineralia*, then sometimes passed as a work of Aristotle.

4 The Natural Sciences section of *Kitāb aš-Šifā'* begins with physics in general, then the heavens, then generation and corruption in the sublunary world, then the qualities, then meteorology, then stones, minerals and chemicals, then psychology, then plants and animals. It is notable that chemistry is connected with the weather, as it was even in Aristotle's *Meteorologica* (although Aristotle did not write Book 4, on the generation of minerals, which is the relevant book for our topic). The reason for the connection with meteorology is that it was believed that, in the order of generation, the subtler, atmospheric qualities came first, and led to the generation of matter. In the context of Arabic-Islamic science, and certainly for the alchemists, the most influential book on this subject was the translation of pseudo-Apollonius, *Sirr al-ḫalīqa* (Secret of the Creation), also known as *al-'Ilal* (Causes). See: Ursula Weisser (ed.), *Buch über Geheimnis der* Schöpfung, 1979. The influence of this book on the Jābir ibn Ḥayyān books was demonstrated by Paul Kraus, *Jābir ibn Ḥayyān* (1942). For a collection of passages on the generation of minerals relevant to this Arabic pseudo-Apollonius tradition, see: Fabian Käs, *Kitāb al-Maqāṣid* (2015), Kommentar.

refutation of the alchemists' main aim, which was transmutation, for example of lead to gold. Ibn Sīnā says that they cannot change one metal into another.[5]

We have said that *Kitāb aš-Šifā'*, written in the early AD 1020s, refutes the main aim of alchemy. This does not mean that at another time, probably earlier, the author did not have different views which were controversial and from which he distanced himself. Could Ibn Sīnā have been engaged in alchemy and been influenced by its claims? In modern scholarship arguments in favour of such an idea have been discredited, although respectable external evidence exists.[6] In the forefront are the various alchemical treatises ascribed to Ibn Sīnā, some clearly false, and only two need attract our attention. *Risala Fī al-Amr al-mastūr* (On the Hidden Matter) is listed as Ibn Sīnā's work in the anonymous Longer Bibliography, written before AD 1192. The work was translated into Latin as a work of Ibn Sīnā within 150 years of the philosopher's death in AD 1036. There is what may amount to internal evidence of an engagement with alchemy in the certainly authentic *Kitāb aš-Šifā'*, so we need to look at the relevant Discourse (*Fann* 1, *Maqāla* 1) in more detail.[7] We can mention also *Fī aṣ-Ṣinā'a al-'āliya* (On the Exalted Art), which is not listed in old bibliographies, but which has strong similarities to *Fī al-Amr al-mastūr.*

I will briefly describe how Ibn Sīnā's views took their place in the polemics which surrounded alchemy from the outset. Most later authors, but not 'Abd al-Laṭīf al-Baġdādī, saw Ibn Sīnā as an opponent of the alchemists. Switching

---

5 Before leaving the subject of the Latin version of the chapters under discussion, we note that Chapters 2, 3, 4, and 6 (on the weather, seas and rivers, and earthquakes, and, in the last chapter, on continents, the sun, and climates). Holmyard/Mandeville describe this passage, which begins "sciant artificies alchemiae. . ." (those who practice alchemy. . .), as 'celebrated' (p. vi). In fact it was a well-known pssage in the context of polemics surrounding alchemy both in the West and in the East.

6 Opponents are Julius Ruska ("Die Alchemie des Avicenna," *Isis* no. 60, 1934), and Manfred Ullmann (*Die Natur- and Geheimwissenschaften*, 'betrachte ich. . . ihre Unechtheit als erwiesen', p. 223.1–2). Dimitri Gutas, in view of testimony in the Long Bibliography, includes *Fī al-Amr al-mastūr* in his list of Ibn Sīnā's works as a 'pseudepigraph, to be authenticated' (*Avicenna and the Aristotelian Tradition*, 2014 revised ed, p. 459). I do not rule out the possibility that Georges Anawati (Encycopedia of the History of Arabic Sciences, Vol. 3, 'Alchemy') was right that Ibn Sīnā could have believed in alchemy, at least at a period some time before AD 1020. The main supporter of the authenticity of *Fī al-Amr al-mastūr* and *Fī aṣ-Ṣinā'a al-'āliya* is Harry E. Stapleton et al. ("Two Alchemical Treatises," *Ambix*, vol. 10.2, 1962, p. 42.14–15).

7 In Latin *Fī al-Amr al-mastūr* was known as *Ad Hasan Regem Epistola de re recta* (the 'straight' thing, a mistranslation).

to a broader perspective, I will suggest that alchemy was a close companion to mainstream science in the Muslim world, closer even than it was to science during the Renaissance in Europe. This fact makes it likely that Ibn Sīnā met many of its practitioners. Whether Ibn Sīnā entirely endorsed the alchemists' enthusiastic claims to mastery over nature is unlikely, but ultimately unknown.

## *AŠ-ŠIFĀ'*, Part I.5: Agreements and Differences with the Alchemists[8]

In the first chapter (*aš-Šifā'*, Natural Sciences, 5.1.1) Ibn Sīnā says that rocks are formed either by a process of pot-baking (*tafaẖẖur*), or by congelation (*jumūd*). As a result one class of rock is earthy, the other watery. While he clearly has sedimentary rocks in mind for the first, the second, that from 'congelation', needs more explanation. This kind of rock is generated from water in a process like distillation (*yuqaṭṭar*). It forms on surfaces, like salt crystals. It is here that Ibn Sīnā gives his theory of 'mineral power' noted at the beginning of this paper: in certain places, he says, earth (*arḍ*) has a power to transform the water into stone by causing an earthy quality to dominate.

Ibn Sīnā then says that this process is also like the compounding of two waters (liquids) into a solid, and he gives the example of alchemists making "what they may choose to call the virgin's milk". [9] This must be a reference to the precipitation of a white solid, interpreted by Ibn Sīnā as a solidification which he goes on to compare with fossilization. We note that the philosopher has some familiarity with alchemical terms, although he describes alchemists as 'errant' and frowns on the phantastical names they use.

This leads to a discussion, in the same terms, of fossilization. This is explained as happening quite quickly, as when an object falls into a salt-pan it is 'mastered' by the substance, so that it becomes salt. Even quicker is when an object falls into fire and becomes fire. Ibn Sīnā mentions a volcanic area in Arabia where he saw a loaf which had thus petrified. One anecdote leads to others, and Ibn Sīnā mentions a meteorite he saw, one seen by his student al-Jūzjānī and Maḥmūd of Ġazna, and a large meteorite seen by Sheikh Abū Manṣūr ibn Mašakzār. Important from our perspective is that the philosopher mentions that in Ḫwārazm he experimented on a 'coppery' meteorite which

8 I am basing this section mainly on the footnotes of Holmyard/Mandeville's edition and translation: *Avicennae De congelatione et conglutinatione lapidum*.

9 شيء يتّخذه قوم ضلّوا في حيلهم يسمّونه لبن العذراء
Madkūr (ed.), Nat. Sciences 5.1.1, p. 4.16.

produced a green smoke and eventually burnt to ash. Again, we take account of the fact that, at some point, Ibn Sīnā experimented with chemical substances. The chapter (5.1.1) concludes with an account of the formation of mountains.[10]

These chapters, all concerning the generation of what is under the heavens, continue with an account of rain and dew. Ibn Sīnā knows that rain is produced by distillation, and he says that mountains 'act like alembics of iron or glass. . . the earth is the pot below it, and springs are like the holes and beak. . .'[11] Mountains, cold because of their lack of stability (*qarār*), cause rainclouds to form. The vapours surrounding mountains also produce more metals than in other places (p. 12.8). Chapter 3 gives an account of water which emerges from the earth in the form of streams, wells, and marshes. Chapter 4 explains earthquakes mainly as disturbances caused by underground gases. Other reasons for earthquakes may come from above, for example eclipses (p. 18.19), or when mountains collapse on the earth. Here the authority of Archimedes is cited (p. 16.6), whereas Anaxagoras' ascription of causality to the motion of waters encircling the earth is rejected.[12] Chapter 5 is on how minerals come into being (*Fī takwīn al-maʿdaniyyāt*), and this is the chapter where we can expect the clearest indications of Ibn Sīnā's study of alchemy. Chapter 6 is a description of the inhabitable world (*al-maskūna*), with a focus on the effect of the sun on the seasons and climes. At the beginning of the chapter, the question of why the waters, which occupy three quarters of the world, do not dissolve the land, is answered by saying that this is the effect of the sun and other heavenly bodies.

Returning to the penultimate chapter, which we said would provide indications of Ibn Sīnā's studies, we find a section which recalls, in its terse schematic style, the beginning of ar-Rāzī's *Kitāb al-Asrār* (Book of Secrets). There

---

10 This section on physical geography is of great interest. It gives an account of both earthquakes and erosion in the formation of mountains. I had occasion to talk with the Turkish geologist Prof. Dr. Celal Şengör, and it was these passages which particularly impressed him. Ibn Sīnā notes that shells in the desert show that the earth had once been under the sea (similar conclusions were drawn by Xenophanes, and, among authors in Arabic, al-Biruni), and that stratified rock were formed over time by layers of petrified riverbed.

11 ويكون الجبل في حقنه الأبخرة وإلجائه إياها إلى فجر العيون مثل الإنبيق الصلب من حديد أو زجاج. . . وقعر الأرض التي تحته كالقرع والعيون كالمثاعب والأذناب التي في الأنابيق والأودية والبحار كالقوابل . . .
Madkūr, ed., Nat. Sc. 5.1.2, p. 11.3–4, 7–8.

12 One of the 'benefits of earthquakes' listed at the end is that they remind the evil of God's wrath.

is a four-part classification of solids in the earth: stones, fusible substances (*ḏā'ibāt*, mainly metals), sulphurs, and salts. These can be further divided into strong and weak, the strong being malleable (metals) or not (stones, etc.), while the weak are soluble in water or 'oily' and not easily dissolved. In this account the status of mercury is unique. Although it is weak, it forms the essential, watery element (*'unṣur*) present in all metals. The most 'earthy' element, sulphur, mixes with mercury to form all the other minerals. This statement shows that the philosopher subscribed to the 'sulphur-mercury theory', which has its roots in Arabic alchemy. The Jābir ibn Ḥayyān authors found and adapted it from pseudo-Apollonius (the *Secret of Creation* mentioned in footnote 4).[13] This passage represents a close connection between Ibn Sīnā and alchemical ideas.

Naturally-occurring white sulphur will be better than the sulphur of "those who have clever devices" (*ahl al-ḥīla*, alchemists), so it can produce silver or gold in the earth.[14] The author makes a clear distinction between natural processes, like the formation of gold in the earth, and natural substances, and the imitations of the alchemists. This is not only the main element of his criticism of alchemists at the end of the chapter, but it is also one point of unity with the other works ascribed to Ibn Sīnā on chemistry, as I will indicate below.

This statement leads directly to Ibn Sīnā's famous rejection of the main aim of alchemy:

> The alchemical qualities are not identical in principle or in perfection with the natural ones... alchemy falls short of nature in this respect and, in spite of great effort, cannot overtake her. As to the claims of the alchemists, it must be clearly understood that it is not in their power to bring about any true change of species. They can, however, produce imitations for the senses [*ḥissiyya*, Holmyard has *ḥasana*], dyeing the red [metal] white so that it closely resembles silver, or dyeing it yellow so that it closely resembles gold... Yet in these [dyed metals] the essential nature remains unchanged; they are merely... dominated by induced qualities... But the possibility of eliminating or imparting the specific difference has never been clear to me. On the contrary, I regard it as impossible, since there is no way of splitting up one combination into another. Those properties which are perceived by the senses are probably not the differences

13 Ibn Sīnā expresses the theory like this: *fa-yušbih 'an yakūn az-zi'baq aw mā yušbihuhū 'unṣur jamī' aḏ-ḏā'ibāt...* (Madkūr, ed., p. 21.15 f.): "It seems, moreover, that mercury, or something resembling it, is the essential constituent element of all the fusible bodies, for all of them are converted into mercury on fusion. Most of them, however, fuse only at a very high temperature, so that their mercury appears red."

14 Madkūr, ed., p. 22.2–5.

> which separate the metals into species, but rather accidents or consequences, the specific differences being unknown. And if a thing is unknown, how is it possible for anyone to endeavour to produce it or to destroy it?... If this is so, one metal cannot be converted into another unless the compound is broken up and converted into the composition of that into which its transformation is desired. This, however, cannot be effected by fusion, which maintains the union and merely causes the introduction of some foreign substance or virtue. [15]

Ibn Sīnā here distinguishes nature from art. As alchemists are not able to intervene deeply enough to know the true specific difference which separates one substance from another, it cannot be removed (*al-faṣl al-munawwi' yuslab*). They can only convince the senses with imitations of gold and silver by adding accidents. Ibn Sīnā does not deny that species can change. His earlier description of generation in nature by sulphur and mercury involved such changes. The experiments of adepts involve fusion, which is not the same.

In spite of this, the author expresses in this chapter ideas which are close to those of the alchemists. Although he expresses hostility to them, what we have seen in *aš-Šifā'* is not enough to conclude that he was never one of their number. Indeed, we have noticed that he knows alchemical terms well, and writes of experiments that he conducted.

We may ask at this point whether later Arab-Islamic writers saw Ibn Sīnā as an alchemist or not. It is striking that the 13th century philosopher 'Abd al-Laṭīf al-Baġdādī thinks of Ibn Sīnā as a believer in alchemy. He writes "the most forcible of those who misled me was Ibn Sīnā, through his book on this Craft

---

15 وإن لم تكن الأحوال الصناعيّة على الحكم الطبيعيّة وعلى صحّتها بل تكون مشابهة أو مقاربة لها إلّا أنّ الصناعة تقصر في ذلك عن الطبيعة ولا نلحقها وإن اجتهدت وأمّا ما يدّعيه أصحاب الكيمياء فيجب أن تعلم أنّه ليس في أيديهم أن يقلبوا الأنواع قلبًا حقيقيًّا لكن في أيديهم تشبيهات حسّيّة حتّى يصبغوا الأحمر صبغًا أبيض شديد الشبه بالفضّة ويصبغوا صبغًا أضفر شديد الشبه بالذهب

إلّا أنّ جواهرها تكون محفوظةً وإنّما يغلب عليها كيفيّات مستفادة

وأمّا أن يكون الفصل المنوّع يسلب أو يكسى فلم يتبيّن لي إمكانه بل بعيد عندي جوازه إذ لا سبيلَ إلى حلّ المزاج إلى المزاج الآخر فإن هذه الأحوال المحسوسة يشبه أن تكون هي الفصول التي بها تصير هذه الأجساد أنواعًا بل هي عوارض ولوازم وفصولها مجهولة وإذا كان الشيء مجهولًا كيف يمكن أن يُقصد قصد إيجاده أو إفقاده وأمّا سلخ هذه الأصباغ والأعراض من الروائح والأوزان أو كسوها فهذا ممّا لا يجب أن يُصرّ على جحده لفقدان العلم به فليس يقوم البتة برهان على امتناعه ويشبه أن تكون النسبة التي بين العناصر في تركيب كل جوهر من هذه المعدودة غيرها فى التركيب الآخر و إذا كان كذلك لم يعدّ إليه إلّا أن يفكّ التركيب إعادةً إياه إلى تركيب ما يراد إحالته إليه و ليس ذلك ممّا يمكن بأدائه حفظ الاتصال و إنّما يختلط به شيء غريب أو قوة غريبة

Madkūr, ed., p. 22.16–23.3, 5–14.

with which he supposedly perfects his philosophy."[16] This is surprising, as other writers consider Ibn Sīnā to be the prime witness against alchemy. In AD 1112, aṭ-Ṭuġrā'ī composed *Kitāb Ḥaqā'iq al-istišhād* (Truths of Citing Authorities), as a rebuttal of the refutation of the occult and alchemy written by Ibn Sīnā. Also al-Jaldakī wrote in reply to the philosopher. Most famously, Ibn Ḫaldūn dismisses alchemy as irreligious and akin to magic. He notes both that Ibn Sīnā states that transmuting metals is impossible, and that al-Fārābī accepted this possibility.[17] One can go so far as to say that in earlier times a lost polemic against the Art by al-Kindī was the leading assault on gold-making, and ar-Rāzī, at the beginning of *Kitāb al-Asrār*, says he refuted it. However, Ibn Sīnā became the most celebrated critic, taking the crown from al-Kindī. As a result, we see that the idea that our philospher could be an alchemist would be rejected by most writers of the Middle Ages in the East. 'Abd al-Laṭīf al-Baġdādī is an important exception.

However, before turning to other evidence, above all in the form of *Fī al-Amr al-mastūr*, an alchemical work ascribed to Ibn Sīnā, I want to introduce what I regard as the historical background to the question in hand. This requires a separate section. As the topic is wide-ranging, I will have to summarize.

## Alchemy's Role in the History of Arabic-Islamic Science

There were two translation movements in the history of Abbasid science. One is well-known, for the translators and scholars involved had access to the caliph, or at least to leading figures at his court. In this context, translators in Baghdad were able to provide the ruling class with works about geometry, notably Euclid, Galenic medicine, and Ptolemy's astrology and geography. Others, on the other hand, shared at a distance the state-sponsored passion for science. These men were gold and silversmiths, cloth-makers, scent and medicine makers, and other skilled craftsmen, in any case men who kept trade secrets. Their connections were more with the bazaar than with the palace. Their interests grew from what they knew; the processes on which their livings were based. They were neither fussy about the quality of the rapidly-accumulating alchemical translations, nor inclined to

---

16 Ibn Abī Uṣaybi'a, *'Uyūn al-anbā'* (1965, p. 685/637.) I have not had the opportunity to consult the new translation by Simon Swain et al., but am basing my information on Shawkat Toorawa, "A Portrait of 'Abd al-Laṭīf al-Baghdādī's Eduction and Instruction" (2004), p. 101.

17 These passages are detailed in the introduction of E. Holmyard and D. Mandeville, *Avicennae de congelatione*, p. 5–7, 11.

be sceptical when impressive authorities were cited, like Moses, Cleopatra, and Hermes. Egypt was the font of wisdom, and the translators could be from Upper Egypt,[18] but science now flourished in Islam.[19] Adepts arose in their ranks, but the works they wrote were typically under false names, and mainly under the name of Jābir ibn Ḥayyān, legendary pupil of the Imam Jaʿfar aṣ-Ṣādiq and mysterious mystics, and of a monk and heir of Morienus, who for years was said to have provided Jerusalem with gold bars at the time of Ḫālid ibn Yazīd.

These works ascribed to Jābir bear witness, from the earliest time, to a tendency to split into sects, ostensibly over such vexed issues as the value of organic elixirs. Jābireans would also branch out, and write about mathematics, Galenic medicine, astronomy, and religion. Opposed to the court, the early Jābireans, and many of the later ones, were Shi'ite. Contentious on many issues, they were nonetheless united in the belief that it was alchemy, as the isolation, manipulation and interpretation of substances, that provided the clues to how the kingdoms of the natural world came into being, and thus the clues to all science.[20]

The mid-9th century represents a development from the earliest period of Jābirean enthusiasm. A number of alchemists emerge as scholars in their own right. Above all there is Abū Bakr ar-Rāzī (m. circa AD 932), who cites Jābir as his authority, but who promoted a focused and precise approach to chemistry and gold-making. Muḥammad ibn Umayl (fl. mid-10th c.) rejected all but three of Jābir's books, and wrote polemics against men who called themselves Jābir,

18 Perhaps the translators were from Greek and Arabic-speaking towns of Egypt. See: Martin Plessner, *Vorsokratische Philosophie und griechische Alchemie...* (1975), p. 129–130, where the Egyptian 'Uṯmān al-Aḫmīmī is suggested as the author of this early book. The endurance of a tradition of alchemy in Aḫmīm is suggested by alchemists from the town and references in alchemical literature (I regret that I do not have my notes on this at present).

19 The attitude that science will flourish most in Islamic lands is clear in the following passage in *Musḥaf aṣ-ṣuwar*, a compilation and adaptation of passages from the Greek alchemist Zosimus, we find: "[Theosebeia] said: Tell me about the words of Maria, quoting her father, that: the nation in which this science will appear is at the end of time... [Zosimus] said: They are the sons of Ibrahim. She asked: The Jews? He said: No, they are the sons of Ismail. After one hundred and sixty years of their reign it will appear among them, though in the past no nation had disbelieved the sages as much as them... Great and glorious God will reveal it to them..." (f. 10a.8–9, 12–13) The reference is surely to Ismaili Shi'ism.

20 Paul Kraus edited *Kitāb al-Ḥudūd*, a classification of the sciences in which the master science is alchemy. See: "Studien zu Jābir ibn Ḥayyān," *Isis*, 1931, vol. 15.1.

or 'brothers of Jābir'.[21] These were among the first whose names are known. Many more are found later who, like ar-Rāzī, travelled in search of patrons, and offered to practice a range of the sciences. As is well known, he rose to fame as a physician throughout the Islamic lands, managing leading hospitals, and welcoming numerous students.

The unity which had characterized those Islamic lands came to an end, particularly after the Civil War of AD 811–813. Regional powers became rivals of the once uniquely blessed city of Baghdad. Scholars who had, like ar-Rāzī, begun their study of science with chemistry, but who had many strings to their bow, could find employment alongside those educated in court circles. What percentage of scientists where educated, and where, is hard to gauge. Certainly, by the time of ʿAbd al-Laṭīf al-Baġdādī (AD 1162–1231), alchemists were found as teachers of the sciences throughout the Muslim world. The standard education in law could be supplemented by reputed teachers who also practiced alchemy, mathematics, or medicine. ʿAbd al-Laṭīf gives his account of the progress of his own education in the *Tārīḫ*, written for his son. It survives in extracts in the work of Ibn Abī Uṣaybiʿa. Pursuing his religious studies in Damascus, the Baġdādī polymath was able to read works of Jābir ibn Ḥayyān, Ibn Waḥšiyya and Ibn Sīnā with the specialist in occult topics an-Nāʾilī. An-Nāʾilī's interest in the gold-making art attracted the enmity of his rivals.[22] Then in the year AD 1189, ʿAbd al-Laṭīf met another teacher in Mosul, Kamāl ad-Dīn Yūnus, a jurist and mathematician who was also interested in alchemy. Shortly after travelling with his Ayyūbid patrons to Cairo, ʿAbd al-Laṭīf studied with Yāsīn as-Simyāʾī, among others. However, a turning point came when he returned to Damascus around AD 1192, for he now found errors in his former spiritual mentor, Ibn Sīnā, stating as a reason for his change of mind that the philosopher was an alchemist, and he found alchemy to be false (*buṭlān al-kīmiyāʾ*).[23]

Earlier, in Muḥammad an-Nadīm's time, it was still possible to group all alchemists together, with most of their writings under the name of Jābir. For the purposes of his annotated bibliography called *al-Fihrist*, the book expert took the easy route, grouping the alchemists (except ar-Rāzī and Ibn Waḥšiyya)

---

21 In contrast to ar-Rāzī, Ibn Umayl's works are often, but not always, in the form of wandering allegorical poems, rather than concise prose. He quotes ar-Rāzī approvingly in *ad-Durra*. As this work shows, he was capable of writing concise recipes. A final note on ar-Rāzī: it seems that he never abandoned alchemy, for at the beginning of his most famous work, *Kitāb al-Asrār*, he notes that his death is near.

22 Toorawa, "A Portrait of ʿAbd al-Laṭīf," p. 103.22.

23 Toorawa, "A Portrait of ʿAbd al-Laṭīf," p. 106.11.

together at the end of his book. An-Nadīm records the legendary stories associated with the rise of alchemy and its transfer to Arab-Islamic science, but adds cautiously "God alone knows it, and, in mentioning them, we are free from blame and slander".[24]

Already before Ibn Sīnā's day alchemists were rubbing shoulders with more classically trained philosophers and men of science. One of an-Nadīm's informants was an alchemist. Contemporary with Ibn Nadīm, the translator and philosopher of the Būyid vizier Ibn Sa'dān, Yaḥya ibn 'Adī, is said to have worn a 'silver' ring made by an alchemist.[25]

Ibn Sīnā must have mixed with alchemists. This is surely made more likely by the fact that his father was an Ismā'īlī. On the other hand, we know that alchemy was a bone of contention among the rival teachers, whose varied background would be questioned and impugned if possible. There must have been a strong motive for writing forgeries defending alchemy, and ascribing them to recognized authorities. The work ascribed to Ibn Sīnā at an early date was either genuine, or can be explained as such a forgery. The same can be said for the apologia for alchemy written, allegedly, by Abū Naṣr al-Fārābī.[26]

The quest for mastery over nature, and the excitement this brought to the lives of those who believed such mastery realizable, must be regarded as a motivating factor in the inception and spread of scientific thought in the Arabic-Islamic world. The Jābireans were reading alchemy, but also Galen and Aristotle, in the 8th century, and according to Ibn Nadīm, Ḫālid ibn Yazīd was responsible for the first translation from Greek. The most obvious example of alchemy being important in the spread of science is the scholar Maslama al-Qurṭubī. This Andalusian scholar travelled to Basra where he became a member of the Ismā'īlī Brethren of Purity. Having contributed work on alchemy to their encyclopedia of science and Neo-Platonic philosophy, towards the end of the 10th century he returned to Spain, where he became the tutor of Caliph al-Ḥakam's son 'Abdullāh. He thus contributed to the beginning of a great flourishing of science in al-Andulus. On a broader scale, the lifetime of Maslama coincided with the rise of the Fāṭimids, whose early Imams claimed to have great knowledge and miraculous powers.

---

24 End of the introduction the the 10th and last section of *al-Fihrist*.

25 At-Tawḥīdī, *al-Imtā'*, 17th evening, Aḥmad Amīn and Aḥmad az-Zayn (eds), vol. 2, p. 38.13–17. His pupils are recorded as having been embarrassed by Ibn 'Adī's gullibility.

26 One edition is by Aydın Sayılı (ed.), "Farabi'nin simyanın lüzümü hakkındaki risalesi," *Belleten*, vol. 15, issue 57, 1951.

We should therefore keep an open mind on whether there was a hidden side to Ibn Sīnā's great contributions to science. We should look at further evidence, above all in the alchemical treatise which the Long Bibliography and 12th century Latin translation ascribe to him, *Fī al-Amr al-mastūr* (On the Hidden Matter).

## *On the Hidden Matter: A Work in the Style of Ar-Rāzī*[27]

In spite of the expressed hostility to alchemists in the *Kitāb aš-Šifā'*, we have picked up indications about Ibn Sīnā's study and practice of chemistry that mean that we cannot rule out the idea that at least one of the two Arabic alchemical works ascribed to him are genuine.[28] However, the style and format of the work *Fī al-Amr al-mastūr* differ from the schematic and summary approach, with occasional digressions, of *aš-Šifā'*. The treatise is terse and practical, setting out the preparatory operations for creating dyes and then the production of elixirs which provide substances with all the qualities of natural gold or silver. This style and format recall the *Kitāb al-Asrār* of ar-Rāzī, and I will give examples of the many dependences on ar-Rāzī's work in both concepts and phrasing that have been detailed by scholars.

The introduction to the treatise is important. The author writes that his studies of the natural sciences in general led him to the works of 'the chemists' (*aṣḥāb al-kīmīyā'*). He found that most virtuous and knowledgable people accused them of trickery. It is true, he says, that they do not offer the evidence on which the branches of science depend (*ẖāliyan min al-qiyās allaḏī huwa 'umdat kull ṣinā'a*), and are mostly ridiculous. However, the arguments of their opponents are likewise weak. Finally, based on abstract thought alone, the writer decides that alchemy, in the strict sense of making a lasting change to silver so that it has the character of gold, or copper so that it has the character of silver, is possible. In spite of this tentative introduction, there is no doubt that this treatise is alchemy in a full sense, and the instructions it gives lead up to the production of gold-making elixirs, as alchemical works normally do. In an age long before the science of chemistry, for a substance to have the characteristics

27 Stapleton et al.'s study of this Arabic treatise and *Fī aṣ-Ṣinā'a al-'āliya* offers a systematic comparison with Persian alchemists of the 10th and 11th centuries, notably the *Kitāb al-Asrār* of ar-Rāzī. I base much of what I write on the notes to these editions.

28 I will only deal in detail with the main one, because what applies to one, applies to *Fī aṣ-Ṣinā'a al-'āliya* also.

of gold allowed it to be called gold. While this treatise allows one to distinguish 'philospher's gold' from 'natural gold', it was a distinction without a difference for many.

What is needed, the introduction concludes, is the correct dye (*ṣibġ*, tincture). The treatise sets out the conditions for defining, then making, effective dyes. They must be fluid enough to penetrate, but stable enough not to run, especially when heated. The first dye described by the author is that which whitens, and then, more importantly, he describes the tincture which reddens to gold.[29] They are prepared by cooking, sublimating, and drying, mainly using sulphur, arsenic, lead and mercury.

One stage in the preparation of a tincture which does not burn requires the author to give an explanation of the cause of fire, so that it can be identified and removed.[30] Then the possibility of transmutation is described in the following terms: "[S]o long as [substances] remain as bodies, with their essences united, nothing can combine with them... We can burn and calcine them, but if it be possible to calcine them without burning them we should do so, until they become reduced to such fine powder that it is almost impossible to divide them any further. A specific form is thus lost to them, for, as Aristotle has shown in his *as-Samāʿ aṭ-ṭabīʿī* (Φυσικὴ ἀκρόασις), subdivision destroys specific form... for us to employ them in realizing our object. "[31] In fact Aristotle had no such doctrine, and it is hard to imagine that Ibn Sīnā could write such a statement.

---

29 The other stage in the alchemical work would be 'blackening', but this is produced by fire, not by dyeing.

30 As this passage has considerable interest in its own right, for the theory can be compared to the 'phlogiston' of 17th and 18th century Europe, I will quote it *in extenso*: "The cause of combustion is the existence of a matured humidity in a body [physical object], mixed with a dryness, which, by the accidental heat that it acquires, gives it the virtue of resembling fire, changing the particles of the body into the substance of fire either before or during evaporation. It will thus separate as pure fire, the residue being the ashes... [H]umidity alone does not burn... [but] if the humidity be mingled with something, it is in its nature to evaporate... becoming viscous and turning into oil, [it] will blaze up and burn away." Translation of Stapleton et al., p. 63.18–64.10. Ahmed Ateş (Arabic ed.), p. 43.13–44.10.

31 وهي ما دامت أجسادًا مجتمعة الذوات لم يمكن أن يخلط فيها شيء
فوجب أن نحرقها ونكلّسها إن أمكن تكليسها بغير الحرق فعملنا حتّى تصير هباء لا تكاد تجزّئ بشيء وقد
بطل عنها صورة نوعها إذ قد بيّن أرسطوطاليس في السماع الطبيعيّ أنّ التجزية تبطل الصورة النوعيّة
فإذا حصلت كذلك أمكننا أن نبلغ منها الغرض فرأينا واستصوبنا أن يُتّخذ للفضّة أبدًا إمّا من الفضّة وهي
أحسن وإمّا من الرصاص وللذهب إمّا من الذهب وهو أحسن وإمّا من النحاس وقد قيل إنّ اللازورد أفضل
كلسًا من النحاس
Translation of Stapleton et al., p. 67.2–67.15. Ahmed Ateş (Arabic ed.), p. 47.4–13.

It would nonetheless be interesting to find which passage was interpreted in this way by alchemists. We note also that the terminology for transmutation is somewhat similar to that in *aš-Šifā'* (*ibṭāl aṣ-ṣūra an-naw'iyya/salb al-faṣl al-munawwi'*). According to his usual method, the author of this treatise derives the practice from principles which he sets out first. He recommends the use of a calx of silver or tin, the former being preferable, to make silver, and a calx of gold or copper to make gold. Lapis lazuli can be used.[32] Similarly, white *isfīdāj* (tin or lead oxide) can be used for silver.

The seventh chapter explains that the elixir can be just as good, 'or better', if made from organic matter like hair, eggs, blood, and animal parts. These are cooked, and the liquid which separates (called 'water') has the same effect as mercury, the oil corresponds to sulphur or arsenic sulphide, and the calx performs the function of the calces of minerals.

The final section contains the assertion: "Among the elements, the analogue of the tincture is fire, the analogue of the oil is air, the analogue of the mercury is water, and the analogue of the calx is earth. The white is formed from three things, fire being excluded, the yellow from all four. And God knows best what is right!" It is a universal theme of alchemists that the elixir of gold is formed from some combination of the four elements.

While the evidence connecting *Fī al-Amr al-mastūr* with other works of Ibn Sīnā is slight, the main conclusion that has been demonstrated by studies is the close connection with Abū Bakr ar-Rāzī. This connection is so pervasive that, if this were a work of Ibn Sīnā, it would indicate a dependency of the philosopher on ar-Rāzī in the area of chemistry. In other words, if we accept this to be the work of Ibn Sīnā, we would have to say that the earlier scholar loomed large in his formation as a scientist: "[It] is a mass of connected quotations from the *Kitāb al-Asrār*. . ."[33] Three examples, taken from many identified by Stapleton et al, will suffice. The method for distillation of animal substances in the treatise attributed to Ibn Sīnā reads:

32 Stapleton et al. note that there is no copper in Lapis lazuli. However, we point out that according to pseudo-Apollonius, an authority for alchemists, lapis is basically copper.

33 Letter of Stapleton, quoted in Stapleton et al., "Two alchemical treatises", p. 42. To give the context, Stapleton says: "Each of them [*Fī al-Amr al-mastūr* and *Fī aṣ-Ṣinā'a al-'āliya*] is a mass of connected quotations from the Kitāb al-Asrār, the chief difference being that while the al-Barqī treatise shows little or no sign of being anything else but a series of extracts from somebody's work, the al-Sahlī one is the much more carefully compiled work of a highly logically minded philosopher. . ."

> We therefore distil them over a gentle fire in a cucurbit and alembic. After the water had distilled, the oil begins to pass over, and (the process of) distillation is carried on until both have been removed, and nothing but the dregs remain. The latter are repeatedly heated in the fire, until they are converted into a calx which is permanent over fire. Furthermore, we know that the tincture is in the oil, so we coagulate the oil, and extract its tincture by subjecting it to gentle coction in nothing but its own water, seeing that its water is sharp...

This derives from *Kitāb al-Asrār*:

> A better method is for you to take the hair, and, after cleaning it in the way previously described, to distil its water and oil. Then re-distil the water until it becomes clear and place it on one side. Next coagulate the oil in a 'blind' (cucurbit)... [Re-mix and] then strain the water from the oil. You will find it (i.e. the water) purple red. Then add a fresh portion of the water and repeat the process till you have removed all the tincture from the oil. (Stapleton et al, p. 70, and footnote 78.)

A second example illustrates the fact that the treatise in the name of Ibn Sīnā describes some of the same instruments as are found in *Kitāb al-Asrār.* In *Fī al-Amr al-mastūr* we find:

> We fit on to its top a round disc from which sufficient of the centre has been removed for the top of the pot to pass into it, and over this disc we fit a rounded cover (*mikabba*) in order that the fumes of the mercury that rise up may be retained therein. In the centre of the cover there is also a hole through which passes a properly fashioned stick, which can be taken out whenever we think that the fumes have ceased to be evolved. We can thus see whether they have really stopped or whether they are still rising up.

In ar-Rāzī this is:

> What is necessary for mercury is the removal of its moisture and its desiccation... A better way (than using an *anbīq*) is to have a hole in the *mikabba* of the *uthāl* large enough for the little finger to enter. (This hole is kept open) until the substance appears in the form of earth, either white or black, by which you learn that the moisture has come to an end. Then the hole is closed with a properly fashioned stick bound round with a rag... (Stapleton et al, p. 57, and footnote 30.)

Finally, there is a close verbal parallel between the five methods of dissolving (*taḥlīl*) mentioned in the later treatise and the eight kinds of dissolution listed by ar-Rāzī. Both mention "burying in dung", suspending in a jar (in ar-Rāzī 'tub') of vinegar, burying in damp earth, hanging them in a well, and in a 'well'. (Stapleton et al, p. 75, and footnote 111.)

The treatise follows ar-Rāzī closely. In this way these alchemical works contrast with Ibn Sīnā's philosophy and medicine. There he seems to show little liking for his predecessor. Nonetheless, we always have to bear in mind that any admiration would need to be hidden or disguised, for ar-Rāzī was a notorious unbeliever. Al-Bīrūnī admired ar-Rāzī, and dedicated a treatise to a survey of ar-Rāzī's works, but al-Bīrūnī draws the line at ar-Rāzī's religious opinions, and says about the *Book on Prophecies*: "he mocks, in a most unsuitable way, the great and the good, and in doing so he pollutes his mind, tongue and pen, with what sensible people avoid and pass over, for it only brings hatred in this world." (*Risala fi Fihrist kutub Muḥammad ibn Zakariyā' ar-Rāzī*).[34] In fact, Ibn Sīnā's learned correspondence with his great contemporary contains letters that insult ar-Rāzī in no uncertain terms: "Muḥammad ibn Zakariyā' ar-Rāzī, who is vain and superfluous in his commentaries on theology and in his going well beyond his abilities on slow expulsions, and the study of urine and faeces, shaming himself and exposing his ignorance in all he attempted."[35] Ibn Sīnā was also a critic of astrology, the cousin of alchemy, judging by his *Refutation of Astrology*. In short, if we says that he was at some time an alchemist, we would need to say he hid this in his biography, and in his known works.

On the other hand, one could argue that such secrecy was only to be expected in Ibn Sīnā's day. Secretive groups, such as that of which his father was a member, were the norm for those who set their hopes in the occult sciences.

Additionally, if one is looking for similarities between *Fī al-Amr al-mastūr* and Ibn Sīnā's acknowledged work on chemistry in *aš-Šifā'*, one could point to the clear distinction found in both works between the natural elements and processes, like the formation of gold in the earth, and the artifice of the alchemists. This is not only the main element of his criticism of alchemists at the end of the chapter in *aš-Šifā'*, but also present in *Fī al-Amr al-mastūr*, which emphasizes that the change is the work of a tincture or dye, and thus somehow external. As we have seen above, a further similarity is that both works distance themselves from the phantastical terminology of alchemy.

To conclude with a general remark on the case for or against *Fī al-Amr al-mastūr*, I would say that we are confronted by a treatise ascribed to a well-known writer which begins with an introduction which places it into a polemical context. Immediately we react by suspecting that the polemical context, rather than the main body of the treatise, as the primary aim of the writer of

---

34 Paul Kraus, ed., Paris, al-Qalam, 1936, p. 3, lines 4–7.

35 Muhammad Tanji (ed.), "Beyrûnî'nin İbn-i Sînâya yöneltti̇ği bazı sorular," (1974), p. 272.18–273.2. I want to thank Prof. Said Sabbagh of the Fuat Sezgin Institute, Istanbul, for pointing this passage out.

the work. This is all the more the case in the short work ascribed to al-Fārābī, *On the Necessity for the Existence of Alchemy* (*Fī Wujūb ṣinā'at al-kīmīyā'*).[36]

## Conclusion

The question of whether Ibn Sīnā was an alchemist boils down to two points. Firstly, there are inconsistencies in *Fī al-Amr al-mastūr* when compared to the philosopher's known works. As noted above, it is hard to believe that Ibn Sīnā would assert that Aristotle taught that physical division of a substance can destroy its specific form. The second is that we must measure the likelihood or otherwise that there was a dimension of the philosopher's life which cultivated alchemy in the tradition of ar-Rāzī. One would have to add that, as it is not evident in his other works, this admiration would have to be secret. This is not impossible because, although the Persian doctor's medical achievements could be openly praised, attachment to his philosophy and theology was forbidden in most polite society. Alchemy was in any case questionable. The complex character of geniuses who lived in dangerous times does not discount a hidden life.[37]

## Bibliography

Agricola, Georg, *De ortu et causis subterraneorum* (Basel, Froben, 1546).

al-Bīrūnī, see: Kraus, *Fihrist*; and Tanji, "Beyrûnî'nin İbn-i Sînâ'ya".

Anawati, Georges, "Arabic alchemy", in Roshdi Rashed, ed., *Encyclopedia of the History of Arabic Science*, Vol. 3 (Routledge, London and New York, 1996), p. 853–885.

Apollonius, Pseudo-, see: Ursula Weisser (ed.).

Ateş, Ahmed (ed.), İbn Sînâ, "Risâlat al-iksîr veya Risala fi amr mastûr," *Türkiyat Mecmuasi* (Istanbul) 10. 1951–53, (1953).

Gutas, Dimitri, *Avicenna and the Aristotelian Tradition* (Leiden, Brill, 2014).

Ibn Abī Uṣaybi'a, *'Uyūn al-anbā' fī ṭabaqāt al-aṭibbā'*, Nizār Riḍā' (ed.) (Beirut, Maktabat al-Ḥayāt, 1965).

36 This treatise (*risala*) has some similarities with the *risala* ascribed to Ibn Sīnā. Both defend alchemy by saying that one can establish its existence by abstract thought, and both deprecate the strangeness of mainstream (Jābirean) alchemy.

37 The classic example from the scientific revolution in Europe would be Isaac Newton, who, in terms of volume, wrote more about alchemy than about physics.

Ibn Sīnā, *Kitāb aš-Šifā'*, Ibrahim Madkūr et al. (ed.), (Cairo, Dār al-Kitāb al-'Arabī li-ṭ-Ṭibā'a wa-n-Našr, 1389/1969).

Käs. Fabian, *Al-Maqrīzīs Traktat über die Mineralien:* Kitāb al-Maqāṣid... (Leiden, Brill, 2015).

Kraus, Paul, *Jābir ibn Ḥayyān: contribution à l'histoire des idées scientifiques dans l'Islam: Jābir et la science grecque* (Cairo, Institut Français, 1942; repr. Frankfurt, IHAIS, 2002; Paris, Belles Lettres, 1986).

Paul Kraus, ed., al-Bīrūnī, *Risala fi Fihrist kutub Muḥammad ibn Zakariyā' ar-Rāzī* (Paris, al-Qalam, 1936).

Kraus, Paul, "Studien zu Jābir ibn Ḥayyān," *Isis*, 1931, vol. 15.1.

Holmyard, Eric John, and Desmond Mandeville (eds), *Avicennae De congelatione et conglutione lapidum, being sections of the* Kitāb aš-Šifā' (Paris, Guethner, 1927).

Martin Plessner, *Vorsokratische Philosophie und griechische Alchemie...* Turba philosophorum (Wiesbaden, Steiner, 1975).

ar-Rāzī, Muḥammad ibn Zakariyā', *Kitāb al-Asrār*, see: Ruska (ed.).

Ruska, Julius, *Al-Rāzī's Buch Geheimnis der Geheimnisse*, in Quellen und Studien zur Geschichte der Naturwissenschaften und der Medizin, vol. 6 (Berlin, Springer, 1937).

Ruska, Julius, "Die Alchemie des Avicenna," *Isis*, no. 60, 1934.

Stapleton, Harry, et al. "Two Alchemical Treatises Attributed to Avicenna," *Ambix*, vol. 10.2, 1962.

Shawkat Toorawa, "A Portrait of 'Abd al-Laṭīf al-Baghdādī's Eduction and Instruction," in Joseph Lowry et al. (eds), *Law and Education in Medieval Islam* (Cambridge, Gibb Memorial Trust, 2004).

Muhammad Tanji (ed.), "Beyrûnî'nin İbn-i Sînâ'ya yöneltti̇ği bazı sorular, İbn-i Sînâ'nın cevapları ve bu cevaplara Beyrûnî'nin itirazları," in *Beyrûnî'ye armağan* (Ankara, Türk Tarih Kurumu, 1974, repr. 2011).

at-Tawḥīdī, *al-Imtā' wa-l-mu'ānasa*, Aḥmad Amīn and Aḥmad az-Zayn (eds) (Cairo, 1953).

Ullmann, Manfred, *Die Natur- and Geheimwissenschaften im Islam* (Leiden, Brill, 1972).

Weisser, Ursula (Arabic ed.), *Buch über Geheimnis der Schöpfung und die Darstellung der Natur von Pseudo-Apollonios von Tyana* (Aleppo, Institute for the History of Arabic Science, 1979).

Weisser, Ursula (summary and study), *"Buch über Geheimnis der Schöpfung" von Pseudo-Apollonios von Tyana* (De Gruyter, Berlin, 1980).

Zosimos of Panopolis, *Muṣḥaf aṣ-ṣuwar, The Book of Pictures*, Theodor Abt (ed.), Facsimile (Zurich, Living Human Heritage, 2007).

## Short Biography of Peter Starr

He is an Assistant Professor at the Humanities department of Istanbul Technical University. He was born in London in 1967, and brought up partly in the Middle East. His Cambridge doctorate was on the philosopher 'Isā ibn Zur'a (2000).

Peter's areas of interest are Arabic-Islamic alchemy and Greco-Arabic studies, in which field he published "Isḥāq ibn Ḥunayn's Version of Περὶ φύσεως ἀνθρώπου: A 'Balance of Alternatives' in Translating ἑαυτοῦ," in *Between the Cross and the Crescent* (Roma, PIO, 2018).

He is working with a colleague on a new edition of the alchemist Muḥammad ibn Umayl's *al-Ma' al-waraqī*. Peter has lived in Turkey since 2004, is married and has a son.

Prof. Dr. Salahaddin Khalilov

# Avicenna and Modern Theories of Self-Knowledge

**Abstract:** Aristotle systematizing the soul, he distinguishes the three parts of it - the sensible, appetitive, and rational. Al-Farabi, Avicenna and Suhrawardi continued this line of thinking in their teachings. But they also tried to reconcile the Platonic and Aristotelian positions by admitting the possibility of eternal existence for the rational part of the soul, of its joining the realm of the intelligences.

Avicenna not only commented Aristotle's views on logic, but also brought some innovations in this field of science. In fact, he is the founder of a new field of logic - the modal logic. In Europe, the examining of this issue was started only in XIII-XV centuries and probably after the getting acquainted with Avicenna's works.

According to Avicenna, the human soul is born by the emanation of Divine Light, by its creative energy. And human life is a way to return to the Light. Human being has also a body and in ontological hierarchy the body stands at a lower level than soul. Therefore, the goal of human being or the way of perfection is considered a return from body to soul, from darkness to light. Thus, Avicenna's teaching is regarded as a bridge between Prepatetism and Sufism and between Neoplatonism and Ishraqism.

**Keywords:** Avicenna, Aristotle, eidos, soul, logic, unity, Islamic philosophy

Aristotle's view on spirit and soul, on the structure of spiritual-intellectual life were taken up and developed by Medieval Islamic philosophers. Al-Farabi and Avicenna are the philosophers who contributed the most to the subject. Avicenna, in particular, took Aristotle's doctrine further in many directions. As is well known, in Aristotle *essence* is not distinguished from substrate and it is consequently understood in terms of the *particular* (Aristotle 1992, 190a20–191b13). Avicenna, in contrast, establishing the modern signification of the term, explained it as a *universal*. He devoted much of his *Metaphysics* to a discussion of these problems and added a special paragraph entitled "*explanation of why essence cannot be individual in the necessary being*" (Avicenna 1980, 140). Mehdi Eminrazavi calls attention to the text and shows that for Avicenna essences do not exist concretely in things; their existence is of an abstract sort (1998, 574).

As to Aristotelian logic, Avicenna did not simply comment on but also brought certain novelties with respect to it. He can in fact be considered as the founder of modal logic which is a special branch of logic. European thinkers started to pay attention to this aspect of logic only in the 13th and 14th centuries, probably after having had acquaintance with the works of Avicenna. Avicenna approaches logic from a wider angle. For Aristotle logic is concerned with syllogisms in general and with proof in particular (Aristotle 1938, 201). Avicenna, on the other hand, takes it to consist in the following: "*The subject matter of logic, as you know, is given by the secondary intelligible meanings, based on the first intelligible meanings, with regard to how it is possible to pass by means of them from the known to the unknown*". Matters of syllogism and proof derive from this as its special cases.

As Tajik M. Dinorşoyev writes, Avicenna's theory of deduction is quite different from that of Aristotle. It is not limited to categorical deduction but includes an analysis of hypothetical deductions as well (Dinorşoyev 1980, 19). Avicenna himself explains their difference as follows: "*This deduction derives from two considerations, each of which, losing their independence, is restricted to the consideration at hand and such deductions are called hypothetico-connective and conditional deductions. If there is discordance between the considerations the contrary holds and in this case deduction is called hypothetico-separative deduction*" (Avicenna 1980, 19).

Aristotle, as we know, despite having criticized Plato's doctrine failed to overcome the separation of matter and idea completely. In Avicenna's thought, by contrast, matter can be understood only through its forms and reflections (Avicenna 1980, 29). He conceived matter as the first necessary being, separating it from things, and thought it impossible for it to have a beginning of existence, so much so that it could have been created not even by God. For any created thing there were a time in which it simple was not, for matter on the other hand, there is neither before nor after. It was this idea that Al-Ghazali found to be an obvious defiance of Islamic dogma and heavily criticized. According to him, who consecrated a whole book to this problem (*Incoherence of the Philosophers*) philosophers are from understanding God in a way that is compatible with the strictures of the Quran. Avicenna, in particular, by arguing that matter is non-created, comes to reject the precept that everything is created by God. Averroes, in his *Incoherence of the Incoherence* argues against Al-Ghazali and does not accept his charge of contradiction. As, he argues, philosophy aims at truth and as Islam calls men to knowledge and truth these two ways cannot be set against each other: "*Truth cannot be opposed to truth, they complement each other*" (Hourani 1961, 50; Skirbekk and Gile 2000, 252). Avicenna sees God as the only necessary being and as the first cause and eternity of matter does not amount to importing it a God-like status. For, matter has only possible, not necessary being. Hence, there is no point, argues Averroes, in accusing Avicenna of renouncing the idea of unity, of professing dualism and deism; there simply is no sufficient ground for such conclusions.

Avicenna was mainly a follower of Aristotle and the Aristotelian tradition, but he did not refrain from referring to the doctrines of Plato and Plotinus as a fruitful source of insight into certain problems and tried to achieve a synthesis of these different schools of thought. For Avicenna human soul is born from the emanation (creative energy) of Divine Light and human life is nothing but the way to return back to Light. In his *Mebde and Mead* (Creation and the Turn) he tackles this problem. As man is bodily and as body stands with respect to soul lower in the ontological hierarchy, the way to perfection consists, for man, in turning from the body to the soul, from the darkness to the light. We can see here that he brings Peripatetic and Neo-Platonic doctrines in contact with Sufi and Israqi traditions. As a philosopher and as the greatest physician of his time Avicenna approached the problem of soul and body in a scientific and systematic manner and developed quite original ideas. If the foundations of psychology were laid down by Aristotle, Avicenna must be seen as the most authoritative figure in the later phase of its development.

The shaping of psychology as a scientific discipline in the 19th century led to some considerable success in the area in the 20th century, as methods and technical potential of natural science came to be employed more and more in investigating the soul, establishing it as an independent are of research. These developments influenced philosophical study of the matter to a certain extent, but no philosophical system that provides a systematic explanation has yet been offered. In a period when the emphasis on consciousness in philosophical investigations on reason, soul and spirit was still relatively new, the emergence of the doctrine of unconscious called for a change in philosophical paradigm. This need for change was after all nothing but a need to return to Eastern intellectual traditions. The problem of soul and body have always been a primary concern for eastern thought which generally presents itself in the form of religious-philosophical systems. In the West, on the other hand, following the separation of philosophy from religious thought, this problem had largely receded into the background. Western philosophy in taking science as its model got more and more away from Eastern intellectual traditions, for science explains nature and the order of material reality without reference to soul, relying on its own posits and methods alone. Even though processes of understanding continued to be the subject matter of philosophy of mind, knowledge concerning material reality were deemed to belong to science, to fall under its jurisdiction, and the only role left to philosophy was to understand and justify this scientific endeavor under the rubric of *philosophy of science.*

In late 19th and early 20th centuries, natural science had reached such a high level of development that, it was only natural that a natural-scientific explanation of consciousness and soul itself be demanded and searched for. Science continued to follow philosophy and stepped onto its field. Most importantly, traditional terms gained new content. The employment of ideas like soul, spirit and consciousness in totally new and different contexts brought with it a need to reconceptualize them, as progress in natural science generally puts pressure on philosophical terms, demanding more specificity in their use.

One should not then be surprised that American philosopher William James took psychology to be a branch of natural science (James 1983, 15). Psychology, as professor Ledd writes, describes and examines states of perception. This means that perception, which is among the principal categories of philosophy, becomes the subject matter of natural sciences. Indeed, according to some philosophers (e.g. Herbert Spencer), there is no essential difference between material and spiritual life. (Spencer explains this in evolutionary terms, that is, in terms of the principle of the dependence of internal relations on external ones.) For William James, it is not possible to learn anything of substance concerning spiritual life outside of the physical milieu in which it exists. He refuses, as a result, rational psychology which considers soul as a non-material being. Modern psychology takes it as established that inner capacities of man develop through adaptation to the forms of the material world (James 1983, 19).

James sees that associating psychical processes with neurological system is clearly a materialistic approach and tries to overcome this implication but fails to find a way of incorporating the basic assumptions of natural sciences within an idealistic framework. He admits that materialism amounts to making what stands higher rest upon that which is lower. The association of soul with brain processes is an example of this sort of understanding. Science though, as of now, is unable to offer another alternative (James 1983, 23).

It would be fitting here to remind ourselves that Avicenna and Suhrawardi showed already in Middle Ages that attempts at explaining psychical phenomena through the body were mistaken. Suhrawardi wrote that what is lower cannot govern what is higher. For him it was not possible that soul be a by-product, an effect as it were, of body. It is the soul that governs the body not the reverse (Suhrawardi 1999, 221). Jung, one of the greatest psychologists of the 20th century, argues that ideas do not originate from an individual human being but a greater being is their source. We are not the author of ideas it is rather ideas that shape us (Jung 1916, 9).

William James and Jung, like Averroes and Suhrawardi before them, understand immediately, in a non-inferential manner, the fact that soul enjoys a higher status with respect to body and that its ground lies in a deeper secret. Nonetheless, James, as a man of the West, cannot ignore the possibilities natural sciences present and cherishes the hope that knowledge attained through scientific means will serve, eventually, providing an understanding of physiological and neurological processes, as the basis of the analysis of the soul. He hopes thereby that what possesses the highest value will reclaim its status once a properly philosophical attitude comes to prevail again.

The scientific stand on the matter in general, on the other hand, is that perceptual processes occur as a result of interaction between the body and external material world. The interaction between these two factors brings with it the production of something with a nature of its own; perception. But it is this very nature that proves hard to grasp and remains thereby outside the reach of science. As a result of its interaction with matter the organism undergoes certain physical effects and these effects are then transmitted to the brain. Other processes take place in the brain, signals act upon the neurons, etc.

Science can certainly master all of these. On the basis of further material processes in the brain, however, acts of perception, acts that are not perceivable through the body, acts that can be neither seen, heard nor touched result and these differ radically from the material world, transcending its limits. Natural science is unable to explain this passage and the emergent new nature. Philosophy itself, insofar as it tries to remain within the limits of scientific knowledge, is also far from being able to shed any light on the issue. As this passage, this leap, this point of crisis, is incomprehensible, the new, spiritual world we step into is as incomprehensible. Science has left the study of this problem to philosophy because in this world space and time do not apply, nor does causality. In fact, none of the laws that are valid in the material world apply here. Man, though, thanks to his reason and moral sense develops another kind of interest with regard to the material world. The region thus determined is still a region for scientific study. The prior world is the world before perception, a world prior to the shape it takes in our perception. As the world prior to perception is inaccessible for us, it is dark. World becomes illuminated for us only after perception. To put it better, the illuminated part of it is the world for us.

Hence, contemporary psychology comprises many different fields and regions of investigation. Experimental and theoretical study of the physical, physiological and neurophysiological processes that occur prior to the point of break and experimental and theoretical study of human behavior, and its functioning as a being that perceives. Analogically cognitive psychology also comprises two branches; one that studies the pre-perceptual processes and another that studies post-perceptual processes.

According to Hegel, idea realizes itself only in its appearance and it is actual, it exists only when it so finds itself (Hegel 1995, 21). For him idea can find itself at the universal scale as well as at that of the individual. This process as a whole is, for mankind, nothing but history of philosophy. For man in general, for man with a capital M, self-understanding is the task of mankind as a whole. For the individual self-perception occurs as a moment of sensuous experience, it does not take place within the domain of ideas. It is only here, at this level that the object of experience is one's own Self, its own moral world. A singular spiritual world characterized not only by intelligence but also by instinct, impulse and soul. Merleau-Ponty writes in his *Phenomenology of Perception* that *"Hitherto the Cogito depreciated the perception of others, teaching me as it did that the I is accessible only to itself, since it defined me as the thought which I have of myself, and which clearly I am alone in having, at least in this ultimate sense"* (Merleau-Ponty 2002, xiv).

Who is the Self then, or what is it? In what measure is one's body, soul and reason related to one's Self? In Medieval Islamic philosophy, especially in Avicenna and Suhrawardi, Self is conceived as equal to the soul. Descartes relates man's being to his thought and reason. Materialistic theories and simple common understanding, by contrast, teach it to consist more in its relation to his body. A closer look, however, reveals that all human bodies operate at a more or less equal level, executing the same functions, and the differences among bodies fail to express the different colors of human life in general. Furthermore, that the body loses its function after death shows that it is neither independent nor prior. Death, on the other hand, is conceived as the end of respiration and the separation of the soul from body. Soul is then what gives life to the body and turns it into a living being. The functioning of reason is of a universal nature and differ, if ever, only slightly among human beings. Everyone may not have the same actual intellectual capacity, nor the possibilities open to anyone at a time is equal for all, but the overall course is nonetheless the same. It is difficult, then, to use reason to characterize the individual Self as such.

How are we then to conceive souls? Are they individual, specific to each person? Plato believes that soul survives death and continues its life in other human beings, or even in animals. He thereby rejects the individuality of the soul, its uniqueness. Any individual is responsible for the perfection of her soul in his own personal life and for bequeathing a better soul to subsequent generations. Education, therefore, if in one way is possible on the basis of interpersonal relations, in another way it is a matter of perfecting one's own Self.

Everyone does not get to know oneself and to build a life in accordance with one's own beliefs and preferences. There have been many men that passed their life without having had the chance of knowing themselves and acting in accordance with their own preferences though they sure interacted abundantly with others, knowing and cooperating with them. However, those that have the chance to converse with themselves all experience the wonder and fright that accompanies their initial feelings. It is possible to keep one's reserve and display a critical attitude towards the demands and ideas of others. It is difficult to remain indifferent to the choices of those dear to oneself, but, indifference towards one's own thoughts and feelings is something altogether impossible. It is well possible for one to live without knowing oneself in the least but then it becomes quite questionable whether this can really be considered as one's own life, whether his life has not become part of someone else's life.

Hegel, in his *Philosophy of History*, takes as his task to rethink history as a history of the ideas man has had on himself, on his identity. He gives the famous inscription on the temple of the goddess Neith as an indication of how Egyptians understood themselves: *"I'm that which is, that which was and that which will be; no one has lifted my veil."* (Hegel 1944, 220). This problem of self-understanding, of self-knowledge, embodied in the formula *Know Thyself*, is expressed in a more explicit manner in the case of Greek thought, which shows a relatively higher level of development. Hegel notes that the meaning conveyed here is not that of the understanding one attains as to his own positive and negative, superior and inferior qualities. What is at issue is man's coming to an understanding of himself *in general* (Hegel 1944, 241). Self-knowledge, in this sense, is not understanding one's own *individual self*, but humanity as such and this is a historical process. This is not of course to say that understanding one's own individual being, as it pertains to his personal self, does not have any importance. This understanding is, to the contrary, important in itself and besides, the process of self-understanding, in this regard, is realized within the very context of feeling and sensibility, lived as a part of one's own life.

Knowing one's true self, coming to know one's innermost feelings generates anxiety. A true self-meeting may lead to a dissolution of the groundless, aleatory image one has of oneself and the true image discovered may be something completely new, something which was a complete mystery before. Schopenhauer writes that only man among beings is astonished at his own existence and that *"at the beginning of his consciousness, he naturally takes himself also as something that is a matter of course. This, however, does not last long, but very early, and simultaneously with the first reflection, appears that wonder which is some day to become the mother of metaphysics"* (Schopenhauer 1969, 60).

Some knowingly refrain from listening to their inner voice, trying to lead their life observing actual social norms, spiritual principles and moral values; without ever noticing the material with which they work. This material is a reality that is created by others and given independently of one's desire. This is such a reality that it is possible to come face to face with it only through meditation or philosophical reduction. In both, one tries to get closer to oneself by distancing oneself from all external influence, acquired qualities and what society and those around him preaches. This is a state of freedom and subsequent activity takes place only in the form of self-realization of one's true self.

Upanishads believe that man can attain freedom and happiness in this world only. *"If man can freed oneself of all the desire and passion in his soul he will reach immortality, attaining Brahman in his life time"* (Güngören 34). They thus brought paradise down to earth and raised men to the level of Gods. Buddhism also shares this understanding. In all Veda hymns, in Brahmanism and Hinduism despite the fact that these belief systems succeeded one another throughout the centuries, the essence remained intact. One should reach such a level in this changing world that is full of pain that it become possible to raise above it and free oneself from it. Only who is free from it can have a control over it. This level belongs to the Brahman, the highest beginning. An ordinary man cannot of course be a *Brahman* but everyone can find this beginning in oneself if he looks for his true self. This high beginning named *atman* at the scale of the individual actually corresponds to the Brahman. In other words, *atman* is the specific manifestation proper to the *Brahman* as the universal principle of the highest beginning and principle. When one, in directing his attention completely to his own self, gets freed from any external influence whatsoever, from *samsara* that comprises the incessant changes of this transient world, the path to the *brahman* is now open for him. *Atman* is the embodiment of the purified individual soul and it is where one attains divine soul, the *Brahman*.

This process of purification, this elevating of oneself over everything worldly leads to ascetism. This road is an endless one though. If purification of the individual soul is realized in the form of separation from the body, what good this can have for human life? Should the victory of the soul be necessarily predicated on the denial of the body?

The purified soul must return to the body and traverse the road of life together with it. Body is not a mere lifeless thing; it has its own inclinations and desires and what is needed is to be able to mastermind these, that is, to cultivate this very body itself. Soul after having entered into the vast of spiritual realm and getting purified returns and connects with *"the soul of the body"* and gets his soul purified. This process goes on and each day the soul, through contact with divine soul, comes to be directed to truth. Soul itself gets purified as a result, it gets illuminated. Even the body, on the whole character of the man changes, becoming luminous. Only a purified man can connect with his true face, with his true being and freedom becomes a possibility only then.

An educational system based on advices and recommendations may suffice, if it turns into habit, for the exigencies of the traditional environment one finds oneself in. In order to be able to make optimal decisions in non-standard extraordinary situations, decisions that are fitting for those situations, however, what is required most of all is free and creative thinking, as it becomes possible only then to bring moral principles in line with statist outlook and interests of the expertise and to incorporate all these into the decision, into its structure. It is well possible to know spiritual principles, to own an expertise and to have digested political and legal knowledge in isolation, but what counts is to be able to arrive at an optimal synthesis of them, relating each to one another. Such relating is possible only at the level of thought and contemplation; never at that of sentiment and custom. It is for this reason that Western world put intellectual education to the forefront. John Locke in his *Some Thoughts Concerning Education* argued that the fundamental duty of education is nothing but disciplining the intellect. The East, nonetheless, is ahead of the West chronologically in that this idea had already been entertained there. That is, Avicenna claimed for this idea eight centuries before Locke and called the intellect that is to be turned into habitual intellect as *material intellect* (Avicenna 1980, 319). What is important, though, is of course not which among the peoples conceived the idea before the others but which employed and put it into practice first.

## References

Aristotle (1985). *Categories. On Interpretation. Prior Analytics.* trans. by H. P. Cooke, Hugh Tredennick. Cambridge, MA: Harvard University Press.

Aristotle (1992). *Physics (Books I and II).* trans. by William Charlton. Oxford: Clarendon Press.

Avicenna (1980). *Izbrannie Filosofiskie Proizvedenye.* Moskova: Nauka.

Dinorşoyev, M. (1980). Ibn Sina i Yego Filosofskie Voozreniya. in Abu Ali İbn Sina. *Izbrannie Proizvedeniye.* vol. 1. Dushanbe: Irfon.

Eminrazavi, Mehti (1998). *Avicenna Velikie Mislıteli Vostoka.* Moscow: Kronn Press.

Hegel, G.W.F. (1944). *The Philosophy of History,* trans. by J. Sibree. New York: Willey Book Co.

Hegel, G.W.F. (1995). *Lectures on the History of Philosophy.* trans. by E.S. Haldane and Frances H. Simson. University of Nebraska Press.

Hourani, G. F. (1961). *Averroes on the Harmony of Religion and Philosophy.* London: Gibb Memorial Trust.

James, W. (1983). *The Principles of Psychology.* Cambridge: Harvard University Press.

Jung, Carl Gustav (1916). *Psychology of the Unconscious.* trans. by Beatrice M. Hinkle. New York: Dodd Mead and Company.

Merleau-Ponty, Maurice (2002). *Phenomenology of Perception.* Routledge.

Schopenhauer, Arthur (1969). *The World as Will and Representation*, vol. II. New York: Courier Dover Publications.

Skirbekk, G. and Gile, H. (2000). *Istorii Filosofii.* Moscow.

Suhrawardi (1999). *Nur Heykelleri.* Baku.

## Short Biography of Salahaddin Khalilov

He defended his PhD thesis titled "Systematic Structural Analysis of Scientific and Technological Progress" in 1976. After completing his postdoctoral research he defended a thesis titled "Logical-gnoseological issues of Scientific and Technological Progress" in 1990. In the same year he became a professor and the head of the Philosophy Department at Azerbaijan State Pedagogical University.

He founded "Azerbaijan University" - the first private university in Azerbaijan in 1991 and was its rector up to 2006. Now he is honorary professor of Azerbaijan University.

Since 1994 he has been leading the Research Center "East and West".

Prof. S. Khalilov is the Chairman of the Presidium of the Azerbaijan Association of Philosophy and Socio-Political Sciences (AFSEA).

The focus of his researches are mainly on the Philosophy of Science, Philosophical Comparativism, Phenomenology, Philosophical Aspects of Eastern and Western Civilizations.

Prof. S. Khalilov was the Member of the Parliament of Azerbaijan in 2000-2005.

In 2015-2020 he headed the UFAD (International Philosophical Research Centre) in Istanbul and now holds the honorary chairmanship.

Hamed Arezaei, Ph.D.

# The Idea of the Suspended Man in Space; from Thought Experiment to Actual Realization

## 1- Introduction[1]

Avicenna (Ibn Sina) made many efforts to understand the existence of the self more than any of the medieval philosophers. The dedication of a detailed section of the books *Elements of Philosophy* ('Uyūn al-Ḥikma), *the Salvation*[2] (*Kitāb al-Najāt)* also known as *Deliverance, Kitāb al-Shifā'* (The Cure), also known as *The Book of Healing* and *Sufficientia*, *al-Ishārāt wa al-Tanbīhāt* (Remarks and Admonitions or Pointers and Reminders), *Dāneshnāme-ye 'Alā'ī*, also known as *Philosophy for 'Alā'-ad-Dawla*[3], and other works, along with numerous independent treatises on philosophical self-consciousness, represent his special attention to these matters. Moreover, his works in the sphere of understanding the existence of the self have initiatives and innovations.

The idea of "the man suspended in space" is regarded as one of the original contributions of Ibn Sina on self-consciousness. Examining Aristotle's *On the Soul* treatise, we do not see such an idea. Ibn Sina himself has written annotations to Aristotle's treatise on the soul, in which, while presenting commentary and criticism on this work, he has expressed his evaluation about this work in such a way that the accuracy of the arguments and the delicacies of the reasoning of the Physics are higher than that of *On the soul* (Badawi 1978, pp. 16–15, 75).

The idea of the Suspended Man in Space or Suspended Man in Air is also known with titles of *Flying Man* or *Floating Man* and *Into Thin Air*[4]. Avicenna

---

1 *I am grateful for helpful suggestions from Glen M. Cooper and Mahdi Alizadeh and Shahrzad Irannejad.*

2 *To see the full translation of the " 'Ilm al-Nafs (psychology)" section of this book, see Fazlur Rahman (1952)*

3 *This work was originally written in Persian*

4 *Peter Adamson employs this name for the elaboration of this idea (Adamson 2016, p. 133). Shams Inati prefers the word free air to translate "الهواء الطلق" (Inati 2014, p. 96). Also, Ibn Sina has used the term "هواء سَجْسَج," i.e., moderate (not hot and not cold) air,*

introduces this idea in *The Book of Healing* (Ibn Sina 1984, p12. P225), and *Remarks and Admonitions* (*Pointers and Reminders* or *Al-Ishārāt wa al-Tanbīhāt*[5]) (Ibn Sina 1996, pp. 80–82), and *A Treatise on Knowledge of the Rational Soul* (Ibn Sina 1952, p. 184), and in the *Risālah aḍḥawīyah fī amr al-mi'ād or Judgment Day* (Ibn Sina 2003, p. 127–128). This repetition reflects the importance of this idea in his mind. He also points out this argument in his two writings, *Al-Ta'līqāt* and *Discussions* (*al-Mubāḥathāt*), which contain his dialogues with his disciples, and provides explanations about some criticisms sustained against the idea. This indicates that, since that time, the idea, which is considered one of Avicenna's innovations, has been debated and criticized.

One of the drawbacks raised from the beginning is that the structure of Ibn Sina's scheme to explain this idea does not fit into the conventional logical reasoning forms. For example, we see these deficiencies in the critiques of Abolghasem Kermani (Reisman 2002. Ibn Sina 2017, p81–89), Fakhr al-Din al-Razi (Zahit Tiryaki, 2020), and Quṭb al-Din al-Razi (Quṭb al-Din al-Din al-Razi 1983, pp. 293–295). Accordingly, commentators on the statements of Ibn Sina have attempted to offer an interpretation of the idea that does not include the listed shortcomings. Ibn Sina himself was the first to mention this idea, both in *Al-Ishārāt wa al-Tanbīhāt* and in *the Book of Healing* when he expresses this argument, and in *Al-Mubāḥathāt* when he seeks to provide explanations in response to the criticisms of this reasoning, not as an argument in the ordinary forms of Aristotelian logic, but as a kind of admonition or reminder that can be employed for people who realize its elegance (See the rest of the article). After him, loyal commentators such as Nasir al-Din Tusi (Tusi, 1983, pp. 141–145) and Fayyaz Lāhījī (Lahiji, 2005, vol. 3, p. 449) have provided similar answers to these problems.

This idea became very conventional among philosophers and theologians in the Middle Ages, and some have even attributed it to Descartes' Cogito

*in the book Al-Mubāḥathāt. (Ibn Sina 2017, p. 88). Al-Farāhīdī in his book Kitab al-'Ayn in the interpretation of the hadith "*الجَنَّة سَجْسَجٌ*" has translated this word to mean neither being cold nor hot: "*لا فيها حَر يؤذي و لا برد*" (al-Farāhīdī, 1989, vol. 6, p. 5). See also Ibn Manzur, The root of* سجج*: "*الهواء المعتدل بين الحر و البرد*", i.e., the moderate air between hot and cold. (Ibn Manzur, 1994, p. 2, p. 295).*

5 *Pointers and Reminders (al-Ishārāt wa al-Tanbīhāt). Text in J. Forget, Ibn Sīnā. Le livre des théorèmes et des avertissements, Leiden 1892, and in M. Zāre'ī, Al-Ishārāt wa al-Tanbīhāt li-l-Shaykh al-Ra'īs Ibn Sīnā, Qum 2002. French translation in Goichon 1951; English translation in Inati 1984, 1996, and 2014).*

Argument (Fakhry 2004, p179. Fazlur Rahman 1963, p487. Benevich & Adamson 2018).

In the tradition of Islamic philosophy, many distinguished philosophers following Ibn Sina have mentioned this argument in their works and analyzed and examined it. Abu'l-Barakāt al-Baghdādī (Abu'l-Barakāt 1994, vol. 2, p. 306), Shahab al-Din Suhrawardi (Marcotte 2004), Shams al-Din al-Shahrazuri (Shahrazuri 2005, vol. 2, pp. 424–425), Quṭb al-Dīn al-Shīrāzī (Shīrāzī 2006, pp. 691–692), Sadr al-Muta'allehin Shirazi (Mulla Sadra 1984, vol. 8, pp. 44–47), Fayyaz Lahiji (Lahiji 2005, vol. 3, p. 449), and Mollahadi Sabzevari (Sabzevari 2004, p. 324) were only some of the prominent philosophers that have noted this argument in their works.

In the tradition of medieval Christian philosophy, as researchers like Étienne Gilson (Gilson 1960), Thérèse-Anne Druart (Druart 1983, 1988, 2005), Dag Nikolaus Hasse (Hasse 2000)[6], and Juhana Toivanen[7] (Toivanen 2015) exhibited, the idea has been welcomed by many scholars.

The attention of post-Avicennian philosophical traditions to this idea caused historians of philosophy and scholars of rational thought to address this idea in the new era and to present schemes in terms of commentary. Most of the people who have dealt with the interpretation of this approach regarded it in the category of a Thought experiment (German: Gedankenexperiment (Perkowitz 2017), Gedanken-Experiment (Stöltzner 2003), or Gedankenerfahrung (Brown 2019). In the meantime, some considered the idea similar and influential to other thought experiments in philosophy.

According to these researchers, the Flying Man appears more similar to Putnam's Brain-in-a-Vat, Kirk's Zulliver's (because of rather bizarre thought experiment premises), and Chalmers' Anti-Materialist Modal Argument (both because of rather bizarre thought experiment supposals and because of the presupposition of a conscious world) (Hertogh 2013)[8].

6 *Hasse presents the most detailed study on this issue in his work entitled "Avicenna's De Anima in the Latin West: The Formation of a Peripatetic Philosophy of the Soul 1160–1300."*

7 *Toivanen also traces the course of this argument in the West in a relatively detailed article as follows: "The Fate of the Flying Man: Medieval Reception of Avicenna's Thought Experiment."*

8 *Another similarity between Ibn Sina's theory and physical theory is mentioned in this way: Because of the contents of the thought experiment premises, the Flying Man is very similar to Einstein's Chasing a Beam of Light, which also suggests a flying man, this time flying on a ray of light (Ibid)).*

In contrast, others have attempted to demonstrate that the Actual Realization of this idea is not far-fetched, and that this idea can also be regarded as an empirical argument. Others have also presented introspective personal formulations or a conceptual and logical image of this idea.

The purpose of the present paper is merely to show possible readings of the idea of the suspended man. We strive to elaborate on four interpretations of Ibn Sina's thoughts about the idea of the suspended man and highlight some descriptions of the first and second interpretations as examples of abstract interpretation and empirical interpretation. Hence, after this introduction, we explain this idea based on the works of Ibn Sina in the second part of the article. In the third part, on the basis of the concept of the thought experiment, we provide an analysis of this idea. In the fourth part, we assess the possibility of an actual realization of this idea based on recent scientific achievements. In the final section, we will briefly explain the other two interpretations.

## 2- The Idea of the Suspended Man based on the Words of Ibn Sina

Here, we present this idea based on two essential books, i.e., *The Book of Healing* and *Remarks & Admonitions*. We know that Abu 'Ali Ibn Sīnā- as he himself stated in the introduction of *Manṭiq al-Mashriqiyyīn*, as well as the introduction of *Healing* - wrote *The Book of Healing* in the official tradition of the philosophy of his time (Ibn Sina 1910; Ibn Sina 1952). On the other hand, the books of *Oriental Philosophy* and *Remarks & Admonitions* (*Al-Ishārāt wa al-Tanbīhāt*) are also considered to contain his specific views. Here, the existence of this idea in the Book of Healing - in two different cases - evidently represents that Ibn Sina paid particular attention to this idea. Even in a book written in the tradition of teaching formal philosophy, Ibn Sina goes beyond Aristotelian thought and presents his own specific scheme to prove the soul and its abstraction.

### 2-1- The Idea of the Suspended Man in the *Book of Healing*

Ibn Sina explains this idea in the chapter ("In Proving and Defining the Soul because it is the Soul") in the soul section of *the Book of Healing* (Ibn Sina, 1996, pp. 14–16). He states the aim of his scheme is to demonstrate the existence of the soul. After explaining the scheme, Ibn Sina asks his audience, "In this case, does the suspended man not prove his existence?" Then, he states that the existence of members - both external and internal - in the above assumption is unproven for the subject, but he understands them himself. So what has been proven and understood is different from what has not been proven. We conclude that the nature and existence of the man are other than the organs of his body. The summary of his argument is in this way:

> Let someone imagine himself as wholly created in a single moment, with his sight veiled so that he cannot see any external object. Imagine also that he is created falling through the air, or in a vacuum, so that he would not feel any pressure from the air. Suppose too that his limbs are parted from each other so that they neither meet nor touch. Let him reflect whether, in such a case, he will affirm his own existence. He will not hesitate to affirm that he himself exists, but in so doing, he will not be affirming the existence of any limb, or external or internal organ such as heart or brain, or any external object. He will be affirming the existence of himself without ascribing to it any length, breadth, or depth. If in this state he were able to imagine a hand or some other bodily part, he would not imagine it being a part of himself or a condition for his own existence. (Kenny 2004, p 225. Druart 2003, p.110)[9]. [10]

As it is evident from these words, Ibn Sina, by illustrating the contrast of soul and body and that the soul is perceived, even in the absence of body perception, intends initially to demonstrate the soul and then to express the abstraction and immateriality of the soul (Ibn Sina, 1996, p. 26).

At the end of the book *De Anima* (on the Soul)- Chapter SIX of the *Physics of the Healing* - Ibn Sina once again raises the idea of the suspended man. Here, he primarily presents his schema and then suggests that man is self-aware in this case while he is ignorant of all his members. It is clear that our knowns are apart from our unknowns. Therefore, the soul cannot be considered the body or its organs. The soul is what we refer to it as "self" and man always understands it. However, the organs of the body – e.g., the brain or the heart - are not always intended by man, and perhaps we need to dissect the body for the detection of the organs. As a result, given that a thing in a sense cannot be both known and unknown, the "self" which is known is different from the "body or its organs" which is unknown. The focus of Ibn Sina here seems to be on proving the abstraction and immateriality of the soul (Ibn Sina, 1996, p 225).

---

9 *Compare this translation with Jon McGinnis 's translation of these words in the article "Experimental thoughts on thought experiments in medieval Islam."*

10 فنقول: يجب أن يتوهم الواحد منا كأنه خلق دفعة وخُلق كاملا، لكنّه حُجب بصره عن مشاهدة الخارجات، وخُلق يَهوى فى هواء أو خلاً هويّا لا يصدمه فيه قوام الهواء صدما مّا يحوج إلى أن يحسّس، وفرّق بين أعضائه فلم تتلاق ولم تتماس، ثم يتأمل أنه هل يثبت وجود ذاته ولا يشك فى إثباته لذاته موجودا ولا يثبت مع ذلك طرفا من أعضائه ولا باطنا من أحشائه ولا قلبا ولا دماغا ولا شيئا من الأشياء من خارج. (Avicenna, *De anima*, 1.1, 16)

## 2-2- Statements of Ibn Sina about the Idea of the Suspended Man in *Al-Ishārāt wa al-Tanbīhāt* (Remarks and Admonitions)

The third class in the philosophy section of *Al-Ishārāt wa al-Tanbīhāt* is related to the soul with the title of "On the Terrestrial and Celestial Souls." In the first sentences of this class, Ibn Sina proposes the idea of the suspended man. In this book, unlike *the Book of Healing*, the self-consciousness topics basically begin with this idea. Thus, the position of this scheme in *Al-Ishārāt wa al-Tanbīhāt* is more central than what is proposed in *the Book of Healing*.

Here, Ibn Sina asks the reader of the book to assume himself to be in a situation in which he was created as a perfect human being with a sound mind and body and was suddenly in a position between heavens and earth where none of his senses work. His eyes do not see the organs of his body, and his sense does not touch an organ. Because he is in thin air and no breeze blows, and the air is not cold nor hot, he does not feel any organ. Similarly, his auditory, taste, and smell senses do not feel anything. In this situation, even though we are unaware of everything, we still understand the soul (Ibn Sina 1983, p. 292).

In this work, it appears, while proving the soul, he seeks to demonstrate or explain two essential matters: the intuitive knowledge of oneself and the immateriality of the soul. Given the significance of Ibn Sina's expressions in *Al-Ishārāt wa al-Tanbīhāt* (Remarks and Admonitions), we here quote his exact statements in this respect[11]:

### Chapter 1. Admonition: Proof for the Existence of the Soul through Intuition

Return to yourself and reflect. If you are healthy, or rather in some states of yours other than health such that you discern a thing accurately, do you ignore the existence of yourself and not affirm it?

To me this [ignoring and not affirming] does not befit one who has mental vision. One's self does not escape even the one asleep in his sleep and the intoxicated in his intoxication, even though its representation to oneself is not fixed in memory.

Further, if you imagine yourself at the beginning of its creation with a healthy intellect and a healthy disposition, and supposedly it is altogether in such a position and disposition as not to perceive its parts nor have its members

11 *In the English translation of the statements, we have mainly exploited the translation of Shams Inati with some minor changes. To see another translation of these words of Ibn Sina, refer to (Marmura, 1986).*

in contact-but separate and suspended for a certain moment in thin air-you find that it ignores everything except the assertion that it is (Inati 2014, p 94).[12]

### Chapter 2. Admonition: Concerning the Non intermediary Manner in which the Soul is Apprehended

With what do you apprehend yourself at that time, prior to that time, and posterior to it?

Also, what is it of yourself that is apprehended?

Is that which apprehends yourself one of your external senses, is it your intellect, or a faculty other than your senses and what belongs to them? If it is your intellect or a faculty other than your senses by which you apprehend yourself, then do you apprehend it by means of an intermediary or without an intermediary?

I do not believe that in that case you are in need of an intermediary. Thus it is without an intermediary [that you apprehend yourself. It remains, therefore, that you apprehend yourself without the need for another faculty or an intermediary. Hence it remains that you do so by means of your external senses or internal faculties without an intermediary. Reflect further! (Inati 2014, p 96).[13]

### Chapter 3. Admonition: Regarding the Nonsensible Nature of the Soul

Do you gather that that which is apprehended of yourself is that [part of] your body that your vision apprehends? No, for if you were stripped of that part of your body, and if it were substituted for you, you remain yourself. Or is it what you apprehend by your touch?

---

12 تنبيه [في وجود النفس الانسانية] ارجع إلى نفسك وتأمّل هل إذا كنت صحيحا بل وعلى بعض أحوالك غيرها بحيث تفطن للشيء فطنة صحيحة هل تغفل عن وجود ذاتك ولا تثبت نفسك. ما عندي أن هذا يكون للمستبصر حتى أن النائم في نومه والسكران في سكره لا يعزب ذاته عن ذاته وإن لم يثبت تمثله لذاته في ذكره، ولو توهمت أن ذاتك قد خلقت أول خلقها صحيحة العقل والهيئة وفرض أنها على جملة من الوضع والهيئة لا تبصر أجزاءها ولا تتلامس أعضاؤها؛ بل هي منفرجة ومعلّقة لحظة ما في هواء طلق وجدتها قد غفلت عن كلّ شيء إلا عن ثبوت إنيتها (Ibn Sina 1996, p 80).

13 تنبيه [في أن الانسان لا يدرك نفسه الا بنفسه] بما ذا تدرك حينئذ و قبله و بعده ذاتك، و ما المدرك من ذاتك. أ ترى المدرك منك أحد مشاعرك مشاهدة، أم عقلك و قوة غير مشاعرك و ما يناسبها. فإن كان عقلك و قوة مشاعرك بها تدرك. أ فبوسط تدرك أم بغير وسط ما أظنك تفتقر في ذلك حينئذ إلى وسط. فإنه لا وسط. فبقي أن تدرك ذاتك من غير افتقار إلى قوة أخرى و إلى وسط فإنه لا وسط. فبقي أن يكون بمشاعرك أو بباطنك بلا وسط ثم انظر.(Ibn Sina 1996, p 80)

Again, no, for this is nothing other than external members of yourself, whose case is the same as that which was discussed above. Further, in the first place, we have supposed that the senses are unaware of their acts.

It is evident, therefore, that that which is apprehended of you is not then one of your organs such as the heart or the brain. How [could it be one of these organs] when the existence of such organs is not revealed to you except through dissection?

Nor is that which is apprehended of you the whole [of your body] inasmuch as it is a whole. This [must be] clear to you from what you observe by yourself and from what you have been warned about.

Therefore, that which is apprehended of you is something other than those things that you may not apprehend when you apprehend yourself and that you do not find necessary for your being yourself.

Thus that which is apprehended of you is not one of the things that you apprehend by the senses in any way, nor one of the things that resemble the senses and that we will mention (Inati 2014, p. 96).[14]

## 3- Thought Experiment and Analysis of Ibn Sina's Idea of the Suspended Man

### 3-1- Definition of Thought Experiment and its Application in Various Fields

Thought experiments are basically devices of the imagination that employed for various purposes such an education, exploration, conceptual analysis, hypothesizing, theory selection, theory implementation, etc. Few would object to thought experiments that serve to illustrate complex states of affairs, or those that are used in educational contexts. The situation is different, however, with respect to the appropriation of imagined scenarios to investigate reality

14 تنبيه [في بيان أن النفس الانسانية ليست محسوسة] أ تحصل أن المدرك منك أ هو ما يدرك البصر من إهابك. لا. فإنك إن انسلخت عنه وتبدّل عليك كنت أنت أنت أو هو ما تدركه بلمسك أيضا، وليس أيضا إلا من ظواهر أعضائك. لا. فإن حالها ما سلف. ومع ذلك فقد كنا في الوجه الأول من الفرض أغفلنا الحواس عن أفعالها. فبيّن أنه ليس مدركك حينئذ عضوا من أعضائك كقلب أو دماغ. وكيف ويخفى عليك وجودهما إلا بالتشريح، ولا مدركك جملة من حيث هي جملة. وذلك ظاهر لك مما تمتحنه من نفسك، ومما نبهت عليه. فمدركك شيء آخر غير هذه الأشياء والتي قد لا تدركها وأنت مدرك لذاتك والتي لا تجدها ضرورية في أن تكون أنت أنت. فمدركك ليس من عداد ما تدركه حسا بوجه من الوجوه، ولا مما يشبه الحس مما سنذكره.
(Ibn Sina 1996, p. 81)

(very broadly conceived to include things like electrons, tables, beliefs, morals, people, numbers, universes, and even divine beings). It should be mentioned that this use of thought experiments that attracts most of the attention inside and outside of philosophical discourse (Brown & Fehige 2019).

As it is discernable by the above instances, there is significant overlap here with many other central philosophical topics, such as the nature of the imagination, the importance of understanding in contrast to explanation, the role of intuition in human cognition, and the relationship between fiction and truth. Moreover, thought experiments are interdisciplinary in two important respects. Firstly, not only philosophers treat them as a topic, but also historians, psychologists, cognitive scientists, etc. Secondly, they can be found in many disciplines, including biology, physics, philosophy, mathematics, history and economics (although, interestingly, not with the same frequency in each) (Ibid).

Although the use of thought experiments practically has a long history, the analytical philosophers examined, analyzed, and criticized thought experiments as an epistemological matter for the first time. In this regard, some scholars have explained the thought experiment in such a way that our mind imagines a kind of order and discipline in a series of affairs and subsequently, in the form to see its results, moves this set so that the desired result is achieved from it (Brown 2006, p 63). Some others have considered the benefits that derive from parallel mental scenarios through the use of thought experiments for the verification or falsification of a theory (Gendler 2002).

## 3-2- Examples of Exploiting Thought Experiments in the History of Philosophy and the Natural Sciences

Although not much time has passed from the naming of the term thought experiment and philosophical-logical analysis[15], the use of thought experiments has a very long history (Rescher 2005, p. 2). Some scholars have revealed multiple examples of employing thought experiment in ancient times (Ierodiakonou 2011 2018, p. 31. Becker 2018. Fuhrer 2007. Rescher 1991 2005, pp. 61–72).

15 *Ernst Mach is commonly credited with introducing the word "Gedankenexperiment" (thought experiment) and thereby coining a term for philosophical discussion (most recently Krauthausen 2015, p. 15). "This view is incorrect, however! [. .] it can be substantiated that it was used [. ] already in 1811." (Witt-Hansen 1976, p. 48. Buzzoni 2008, pp. 14-15. 61–65. Kühne 2005, pp. 92–224; Moue et al. 2006, p. 63). The conceptual history of "thought experiment" goes back at least to the Danish "Tankeexperiment, as it was used by Hans-Christian Ørsted (Ørsted 1998. Brown & Fehige 2019)).*

Because some thinkers, taking into account the difficulty of defining the thought experiment, have considered the best way to get acquainted with it is to represent its examples, we here reflect on some cases of the use of thought experiment in the history of philosophy and the natural sciences. Of course, our focus will be on the Islamic period and afterward.

**3-2-1- Parallel and Collimation Experiment:** This experiment is exploited by Ibn Sina and Avicennian commentators to prove the finitude of dimensions (Tusi 1996, pp. 217–218).

**3-2-2- The Ladder Paradox Thought Experiment** (For example, see: Mulla Sadra 1984, vol. 4, p. 23): This experiment has also been applied in the philosophical tradition to prove the finitude of dimensions.

Generally, we see some examples of thought experiments in the finitude of dimensions of the universe, which has been accepted by the classical philosophers of the Islamic period. It is evident that reaching the boundary point of the universe - if we consider it to have a boundary point? - is beyond human empirical and sensory perception. Hence, Muslim philosophers have attempted to design thought experiments such as these two listed examples to speak about the issue (To observe the arguments that are intended for the impossibility of the finitude of dimensions of the universe, see Shahrzuri, 2005, vol. 2, pp. 88–102).

### *3-2-3- Motion in the Category of Position*

In order to demonstrate that an object may have a motion in the category of position while not moving in the category of this (place), Ibn Sina designs a thought experiment (Ibn Sina 1996, p. 104. Ibn Sina 2010, p. 206).

### *3-2-4-Mentally Positedness of the Numbers*

Suhrawardi - Iranian illumination philosopher and founder of Illumination Wisdom in the East of the Islamic World (See Marcotte 2019) resorts to a thought experiment to present his views on the theory of numbers and concludes that numbers are mentally posited things. In his view, the fact that a man can be considered in the East and another in the West of the world and that they can be taken into account as two persons represent the fact that the number two can be mentally posited. Besides, in a human set, subjects can make various divisions and consider groups of 5 or 6 human beings concerning the mentally positedness of diverse attributes. These categories have generality and peculiarity in some respects and can be multiplied by the number of subjects. This also implies that the numbers are mentally posited (Suhrawardi, 2001, vol. 2, p. 68).

### *3-2-5- Infinite Regress by Applied Proof*

This proof is one of the well-known arguments for infinite regress. It regresses the infiniteness based on indicating the states that lead to contradiction or demonstration *per impossible* (For example, see: Sabzavari, 2005, vol. 2, pp. 450–451; Khademzadeh & Saeedimehr2010; Dirbaz & Saydi 2014).

### *3-2-6- Infinite Regress by Argument of Ones and Thousands*

This argument, which is considered an argument against infinite regress, can be regarded as an example of a thought experiment (To examine this argument, see: Taftazani, 1992, vol. 2, pp. 129–130; Khademzadeh & Saeedimehr 2010).

These examples were cases of thought experiments in the Muslim world. However, thought experiments in the medieval Islamic period do not end there. In addition to mentioning more examples from Ibn Sina, Jon McGinnis refers to other instances of thought experiences of Ibn al-Haytham on optics or before philosophers such as Ibn Rushd or theologians such as al-Ghazali (McGinnis, 2018).

### *3-2-7-Theory of Free Fall*

This argument is the most famous example of a thought experiment designed by Galileo Galilei (1564–1642). Aristotle believed - assuming the existence of a vacuum - that the speed of free fall of objects is proportional to their weight. In this way, the object with more weight falls faster than the object with less weight. In opposition to this view, Galileo designed a thought experiment. Thus, if we connect two metal spheres and drop them from the top of a high place – e.g., the Leaning Tower of Pisa - the lighter sphere moves with less acceleration and prevents the movement of the larger sphere. As a result, the larger sphere will reach the Earth in more time relative to the normal case. However, we know that the total weight of the large and small spheres is higher than only a big sphere (the whole is greater than the part). So the sum of the two should fall sooner than just the big sphere. This paradox, from the view of Aristotle, would invalidate Galileo's view (Cohen, 2005, p. 33).

### *3-2-8- Wittgenstein's Beetle*

Like the finitude of dimensions experiments, this experiment is an example of the thought experiments employed to prove philosophical propositions. The experiment is designed to defend Wittgenstein's idea based on the lack of meaningfulness of words associated with specific objects in the external world (For information on the content of the argument, see: Cohen 2005, p. 87).

### *3-2-9- Twin Earth*

Putnam, with the design of this thought experiment, intends to put into question the idea that meaning is a matter relying on mental states (For information on the content of the argument, see: Putnam 1973, pp. 701–703).

### *3-2-10- The Gettier Problem*

This experiment is also among the famous thought experiments in the domain of epistemology. In particular, it seeks to challenge the definition of knowledge as justified true belief by designing a kind of thought experiment of the Platonic idea (See Sorenson 1992, pp. 136–137).

These are merely the representations of some examples through which we can achieve an elucidated picture of the concept of the thought experiment and its application in miscellaneous areas. Meanwhile, some famous thought experiments in philosophy, e.g., René Descartes' Cogito and philosophy of mind, e.g., Hilary Putnam's *Brain-in-a-Vat* (Putnam 1982. Wright 1992), and philosophy of religion, e.g., Robert Kirk's *Zulliver* (Kirk 1974, p. 135–52) and David Chalmers' *Anti-Materialist Modal Argument* (Chalmers 1996 2009), and physics, e.g., Albert Einstein's Chasing a Beam of Light, are considered to have similarities with Ibn Sina's idea of the suspended man (Hertogh 2013).

## 3-3- The Argument of the Suspended Man as a Thought Experiment

In fact, the case has been made "that Ibn Sina is the first philosopher in the Aristotelian tradition, and thus perhaps the first in Western philosophy overall, to try to identify the psychological processes that go into postulating a hypothetical scenario. Ibn Sina also exhibits an interest in accounting for why, and to what extent, such psychological acts are thought to carry weight in our study of nature." (Kukkonen 2014, p. 434).

The idea of the Suspended man in air proposed by Ibn Sina is regarded as a perfect example of the thought experiment (McGinnis 2018). Some strived to evaluate the idea concerning the standard formulations of thought experiments in analytic philosophy (Saeedimehr & Khademzadeh 2009). In this way, they employed Sorenson's logical model called Necessity Refuter (See Sorenson

1992, pp. 136–152) to formulate, analyze, and critique the idea of Ibn Sina's suspended man.

Here, by exploiting this study, we present the formulation of Ibn Sina's thought experiment for the two purposes mentioned in the book of *Al-Ishārāt wa al-Tanbīhāt*, i.e., demonstrating the intuitive knowledge of yourself and proving the immateriality of the soul. Accordingly, the rational formulation of Ibn Sina's thought experiment to prove the immateriality of the soul can be expressed as follows:

1- Soul is a part of the body or the whole body
2- If the soul is a part of the body or the whole body, then necessarily when a man neglects the body, he is also unaware of his soul.
3- If man, while neglecting the body, is also unaware of his soul and the suspended man in space is unaware of his body, then the suspended man has no knowledge of his soul.
4- It is impossible that the suspended man in space has no knowledge of his soul.
5- It is possible that the suspended man in space to be suspended so that he is unaware of his body (Saeedimehr & Khademzadeh 2009).

Thus, the introduction is nullified, and Ibn Sina indicates that the soul is apart from the body and, accordingly, is immaterial.

Furthermore, another formulation of this thought experiment can be organized to prove the intuitive knowledge of man on oneself:

1- Man's knowledge in relation to his soul is a piece of empirical knowledge.
2- If man's knowledge in relation to his soul is a piece of empirical knowledge, then man necessarily acquires knowledge of his soul with the mediation of cognition.
3- If the man acquires knowledge of his soul with the mediation of cognition, and the suspended man in space lacks a cognitive form, then the suspended man has no knowledge of himself.
4- It is impossible that the suspended human has no knowledge of his soul.
5- It is possible for the man to be suspended in space so that he has no cognitive form (Ibid).

Thus, introduction 1 is invalidated, and Ibn Sina indicates that the soul has intuitive knowledge.

## 3-4- A Study and Critique of Ibn Sina's Thought Experiment of the Suspended Man

There has been an extensive debate among analytic philosophers on the knowledge or lack of knowledge of thought experiment insofar as, in the past decades, some considered thought experiments as types of arguments, and some have considered it as a kind of Platonic Seeing (Brown & Fehige 2019).

Arguably, the ongoing discussion took off in light of a debate between James Robert Brown and John D. Norton (for a concise statement of each position, see Brown 2004; Norton 2004), which many have found useful to establish a contrast with their own alternative accounts of thought experiments. These views "represent the extremes of Platonic rationalism and classic empiricism, respectively." (Moue et al. 2006, p. 69).

In this conflict, Robert Brown believes that thought experiments allow the man to discover facts without relying on sensory experience pre-empirically, and hence have a supra-empirical place (Brown 1991, 1993, 1999, 2002, 2004). In contrast, Norton argues that thought experiments cannot go beyond experience. He believes that thought experiments deal with argument formulation by making certain assumptions, the result of which is not acceptable without recourse to sensory experience (Norton 1991, 1993, 1996, 1996, 2002, 2004).

From the time of Ernst Mach (Mach 1976) onwards, many people have commented on the epistemology of thought experiments. In the meantime, Sam Scott, Kathleen Vaughan Wilkes, and David Sorenson have made extraordinary contributions and have dealt with the critique (Wilkes 1988) or proving (Sorenson 1992) of the epistemology of these experiments.

Addressing these views takes us away from the purpose of this paper. Here, we only point out that some new studies on epistemology, e.g., (McGinnis 2010, 2018. Saeedimehr & Khademzadeh 2009), have demonstrated this argument of Ibn Sina with respect to some of the peripheral matters. For example, in a study that assessed Ibn Sina's idea of the suspended man as a thought experiment in accordance with the Sorenson's logical model, it is concluded:

> Based on Sorensen's model, however, the experiment of suspended man keeps aspect of it, and giving knowledge, but, we can't make uttermost use, rather, its effective extent should be adjusted. In this article, it will be shown that this idea can be applied to prove the immateriality of the soul; however, this application will depend on the acceptance of some additive assumptions and assistive hypotheses (Saeedimehr & Khademzadeh 2009).

Overall, as some researchers pointed out (Grant 2007, p. 201), the pattern of a thought experiment can hardly be explained by forms of Aristotelian logic.

It is interesting here that the critiques raised about this Avicennian idea in the Islamic period are also from the perspective of fitting this idea to the four statements of argument in Aristotelian logic. In the meantime, the critiques of Abolghasem Kermani (Reisman 2002. Ibn Sina 2017, p. 81–89), Fakhr al-Dīn al-Rāzī (Zahit Tiryaki 2020), and Quṭb al-Din al-Rāzī (Quṭb al-Din al-Razi 1983, pp. 293–295) are worth noting.

The point is that Ibn Sina himself is aware of the difficulty of formulating the idea of the suspended man and expresses detailed explanations in response to the criticisms of Abu l-Qasim al-Kirmani and the letter of Bahmanyar ibn al-Marzuban or Ibn Zayla in the book of *Al-Mubāḥathāt* (Ibn Sina2017, p81–89). Besides, the explanations of Ibn Sina in the book of *Al-Ishārāt wa al-Tanbīhāt* (Ibn Sina 1996, p. 80–85) and the descriptions of his commentators such as Nasir al-Din al-Tusi (al-Tusi, 1985) can well represent that, given the unknown nature of the concept of thought experiment, drawbacks were expressed by loyalists of the patterns of formal logic. To get out of these problems, they considered this argument useful to those who believed in its basics with some explanations and brought forward other arguments.

In the book of *Al-Mubāḥathāt*, Ibn Sina in response to Abu l-Qasim al-Kirmani writes that,

> during the conversation, I told him this argument to prove the soul is not suitable for you since it has mental preparations that its acceptance is not possible except for intelligent people and those with the power of conjecture (imagination). This is while you would like to refute these basics from the beginning, and hence, you will have nothing but doubt. . .. All in all, this argument is either inappropriate or convincing. It is inappropriate for those whose minds are not smart enough to realize those basics and find themselves apart from their senses, and arguments that employ type and material should be used for them. However, this argument is convincing for people who have a clear understanding of the image of the dilemma (the enlightened persons)[16].

16 «فأمّا الكلام في الحجّة المثبتة للنفس، المبنيّة على فرض يلزم فيه شعور بالذات، فقد كان ذلك الشيخ ذاكرني ذلك- وهو في أن يقرأ علي كتاب النفس من الشفاء، وأنا في أن أمتنع- فقلت له: هذا الواحد ليس من الحجج التي يلزمك، لأنّ ذلك البيان مبنيّ على مقدمة اعتباريّة ليس التصديق بها ممّا يتيسّر إلا لأهل الفطانة ولطف الإصابة، وإذا كان مع عدمهما يلحظ المقدمة بعين السخط، كان الشك أسرع إليه من الماء إلى الحدور. وهنا قياسات مبنيّة على مقدّمات إنّما يقع التصديق بها لبعض دون بعض؛ مثل أن تكون مقدّمات حسيّة وتجربيّة رصديّة وغيرهما . . . وقد يتهيّأ أن ينبّه المنصف على هذا الاعتبار إذا لم يبادر إليه بذهنه.وبالجملة فهذه الحجّة إما ضائعة وإما قاطعة؛ فإنّها ضائعة بالقياس إلى من يتوقّف ذهنه عن التفطّن لهذا الاعتبار حتّى يكون مجوّزا أن يكون الإنسان موجودا كامل الخلقة والعقل، غير مبلوّ بآفة- وقد فرض ذلك الفرض- فيكون حكمه حكم الجماد في أنّه لا يشعر بذاته حتّى يفتح عينيه مثلا، فيلقى بصره على سطحه الظاهر، فيكون ما أدركه هو ذاته التي يشعر بها؛ فإنّه لا مدرك لشيء إلا وهو يدرك ذاته مدركة. فأمثال هؤلاء لا تجدي في بابهم هذه الحجّة؛ بل تكون ضائعة- أعني الحجّة التي تستنبط من اعتبار الشخص حال نفسه- ويحتاجون

As we see in Ibn Sina's words, he considers this argument to be a suitable one for those who have sufficient intelligence to perceive the basics and proposes others to address other arguments. Some contemporary thinkers have emphasized the importance of introspection and intuitive experience of understanding the essence as an explanation of this argument. Hence, they did not consider the validity of this argument to depend on the practical experience of the listed conditions and related it to the intuitive ability of the individual to understand his nature (Mesbah Yazdi, 1996, pp. 212–215). However, some scholars have spoken about the possibility of actually realizing this idea today. They have attempted to demonstrate that not only is the realization of this idea possible, but also that scientific experiences have provided a space for generating the conditions of this idea and thus proving it in the past few decades (Anvari & Ahanchi 2012). They will be described below.

## 4- The Possibility of Actual Realization for the Idea of the Suspended Man in Space

From the original presentation of the idea of the suspended man in space up to now, there have been several discussions about it. As seen earlier, the majority of theoretical interpretations have regarded the idea as a thought experiment. However, some researchers have recently striven to show that the conditions of this idea have been realized today to some extent, with the progress of modern science, and, consequently, that this idea can be considered as something beyond a mere thought experiment (Anvari & Ahanchi 2012). Here, we will somewhat investigate this scheme.

### 4-1- Experimental Conditions of Sensory Deprivation Similar to the Conditions of the Idea of the Suspended Man

As we have observed in the presentation of the idea of the suspended man, the main scheme of this idea is based on depriving a man of all states of sensory perception. One of the examples given by Ibn Sina is the idea of the suspended man discussed here, and the other is the state of sleep and drunkenness (Ibn Sina 1996, pp. 81–82). The basic claim is that it is possible to deprive the man of all states of sensory perception, while he himself can achieve such outcomes as

---

وما «إلى الحجج النوعية والجنسيّة القائلة: «لما كان للأجسام أفعال كذا حيوانيّة، فلها مبدأ كذي هو نفس يشبه هذا؛ لكنّها بالقياس إلى المستبصرين قاطعة.» Ibn Sina2017, p81–82)

proving the existence of the soul, intuitive knowledge of man on oneself, and immateriality of the soul.

Previously, we have shown that some regarded this state of sensory deprivation as a thought experiment. However, some new scientific achievements have provided conditions similar to those mentioned above that can be employed for the actual realization of this idea. For example, experimental conditions of sensory deprivation have similarities to the hypothetical state of the idea of the suspended man.

Sensory deprivation, also called perceptual isolation, is the deliberate reduction or removal of stimuli from one or more of the senses. Simple devices such as blindfolds or hoods and earmuffs can cut off sight and hearing, while more complex devices can also cut off the sense of smell, touch, taste, thermoception (heat-sense), and the 'feeling' of gravity (Hebb 1980). Sensory deprivation has been used in various alternative medicines and in psychological experiments. When people are kept in isolation, sensory deprivation (e.g., with an isolation tank), information input via the senses (such as hearing and sight) is reduced. Also, a related phenomenon is a perceptual deprivation, also called the Ganzfeld effect. In this case, a constant uniform stimulus is used instead of attempting to remove the stimuli; this leads to effects that resemble sensory deprivation. (Wackermann 2008).

In the first half of the twentieth century, sensory deprivation was exploited for applications such as hypnosis and brainwashing.

Brainwashing, also known as mind control, coercive persuasion and thought control, is the concept that the human mind can be altered or controlled by certain psychological techniques.

Usually, three phases are considered in brainwashing:

1. Unfreezing phase, which means breaking the personality and destroying the balance of human personality and creating a state of instability in him.
2. Changing phase, in which the desired information is instilled in the person.
3. Refreezing phase, which means the rebalancing of the person's personality and the consolidation of the information transferred to him (Sargant 1966, p 18).

The basis of the first phase is dependent on Sensory deprivation. In this case, the person loses his information, which is the result of the function of the outer and inner senses, but he does not lose the knowledge of himself. This is the idea that has been considered in the suspended man by Ibn Sina and his followers.

For further elucidation of the second and third phases, it can be stated that experimenters are able to alter the substantial traits of the subject being tested in the brainwashing process, but they cannot convince him or her that he or she does not exist. The perception of the essence in this case - as Ibn Sina proposes in his idea - is a genuine thing that is not cut by the elimination of sensory perceptions and still remains.

In addition to brainwashing, other applications for the Sensory deprivation were reported. Sensory deprivation techniques were developed by some of the armed forces within NATO, as a means of interrogating prisoners within international treaty obligations (Jeffery 1985, p 58). Furthermore, employing this method has been reported alongside Deep-Interrogation techniques.

At this point, the extensive applications in psychology with the goal of relaxation and relieving stress, forgetting bad memories, and quitting abnormal habits (such as smoking or alcohol addiction) can be pointed out. Moreover, other therapeutic purposes, such as obesity, pain reduction, and insomnia, were mentioned. The cases, such as lowered blood pressure, lowered levels of cortisol, and maximal blood flow, are other benefits have been reported from the experience of sensory deprivation (Van Dierendonck & Nijenhuis, 2005).

Restricted environmental stimulation therapy (REST) is one of the most famous examples of therapeutic applications. There are many different kinds of basic methods of restricted environmental stimulation, including therapy (REST), chamber REST, and flotation REST (Suedfeld 1999).

In studies carried out in connection with individuals in experimental isolation chambers, various states of illusion, slow or fast perception of time, varying emotions such as feelings of depression and sadness or intense joy (Zukherman, 2007) and even in some cases - primarily when a flotation tank is used - states of the feeling of gravity have also been reported. In these studies and the aforementioned therapeutic experiences, the person is placed in an isolation tank.

An isolation tank, often referred to as a sensory deprivation tank (also known as float tank, float pod, float cabin, or flotation tank), is a pitch-black, light-proof, soundproof environment heated to the same temperature as the skin.

Another type of isolation tank is the flotation tank, in which this flotation is attempted to be maximal. In this regard, studies conducted seek to increase this state up to its maximum by creating breathing a liquid instead of air. This idea, known as Liquid breathing or Liquid ventilation, is being experienced in the form of biological models (Janke et al. 2017), although its human state has not yet been realized. However, it is expected, in the event of the success of this project - which is currently being worked on, for example, by German researchers from TU Bergakademie Freiberg - this condition also involves a loss of sensation in the body along with a feeling of weightlessness. Of course, the experiences of space agencies such as NASA can also contribute to this feeling of gravity if coupled with the isolation conditions.

Although the experience of being in these isolation tanks is associated with the aforementioned mental states, the self-perception has always been an essential component of it. Accordingly, the experience of being in this situation matches very well with Ibn Sina's hypothetical state in the idea of the suspended man[17].

It is worth noting that the experience of sensory deprivation in the states mentioned earlier has hierarchical degrees and levels, and sensory deprivation is a relative thing. Ibn Sina was also familiar with this hierarchy. Hence, he cites examples such as sleep - in which only the outer senses are disturbed - and drunkenness - in which part of the inner senses are also impaired - in his works (Ibn Sina 1996, p 81–82)[18].

He intends the state of the suspended man to be the highest state of the lack of sensory perception. Therefore, the hierarchy of sensory deprivation has similarities with Ibn Sina's idea of the suspended man, and the higher the sensory deprivation, the closer it is to Ibn Sina's hypothetical state. In some cases of the abovementioned states, it has also been reported that emotional, psychological states and audiovisual illusions decline with more prolonged exposure to isolation tanks, and the person's sensory deprivation state becomes closer to Ibn Sina's desired state.

In addition to the thought experiment that included one of the significant interpretations of Ibn Sina's argument on the contrast between the soul and the body, and therefore, the immediate perception of the soul and the abstraction of the soul, this report shows that, according to some studies, it could be stated that sensory deprivation experiments based on the placement of individuals in experimental isolation chambers have brought Ibn Sina's idea closer to actual realization nowadays. It is worth mentioning that one might claim that this actual realization happens merely for the outer senses and that these

---

17 *In addition to the general similarities, some more detailed similarities can also be listed. For example, the flotation medium consists of a skin-temperature solution of water. Ibn Sina, as I have pointed out, also uses the term moderate (not hot and not cold) air, which means air that agrees with the degree suitable for human skin (Ibn Sina 2017, p 88).*

18 *Ibn Sina mentions in the book Al-Mubāḥathāt other conditions besides the sleeping man (asleep) and the drunken man (drunken) for the sensory disorder, which he refers to as "al-Masbut wa al-Maskoot wa al-Masrou'a wa al-Mamrour ("المسبوت و المسكوت والمصروع و الممرور")" (Ibn Sina 2017, pp. 88–89)).*

experiments cannot remove the inner senses and human memories, which constituted part of the introduction of Ibn Sina's argument. Hence, we are speaking here about the fact that these experiments approached the actual realization of Ibn Sina's idea, but have not yet reached it completely.

## 5- Two Other Interpretations for the Idea of the Suspended Man Proposed by Ibn Sina

It is worth noting that the idea of the suspended man in space introduced by Ibn Sina has other analyses in addition to the two listed analyses (thought experiment, empirical actual realization).

**5-1-** An analysis, which is on the basis of inner intuition, considers the basics of this argument as an intuitive thing and the outcome of introspection. Accordingly, if the first premise - based on self-awareness without finding body - is achieved by personal intuition, the rest of the argument follows the rules of formal logic, then the reasoning will be causing. The only problem that arises is that this argument - in the introduction mentioned above - becomes a personal matter and depends on a person's introspective ability and talent. The statement of Ibn Sina in the book *Al-Mubāḥathāt* also supports this interpretation. Ibn Sina explicitly states that this argument is appropriate for a one who is intelligent (*Ahl al-Faṭanah*) and has the power of conjecture (*Luṭf al-Iṣabah*) (Ibn Sina 2017, p81–82), and for those who have difficulty in this self-awareness, conceptual arguments can be presented based on type and genus (al-ḥujaj al-nu'eiyah wa al-jinsiyah) (Ibid). Some contemporaries have even spoken that this idea is a kind of invitation to reflect on oneself and practice with introspective states (Mesbah Yazdi 2014, p 213).

Perhaps Ibn Sina's use of imperative verbs in the book of *Al-Ishārāt wa al-Tanbīhāt* (refer to yourself) is a proof of this interpretation. Moreover, in the book of *Al-Ishārāt wa al-Tanbīhāt*, dissimilar to *the Book of Healing*, Ibn Sina presents this argument immediately and directly at the beginning of the chapter without setting any conceptual premise, which can reinforce the view that this idea is a kind of departure from the conceptual course of conventional logic in formal philosophy and somehow brings the beginning of self's existence with introspection and intuitive attitude.

**5-2-** The fourth analysis is that this idea is not only an idea based on one of the three previous interpretations, but can also be adequately provided in the form of Aristotelian logic statements. By the acceptance this interpretation, not only is this idea a useful argument for specific individuals or in terms of the conditions mentioned in empirical or thought experiments, but even as some prominent philosophers have inclined to it, the immateriality of the souls of animals can be proved (Mulla Sadra 1984, vol. 8, p. 44)[19]. Such an interpretation requires delivering a sort of conceptual reading of the basics of the idea that is consistent with the foundationalism approach. Saeed Anvari and Omid Ahanchi have attempted to demonstrate such an interpretation that is justifiable alongside the past listed possibilities (Anvari & Ahanchi 2012). In this regard, by referring to the criterion explained in logic for distinguishing the fundamental theorems - according to Ibn Sina and his commentators - they have represented that the idea of the suspended man is a logical idea, and its first introduction is based on rational axioms. With this explanation, by scrutinizing the criteria for the detection of basic theorems in logic books, we find that the proposition "everyone understands his own soul" is an axiom theorem[20]. Hertogh likewise - albeit more cautiously - attempted to make a logical analysis of the idea of Ibn Sina (Hertogh 2013).

## 6- Conclusion

At the end, we should point out that the idea of the suspended man in space proposed by Ibn Sina, which has had extensive applications in the Muslim world and the Western world to the present time, intends to demonstrate an immaterial soul for man; the soul that perceives itself as intuitive knowledge and is not a body or a part of the body. In this paper, four different interpretations of this idea were presented. For any further critique and analysis of the Avicennian idea of the suspended man, these four readings must be initially taken into account. Among these readings, some considered philosophical and abstract aspects and some considered empirical aspects. With the simultaneous attention to these interpretations, we can gain a more comprehensive view of this argument and, thus, take a more in-depth look at the vital matter of the human soul and its immateriality.

---

19 *As an example of critiques, see Mulla Sadra on this problem (Mesbah Yazdi 2014, 214).*

20 *The authors of the mentioned article also believe that the lack of attention to axiomatic nature of this theorem by Fakhr al-Din al-Razi (al-Razi 1984, vol. 1, p. 122) has caused him not to accept this argument and a lot of debates have arisen in the tradition of writing commentaries on the Book of al-Isharat wa-l-tanbihat).*

## Bibliography

### Editions, commentaries, translations

Al-Baġdādī, Abu'l-Barakāt. (1994). *Ketāb al-moʿtabar.* Isfahan: University of Isfahan.

Al-Rāzī, Fakhr al-Dīn. (1984). *Sharḥ al-Isharat wa-l-tanbihat or commentary on Ibn Sina's Pointers and Reminders.* Qom, Iran: Ayatollah Mar'ashi's Library.

Al-Rāzī, Quṭb al-Dīn. (n.d.). *Lawami' al-asrar "ala Sharḥ Matali" al-anwar.* Qom, Iran: Kotobi Najafi.

Al-Shirazi, Quṭb al-Dīn. (2006). *Dorrat al-tāj fi ğorrat al-dabbāj.* Tehran: Hikmat.

Al-Taftazani, Saʿd al-Din. (1992). *Maqaṣıd al-Ṭalibin fi 'Ilmi Uṣul al-Din.* Qom, Iran: Sharif al-Razi.

Al- Ṭūsī, Naṣīr al-Dīn. (1996). *Sharḥ al-Isharat wa'l-tanbihat.* Qom, Iran.

Badawi, A. R. (1978). *(Aristotle in Arabic Civilazation) Arasṭū ʿinda l-ʿArab.* kuwait: Wikalat Matbuat.

Ibn Sina. (1892). *Le livre des théorèmes et des avertissements.* Brill.

Ibn Sina. (1910). *Manṭiq al-mashriqiyyīn wa-l-Qaṣīda al-muzdawija, taṣnīf al-Raʾīs Abī ʿAlī Ibn Sīnā.* Cairo: al-Maktabah al-Salafīyah.

Ibn Sina. (1951). *Livre des directives et remarques (Kitāb al-Ishārāt wa al-Tanbīhāt).* (A. M. Goichon, trans.). Paris: Vrin.

Ibn Sina. (1953). *Logic of The Cure or Manṭiq al-Shifāʾ.* Cairo: Ministry of Education.

Ibn Sina. (1959). *Avicenna's De anima: being the psychological part of Kitab al-Shifa'.* London: Oxford University Press.

Ibn Sina. (1981). *Avicenna's Psychology: An English Translation of Kitāb Al-najāt, Book II, Chapter VI, with Historico-philosophical Notes and Textual Improvements on the Cairo Edition.* (F. Rahman, trans.). Hyperion Press.

Ibn Sina. (1996). *al-Isharat wa-l-tanbihat maʿ sharḥay al- Ṭusi wa-l-Razi.* Qom, Iran: Nashr al-Balagha.

Ibn Sina. (2003). *Risālah aḍḥawīyah fī amr al-miʿād or Judgment Day.* Tehran: Shams Tabrizi.

Ibn Sina. (2014). *Ibn Sina's Remarks and Admonitions: Physics and Metaphysics. An Analysis and Annotated Translation.* (Shams Inati, trans.). New York: Columbia University Press.

Ibn Sina. (2016). *On the Soul from Book of Healing.* Qom, Iran: Bostan ketab.

Ibn Sina. (2017). *Al-Mubāḥathāt (Discussions).*(M. Zāreʿī ed.) Tehran: Iranian Institute of Philosophy.

Lahiji, F. (2005). *Šawāreq al-Ilhām*. (Asad'Ali Zade A. ed.). Qom, Iran: Imam Ṣadiq Institute.

Mulla Sadra. (1984). *Al-Ḥikma al-Muta'aliya fi-l-Asfar al-'Aqliyya al-Arba'a [The Transcendent Philosophy of the Four Journeys of the Intellect]*. Beirut - Lebanon: Dar Ehya l-Turath al-Arabi.

Sabzavari, M. H. (2004). *Sharḥ al-Manzumah or Šarḥ ḡorar al-farā'ed, ma'rūf be-manẓūma-ye ḥekmat*. Tehran: Nashre Nab.

Shahrazuri, S. al-Din. (2005). *al-Shajarah al-Ilahiyyah (The Divine Tree)*. Tehran: Iranian Institute of Philosophy.

Suhrawardī, Shahāb ad-Dīn" Yaḥya. (2001). *Kitab Ḥikmat al-Ishraq* (The Philosophy of Illumination). Tehran: Institute for Humanities and Cultural Studies.

## Secondary literature

Adamson, P., & Benevich, F. (2018). The Thought Experimental Method: Avicenna's Flying Man Argument. *Journal of the American Philosophical Association*, *4*(2), 147–164.

Anvari, S., and Ahanchi, O. (2012). The Argument of Suspended Man in Ibn Sina's Philosophy and the Study of its Actual Realization. *Avecinnian Philosophy Journal*, *15*(46), 79–94.

Becker, A. (2018). Thought Experiments in Plato. In *The Routledge Companion to Thought Experiments*. London: Routledge.

Brown, J. R. (1986). Thought Experiments Since the Scientific Revolution. *International Studies in the Philosophy of Science*, *1*(1), 1–15. https://doi.org/10.1080/02698598608573279

Brown, J. R. (1991). *The Laboratory of the Mind: Thought Experiments in the Natural Sciences*. Routledge.

Brown, J. R. (2004). Why Thought Experiments Do Transcend Empiricism. In *Contemporary Debates in the Philosophy of Science*. Oxford: Blackwell.

Brown, J. R. (2005). *The Laboratory of the Mind: Thought Experiments in the Natural Sciences*. Routledge.

Brown, J. R. (2007). Thought Experiments in Science, Philosophy, and Mathematics. *Croatian Journal of Philosophy*, *7*(1), 3–27.

Brown, J. R., & Fehige, Y. J. H. (1995). Thought Experiments. *Canadian Journal of Philosophy*, *25*(1), 135–142.

Brown, J. R., & Fehige, Y. (2019). Thought Experiments. In E. N. Zalta (ed.), *The Stanford Encyclopedia of Philosophy* (Winter 2019). Metaphysics Research Lab, Stanford University.

Brückner, T. (2008). Ulrich Kühne, Die Methode des Gedankenexperiments. *Journal for General Philosophy of Science, 39*(1), 161–165.

Brueckner, A. L. (1986, March 1). Brains in a Vat. https://doi.org/10.2307/2026572

Buzzoni, M. (2008). *Thought Experiment in the Natural Sciences. An Operational and Reflective-Transcendental Conception.* Würzburg, Germany: Königshausen+Neumann.

Chalmers, D. J. (1996). *The Conscious Mind: In Search of a Fundamental Theory.* UK: Oxford University Press.

Chalmers, D. (2009). The Two-Dimensional Argument against Materialism. In B. P. McLaughlin & S. Walter (eds.), *Oxford Handbook to the Philosophy of Mind.* Oxford University Press.

Cohen, M. (2008). *Wittgenstein's Beetle and Other Classic Thought Experiments.* John Wiley & Sons.

Dierendonck, D., and Nijenhuis, J. (2005). Flotation restricted environmental stimulation therapy (REST) as a stress-management tool: A meta-analysis. *Psychology & Health.*

Druart, T.-A. (1983). Imagination and the Soul—Body Problem in Arabic Philosophy. In A.-T. Tymieniecka (ed.), *Soul and Body in Husserlian Phenomenology: Man and Nature* (pp. 327–342). Dordrecht: Springer Netherlands. https://doi.org/10.1007/978-94-009-7032-8_28

Druart, T.-A. (1988). The soul and body problem: Avicenna and Descartes. *Arabic Philosophy and the West: Continuity and Interaction.*

Druart, T.-A. (2003). Philosophy in Islam. In *The Cambridge Companion to Medieval Philosophy.* UK: Cambridge University Press.

Druart, T.-A. (2005). Metaphysics. In *The Cambridge Companion to Arabic Philosophy.* UK: Cambridge University Press.

Fakhry, M. (2004). *A History of Islamic Philosophy.* Columbia University Press.

Fuhrer, T. (2007). Der Geist im Vollkommenen Körper: Ein Gedankenexperiment in Augustins De civitate 22. In *Body and Soul in Ancient Philosophy.* Berlin: De Gruyter.

Gendler, T., & Hawthorne, J. (2002). *Conceivability and Possibility.* Clarendon Press.

Gilson, É. H. (1960). *History of Christian Philosophy in the Middle Ages.* USA: Catholic University of America Press.

Grant, E. (2007). Thought Experiments and the Role of the Imagination. In *A History of Natural Philosophy: From the Ancient World to Nineteenth Century.* Cambridge: Cambridge University Press.

Hasse, D. N. (2000). *Avicenna's De Anima in the Latin West: The Formation of a Peripatetic Philosophy of the Soul 1160–1300*. Warburg Institute.

Hebb, D. O. (1980). *Essay on Mind*. L. Erlbaum Associates.

Hertogh, C. P. (2013). Ibn Sīnā's Flying Man: Logical Analyses of a (Religious) Thought Experiment. *Journal of Islamic Philosophy*.

Ierodiakonou, K. (2011). Remarks On The History Of An Ancient Thought Experiment. *Thought Experiments in Methodological and Historical Contexts*, 35–49.

Ierodiakonou, K. (2018). The Triple Life of Ancient Thought Experiments. In *The Routledge Companion to Thought Experiments*. London: Routledge.

Janke, T., Schwarze, R., & Bauer, K. (2017). Measuring three-dimensional flow structures in the conductive airways using 3D-PTV. *Experiments in Fluids*, *58*(10), 133. https://doi.org/10.1007/s00348-017-2407-x

Janssens, J. (2016). Ab Al-Barakat Al-Baġdādī and His Use of Ibn Sina's al-Ḥikma al-ʿArūḍiyya (or Another Work Closely Related to It) in the Logical Part of His Kitb Al-Mu'Tabar. *Nazariyat, Journal for the History of Islamic Philosophy and Sciences*, *3*(1), 1–22.

Jeffery, K. (1985). *The Divided Province: The Troubles in Northern Ireland, 1969–1985*. Orbis.

Karin Krauthausen. (2015). Ermittlung der Empirie. Zu Ernst Machs Methode des Gedankenexperiments. *Bild Wissen Gestaltung | Hermann von Helmholtz-Zentrum für Kulturtechnik*.

Kenny, A. (2004). *Medieval Philosophy: A New History of Western Philosophy, Volume 2*. Oxford University Press, UK.

Kirk, R., & Squires, R. (1974). Zombies v. Materialists. *Proceedings of the Aristotelian Society*, (48), 135–163.

Kühne, U. (2005). *Die Methode des Gedankenexperiments*. Suhrkamp.

Kukkonen, T. (2014). Ibn Sīnā and the Early History of Thought Experiments. *Journal of the History of Philosophy*, *52*(3), 433–459.

Marcotte, R. (2019). Suhrawardi. In E. N. Zalta (ed.), *The Stanford Encyclopedia of Philosophy* (Summer 2019). Metaphysics Research Lab, Stanford University.

Marmura, M. (1986). Avicenna's "Flying Man" in Context. *The Monist*.

McGinnis, J. (2010). *Avicenna*. Oxford University Press.

McGinnis, J. (2018). Experimental thoughts about thought experiments in medieval Islam. In *The Routledge Companion to Thought Experiments*. Routledge.

Mesbaḥ Yazdi, M.T. (2014). *Commentary on Mullā Ṣadrā's al-Ḥikma al-Muta 'aliya fi-l-Asfar al- 'Aqliyya al-Arba 'a* (2nd ed.). Qom, Iran: the Imam Khomeini education & research institute.

Moue, A. S., Masavetas, K. A., & Karayianni, H. (2006). Tracing the Development of Thought Experiments in the Philosophy of Natural Sciences. *Journal for General Philosophy of Science, 37*(1), 61–75.

Nersessian, N. J., Jutronic, D., Puskaric, K., Miscevic, N., Georgiou, A. K. A., and Brown, J. R. (2007). James Robert Brown: Thought Experiments and Platonism. Part Two. *Croatian Journal of Philosophy, 7*(20), 125–268.

Norton, J. D. (1996). Are Thought Experiments Just What You Thought? *Canadian Journal of Philosophy, 26*(3), 333–366.

Norton, J. D. (2002a). *On Thought Experiments: Is There More to the Argument?* University of Chicago Press.

Norton, J. D. (2002b). Why Thought Experiments Do Not Transcend Empiricism. In C. Hitchcock (ed.), *Contemporary Debates in the Philosophy of Science* (pp. 44–66). Blackwell.

Ørsted, H. C. (1998). *Selected Scientific Works of Hans Christian Ørsted.* (Karen Jelved, A. D. Jackson, & O. Knudsen, trans.). Princeton, New Jersey: Princeton Legacy Library.

Perkowitz, S. (2017). Gedankenexperiment. In *Encyclopedia Britannica.* UK: Britannica.

Putnam, H. (1973). Meaning and Reference. *Journal of Philosophy, 70*(19), 699–711.

Rahman, F. (1963). Avicenna. In *A History of Muslim Philosophy.* Kuala Lumpur: Islamic Book Trust.

Reisman, D. C. (2002). *The Making of the Avicennan Tradition: The Transmission, Contents, and Structure of Ibn Sīnā's al-Mubāḥaṭāt (The Discussions).* Brill.

Rescher, N. (1991). Thought Experiments in Presocratic Philosophy. In *Thought Experiments in Science and Philosophy.* Lanham: Rowman & Littlefield.

Rescher, N. (2005). *What If?: Thought Experimentation in Philosophy.* Transaction Publishers.

Saeedimehr, M., & Khademzadeh, V. (2010). Analysis of Idea of «the Suspended Man in Space» Based on Sorensen's Logical Model. *Philosophy of religion Research, 7*(2), 129–152.

Sargant, W. W. (1966). *Battle for the Mind: A Physiology of Conversion and Brain-washing.* Pan Books.

Sorensen, R. A. (1992). *Thought Experiments.* USA: Oxford University Press.

Stöltzner, M. (2003). The Dynamics of Thought Experiments-Comment to Atkinson. In *Observation and Experiment in the Natural and Social Sciences.* Dordrecht.

Stuart, M. T., Fehige, Y. J. H., & Brown, J. R. (2018). *The Routledge Companion to Thought Experiments.* London: Routledge.

Suedfeld, P., & Bow, R. A. (1999). Health and therapeutic applications of chamber and flotation restricted environmental stimulation thrapy (REST). *Psychology & Health, 14*(3), 545–566.

Tittle, P. (2005). *What If?: Collected Thought Experiments in Philosophy.* USA: Pearson/Longman.

Toivanen, J. (2015). Fate of the Flying Man: Medieval Reception of Avicenna's Thought Experiment. *Oxford Studies in Medieval Philosophy, 3,* 64–98.

Van Dierendonck, D., & Te Nijenhuis, J. (2005). Flotation restricted environmental stimulation therapy (REST) as a stress-management tool: A meta-analysis. *Psychology & Health, 20*(3), 405–412.

Wilkes, K. V. (1988). *Real People: Personal Identity without Thought Experiments.* Oxford: Oxford University Press.

Witt-Hansen, J. (1976). HC Ørsted, Immanuel Kant and the Thought Experiment. *Danish Yearbook of Philosophy, 13,* 48–65.

Wright, C. (1992). IV—On Putnam's Proof that we are not Brains-in-a-Vat. *Proceedings of the Aristotelian Society, 92*(1), 67–94.

Zahit Tiryaki, M. (2020). The Flightless Man: Self-Awareness in Fakhr al-Din al-Razi. - *Nazariyat Journal for the History of Islamic Philosophy and Sciences.*

Zuckerman, M. (2007). *Sensation Seeking and Risky Behavior.* American Psychological Association.

## Short Biography of Hamed Arezaei

*He is Ph.D. in Islamic Philosophy,* Faculty Member at Imam Sadiq University(ISU), and member of Academy of Medical Sciences, Iran. *He studies* BA in Arabic Language and Literature at Tehran University and *obtained his* BA and MA in Islamic Theology and Philosophy at Imam Sadiq University (ISU), Tehran (2011), and a *Ph.D. in Islamic Philosophy at Tarbiat Modarres University (TMU), Tehran (2017).*

*His areas of research are on the fields of history of philosophy and Sciences in the Islamic age,* focusing on Ibn Sina's heritage. He has published articles on the classification of knowledge and natural philosophy in Islamic thought, especially Avicennian tradition and the relationship between philosophy, medicine, alchemy, and other natural sciences. He has a keen interest in the philosophical approaches of Islamic medicine.

ORCID ID: 0000-0003-2236-350X
HamedArezaei@yahoo.com
https://modares.academia.edu/hamedarezaei

Prof. Dr. Kadircan H. Keskinbora, M.D., Ph.D.*

# Ibn Sīnā's Contributions to Ophthalmology

*"Medicine was absent until Hippocrates created it, dead until Galen revived it, dispersed until Rhazes (al-Rāzī) collected it, and deficient until Ibn Sina (Ibn Sīnā) completed it."*

**De Poure, European Physician** [1]

Ibn Sīnā (980–1037) was a great scholar, physician, poet and statesman, the "Father of Science" and an encyclopaedist who wrote about all the major problems of the second half of the middle ages. He authored over two hundred works, the most prominent of which is the Canon of Medicine. Above all, Ibn Sīnā was a scientist who made important contributions to various fields. He was recognized as an authority especially in the field of medicine during his lifetime and well after. He was an astute observer. It was his habit to base his work on his personal endeavors rather than those who came before him. A glance at his understanding of medicine, his philosophy and the state of medicine in at the time may offer a better understanding of his work. Ibn Sīnā has been called the greatest medical writer in the Islamic world. In fact, it is claimed by Pollock that the Canon, by its arrangement and exactness makes a magnificent, complete and large textbook of all branches of medicine, including surgery.[2, 3]

---

* ORCID ID: 0000-0003-1940-1026; Google Scholar: https://scholar.google.com/scholar?hl=tr&lr=lang_tr&as_sdt=0%2C5&q=%22Kadircan+Keskinbora%22&btnG=

1 Al-Hassani STS, ed. 1001 Inventions: The Enduring Legacy of Muslim Civilization, 3rd ed. Washington DC: National Geographic Society 2012. p. 168–169

2 Pollock, W.B. Inglis. Arabian Ophthalmology. Downloaded from http://bjo.bmj.com/ on December 11, 2015

3 W. B. Inglis Pollock Arabian Ophthalmology. *Br J Ophthalmol* 1946 30: 445–456. doi: 10.1136/bjo.30.8.445

# I. THE ISLAMIC SCHOOL OF OPHTHALMOLOGY (9TH CENTURY - 13TH CENTURY)

It is not possible to enter into details of the life of each of the Arabic eye surgeons who produced a treatise nor even a full description of their textbooks, but reference must be made to Hirschberg's (1843–1925) brilliant History of Ophthalmology.[4] He was a famous Greek and Latin scholar and translated a number of the Arabic writings with the aid of two orientalists, Lippert and Mitwoch after working at Arabic for twenty years.

In July 1905, Prof. J. Hirschberg mentioned the points below in his talk at the American Medical Association conference:

> *"From 800–1300 C.E. the World of Islam produced not less than 60 renowned Eye Specialists or Oculists, authors of textbooks and producers of monographs in Ophthalmology. Meanwhile in Europe prior to the 12th century an Oculist was unheard of. (.) It was not until the 18th century that the method of removal of cataract by a hollow needle was employed in Europe. (.) During this total darkness in medieval Europe [the Muslims] lighted and fed the lamps of our science (ophthalmology) - from the Guadalquivir (in Spain) to the Nile (in Egypt) and to the river Oxus (in Russia). They were the only masters of ophthalmology in medieval Europe."*[5]

The first systematic textbook of Ophthalmology was written by Hunain a well-known scientist. Between 830 and 870, Hunain collected all of the notes he had made on subjects related to the eyes and brought them out as "The Book of the Ten Treatises on the Eye". Another great scientist was Abul Kasim bin Abbas al Zahrawi (Albucasis), a Spaniard (died 1013) whose great work on medicine called "*Al Tasrif*" (The Explanation) contained excellent surgery, including ophthalmic surgery, done by the Muslims.[6]

Notably, Hirschberg (Leipzig, 1902) translated the eye diseases (ophthalmology) section of the Canon with the aid of J. Lippert. He found that the Latin translations had many mistakes and that to get a truer translation he had continually to work with the Greek sources, namely Oribasius and Aetius and Galen. At the same time Hirschberg produced a glossary of Arabic in Greek and

---

4 Ibn Sina (Ibn Sina). *Die Augenheilkunde des Ibn Sina*. Hirschberg J, Lippert J, translators. Leipzig: Verlag von Veit. Available from: https://archive.org/details/dieaugenheilkund00avic. Accessed September 5, 2014.

5 Pollock WBI. Arabian Ophthalmology. Br J Ophthalmol 1946;30(8):445–456.

6 Albucasis Methodus Medendi, 4to. Basiliae 1541. Lent by R.F.P.S.G. Latin Edition same as used by Wm. Mackenzie.

German. He was able to find both what Ibn Sīnā owed to the Greeks and what was added by Islamic thought and experience.[7]

Hirschberg's contemporary Meyerhof agrees with Hirschberg when he says that no better ophthalmological text-book was written either in the "Orient" or the "Occident" until the beginning of the eighteenth century.

## II. IBN SĪNĀ'S APPROACH TO MEDICINE

### A. Humors, temperaments and degrees of medicines

In the west, following Hippocrates' description of the four humors and Galen's development of the first typology of temperament, Galen "mapped" the four humors to the natural qualities of hot/cold and dry/wet of the four elements. He then went one step further and tied the natural qualities to temperamental categories that he named after the humors, i.e., sanguine, phlegmatic, choleric and melancholic. After Galen, for the next seven hundred years, medicine continued to evolve and reshape itself as new discoveries were made, yet it maintained the distinct characteristics given to it by Hippocrates, Aristotle, and Galen. Just before the turn of the millennium Ibn Sīnā, as a new philosopher and physician, reshaped medical thought, using the basis that those thinkers provided.

Ibn Sīnā appreciated, yet in some ways diverged from, Greek medicine. Like many Muslim philosophers and scientists, he welcomed Greek knowledge and was a faithful translator of many of the Greek works into Arabic. However, he defined temperament differently. Ibn Sīnā often referred to the work of Roman physician Pedanius Dioscorides' Materia Medica.[8] Also, he did not follow Galen's typology.

In the main text of his work, Ibn Sīnā described the individual, specific qualities of simple drugs.[9]

In Volume 1 of the Canon, Ibn Sīnā explains what he means by the degrees.

> *"There are four degrees of medicines—whether eaten, taken in the fluid state, or used as an ointment: The first degree drugs are those whose action is not ordinarily felt by the body, i.e., the heat or cold produced by them is not appreciated unless the drug is taken*

7 J. Hirschberg und J. Lippert, *Die Augenheilkunde des Ibn Sīnā*, Leipzig (1902) S. 19–24.

8 Bakhtiyar Laleh. Ibn Sina On Treating the Visual Organs. Abu 'Ali al-Husayn Ibn Sīnā (Author). Chicago: Kazi Publications, Inc., 2013, pp 16.

9 Bakhtiyar, 2013, ibid. P.18–19.

> *repeatedly or in a larger quantity. The second degree drugs are a little more potent but unless taken repeatedly or in larger doses they do not disturb the normal functioning of the body and even when they do so it is only indirectly. The third degree drugs directly impair the normal functioning of the body but not to the extent of causing disease or death. The fourth degree drugs are those that cause death or damage to the body. These are the poisonous medicines that act on account of their quality. The poisons of course kill by their very nature and are thus specific."*[10]

Ibn Sīnā speaks of degrees of hot, cold, wet and dry temperaments. The iris, for example, is hot and dry in the second degree. The reader has to return to Volume 1 of the Canon where Ibn Sīnā explains what he means by the degree.

Temperaments for Ibn Sīnā are based on the natural qualities in opposite pairs: cold and wet, cold and dry, hot and wet and hot and dry, a point Galen had reached as well, but then went beyond by relating these natural qualities back to the humors. In effect, according to Galen, the humors are the same as the temperaments. For Ibn Sīnā, on the other hand, the natural qualities hidden within substances form what he calls temperament whether the substances be the four elements of air, water, fire or earth or the four humors of sanguine, phlegmatic, choleric or melancholic. This is why his medicine, or the law of natural healing works because healing plants, herbs, animals and minerals also include natural qualities. One cannot, for instance, refer to the iris or saffron as having a choleric temperament. Ibn Sīnā refers to both as having a hot and dry temperament. Therein lies the healing property of the iris and saffron for treating a person who is suffering from a cold disease.[11]

According to Ibn Sīnā, a temperament, as understood by medicine, is never strictly equable or strictly unequable. The physician should abide by the philosopher who is aware that the really 'equable' temperament does not actually exist in the human being any more than it exists in any 'member'.[12] The temperament of a person or member is the elemental composition of that object; the ratio of the elements has a direct relation to how that object behaves, even if that object is a human being. It was thought that people with more fire in them were more courageous and could be prone to anger. Consequently, no person or part of a person was ever truly equal in ratio of all elements. A person who was completely equal with regards to all elements would never become ill, as no

10 Ibn Sina. The Canon of Medicine; Al-Qanun fi' al-tibb. Vol. 1. Chicago: Great Texts of the Islamic World, 1999. The Canon of Medicine, Volume 1, p. 221.

11 Bakhtiyar, 2013, ibid. p.19.

12 Ibn Sina, ibid, p.58.

imposed imbalance would upset the ratios. However, humans are more equally balanced than any other creatures, a trait that allows us to rule over the rest of nature.

## B. The Interrelation of Medicine and Philosophy

Ibn Sīnā saw medicine and philosophy as deeply connected, as is shown throughout his *Canon of Medicine*. Philosophy provides the support and much of the proof for many of the claims that he makes, and he frequently directs readers seeking proof to works of philosophy. For example, in Volume 1 paragraph 44, Ibn Sīnā states that "*the physician is again reminded that he must seek an explanation of the deepest intricacies of his subject in [esoteric] philosophy, for they are not self-evident.*"[13] This also shows that Ibn Sīnā believes that natural philosophy is not self-evident and must be reached though applied reason. In paragraph 16, Ibn Sīnā also clearly defines the limitations of medicine, saying the doctor must rely on precepts gained through the natural sciences and philosophy.[14] For knowledge of some things, the physician depends on the Doctor of Physical Sciences; in the case of other things, knowledge is derived by inference [reasoning]. One must presuppose knowledge of the accepted principles of the respective sciences of origins, in order to know whether they are worthy of credence or not [criteriology]; and one makes inferences from the other sciences which are logically antecedent to these. Hence, if a doctor undertakes the proofs of existence of the 'elements' and the 'constitutions' and their derivatives from medicine itself he errs, for medicine cannot make these things clear, belonging as they do to the domain of natural science.

## C. A Holistic View of Medicine

Ibn Sīnā's application of medicine, especially his belief in the temperaments and humors, led him to a more holistic view of medicine than mainstream healthcare has adopted today. If a patient is viewed as a complex collective, with each part influencing the whole in a different manner, the methodology of treatment is enacted differently than if the patient is seen as having a specific, isolated issue. Health is a complex property for Ibn Sīnā, and each organ or system of organs can influence the other systems both positively and negatively.

13 Ibn Sina, ibid, p.15.
14 Ibn Sina, ibid, p.31.

Ibn Sīnā thinks of the emotional states, which are linked to the temperament of the nervous system and brain, as having a reliable and predictable influence on the pulse of blood, which in turn has a direct influence on many other systems such as digestion.[15] Looking at the Canon in light of today's medical knowledge, we see that some of the methods and theories were the folk medical wisdom of the time. However, we also see that many of Ibn Sīnā's hypotheses were remarkably accurate, such as the function of salt in the body[16] and the role of different nerves.[17]

## D. The Importance of Anatomy

Ibn Sīnā always highlighted the importance of anatomy, or knowledge of structure, recognizing how crucial the structure, positioning and placement of organs were, especially for operating on the body. Therefore, whenever discussing a medical topic, he first makes an anatomical introduction.

Ibn Sīnā's contributions to anatomy as a physician, teacher and researcher represent the most important advances in the subject between those of Claudius Galen (120–200) and Andreas Vesalius (1514–1564 AD). Following the footsteps of previous traditions, the Canon also presented genuine observations and descriptions of diseases that had not been published before, showing Ibn Sīnā's ability for synthetizing existing knowledge with his own view in such a way as to influence the practice of medicine for centuries.[18] Although it is controversial whether or not Ibn Sīnā directly undertook human dissection, most of his descriptions of the structures of the body were novel for his time. Some authorities believe that Ibn Sīnā performed human dissection in secret.[19] In the Canon, he introduced anatomy in a systems-based approach at the beginning of each chapter followed by a discussion on the diseases of that system. This approach, pioneered by Ibn Sīnā, became the template for modern clinically

15 Ibn Sina, ibid, p.321.

16 Ibn Sina, ibid, p.323.

17 Ibn Sina, ibid, p.68.

18 Keskinbora KH, Keskinbora K. A systematic review of Ibn Sina's studies: reflections on anatomy. Eur J Anat. 2016;20(1):99–105.

19 Farhadi M, Behzadian Nejad G, Bagbanzadeh A. Papers of the International Congress of the History of Medicine in Islam and Iran [in Persian] Vol. 2. Tehran: Iranian Institute for Science and Research Expansion; 1996.

orientated anatomy. He stated that 'pupils should learn the general principles of medicine, analyze the diseases that affect different organs and to do so, must first study the anatomy of these organs.[20]

## III. IBN SĪNĀ'S CONTRIBUTIONS TO OPHTHALMOLOGY

As everyone will agree, the eyes are one of the most important organs of our body, allowing us to recognize our surroundings and accordingly ensure our own safety and manage the environment. Therefore, since ancient times, people have been interested in their structure and function and tried to treat their illnesses. Eye related illnesses were especially common in Middle Eastern countries, which compelled ancient civilizations in this region to understand the eyes better, as in the example of Egyptians' success in the treatment of trachoma.[21]

As a polymath, Ibn Sīnā did extensive research on the eye, as he did on many other subjects, delving into the anatomy, physiology and diseases of the eye in great detail. He described sight as one of the five external senses,[22] and presented detailed discussions of ophthalmic anatomy and diseases in volumes one and three of his Canon.[23] The portion of the "Canon" which deals with the eye and its diseases has been mentioned as being superior to its Greek sources.[24] In fact, Ibn Sīnā gave for the first time a correct detailed description of the eye, its different components like the conjunctiva, sclera, cornea, choroid, optic nerves, iris and their functions, and central and peripheral facial paralysis.[2526] He was also the first to speak of the optic nerve rather than the lens being responsible for vision, and noted important functions of the parts of the eye. Ibn Sīnā's

20 Naderi S, Acar F, Mertol T, Arda MN (2003) Functional anatomy of the spine by Ibn Sina in his eleventh century treatise Al-Qanun fi al-Tibb (The Canons of Medicine). *Neurosurgery* 52, 1449–1453.

21 Sayılı, Aydın. Mısırlılarda ve Mezopotamyalılarda Matematik, Astronomi ve Tıb, Ankara: Türk Tarih Kurumu, 1982, s. 149.

22 Finger, Stanley (1994), Origins of Neuroscience: A History of Explorations Into Brain Function, Oxford University Press, p. 71

23 Amr SS, Tbakhi A. Ibn Sina (Ibn Sina): the prince of physicians. Ann Saudi Med 2007;27:134–5.

24 Harry Sobotka, Ophthalmology During the Middle Ages. AMA Arch Ophthalmol. 1957;57(3):366–375.

25 Ibn Sina, Al-Qanun fi' l-tibb. Research and description by Prof. Hesan Ja`far, Al-Hilal, Beirut: Dar-ol-Behar; 2009.

26 Aydin IH. Ibn Sina and modern neurological sciences. *Journal of Academic Researches in Religious Sciences*. 2001; 1: 1–4.

writings on eye disorders in the Canon of Medicine suggest a rigorous approach to the diagnosis and management of patients suffering from eye disorders. The contributions he made to ophthalmology are quite considerable.

Below is a list of topics covered in the 3rd volume of the Canon:

3rd Fen[27] 1st Article:

- The anatomy of the eye
- The characteristics of the eye and all its diseases
- The states of the eye
- All of the eye diseases
- The hygiene of the eye and the features
- Eye inflammation/infections and tearing (Ramed - Ophthalmia - eye infections/inflammations) and Dem'a (tearing - epiphora)
- The common treatment for eye infection and the common cold
- Treatment of eye infections caused by "Humor of blood" and "Humor of Yellow Bile"(see Four Humor Theory of Diseases)
- Treatment of "cold" eye infections (see Four Humor Theory of Diseases)
- Medication for melancholia (Humor of black bile) caused infections of the eye (see Four Humor Theory of Diseases)
- Medications for the infected eye

3rd Fen 2nd Article

- Corneal Edema
- Eye wounds and Corneal Erosions
- Corneal perforation
- Swelling in the eye
- Under the cornea
- Cancer of the eye, malignant tumors
- Swollen eyelids and Chemosis
- Infection/inflammation of the lachrymal glands
- Eyelid skin (excess or scantness of the flesh/muscle)
- Corneal ulcers
- Pannus
- Pterygium

27 In the tradition of Arabic science writing, the sections classified according to their subjects are called "*Fen*". In the translations of the Canon, translators have chosen to use this word as is.

- Subconjunctival hemorrhage
- Tearing
- Strabismus
- Proptosis
- Enophthalmos (Deep-set eyes)
- Glaucoma

3rd Fen 3rd Article

- Eyelid related problems
- Eyelid lice
- Eyelid ulcers
- Cutaneous horns (*cornu cutaneum*)
- Severe eyelid infections
- Blinking and Ticks
- Heavy eyelids
- Sticky eyelids
- Turned eyelids - 3 types
- Hard mass under the eyelids
- Hairs
- Stye
- Verrua
- Conjunctival concretions
- Dryness of the eyelids
- Psoriasis of the eyelids
- Swelling
- Blinking
- Loss of eyelashes
- Turned eyelashes (Trichiasis, Distichiasis)
- Narrow eyelid opening due to anomaly in the eyelids (Blepharal anchylose)

3rd Fen 4th Article

- The power and function of vision
- Impaired vision
- The Function of the eye membranes
- Night blindness
- Day blindness
- Having visions / the intersection of visions and dreams (Illusions and hallucinations)

- Enlarged pupillae, recommended medications
- Narrowing of pupillae
- Cataracts
- Loss of vision
- Seeing flashing lights (flashes)
- Snow blindness

## A. HIGHLIGHTS FROM THE CANON'S OPHTHALMOLOGY ARTICLES

### *1) Anatomy, Physiology and Function of the Eye*

- Ibn Sīnā, in The Canon of Medicine, described sight as one of the five external senses.[28]
- He was the first to define the:
  - conjunctiva
  - sclera
  - cornea (4 layers)
  - choroid
  - iris
  - retina layers
  - lens
  - humor aquose of the anterior chamber of the eye
  - optic nerve
  - optic chiasm
- Describing the position and general structure of the eye in the Canon, Ibn Sīnā says that it is located inside the eye socket (orbita). It is protected by the eyelids and the lashes. He describes the upper lid as being made up of sections such as skin, the conjunctiva, first cushion (superficial lipoid tissue), fatty section, muscle and the second cushion (deeper lipoid tissue). The lower eyelid does not have any muscles. Our present knowledge confirms the accuracy of most of this description.
- He precisely described the trigeminal nerve (Ibn Sīnā distinguished nerves and tendons as different anatomical structures, in contrast to previous interpretations.)

28 http://www.worldheritage.org/articles/Ophthalmology_in_medieval_Islam#cite_note-3

- He also described the dilation and contraction of the pupils and iris of the eye and their diagnostic value.
- He discussed the functions of the tear ducts.[29]
- Ibn Sīnā was the first to describe the exact number of extrinsic muscles of the eyeball or identified the six motor muscles,[30] and the physiology of eye movements. There are 6 muscles, four of these are the superior, interior, medial and lateral [recti] muscles, which are attached to eyeball to elevate, depress, adduct and abduct the eye. The remaining two [superior and inferior oblique] are attached to eyeball obliquely and rotate the eyes. The muscle [levator palpebral superioris] which opens the eye spreads into the upper lid from the center outwards and opens the eye by contraction.
- Ibn Sīnā states that the eyelashes function as a barrier against particles in the air or dropping from the head. He also says that black lashes serve to screen incoming light due to their color. Ibn Sīnā also mentions that the lashes are embedded in a membrane in the eyelid like cartilage, which strengthens the eyelashes and is where the eye muscles are attached. This structure was previously brought up by Galen, who held, though, that this structure was made of cartilage and contained holes from which eyelashes protruded.[31]
- For Ibn Sīnā, the outer membrane of the eye, the sclera, is relatively thicker than the other layers of the eye. This front layer is the most anterior part, in front of the pupilla. This section (cornea) is transparent and does not impede vision; it is as if polished. Actually, the cornea comprises four thin stacked layers. Ibn Sīnā explains the presence of four layers of the cornea saying if a layer is damaged, it can be removed to prevent the lesion from spreading to the other parts.
- Ibn Sīnā takes the part called the conjunctiva as one of the eye's individual layers, which is where the muscles that move the eye are located. The glands of this layer serve to keep it moist and soft.
- Ibn Sīnā defines the choroid layer inside the sclera as the second layer of the eye. He describes it as a web of thin veins like a spider web. This layer is

---

29 Safiya Lokhande, Jaleel Ahmad, Ayesha Fatema. Contributions of Ibn Senna in ophthalmology. International Journal of advances in health sciences (IJHS) 2015;2:108–112.

30 Chams H. [History of Ophthalmology in Iran]. Iranian Journal of Ophthalmology 2006;19(1):1–13.

31 Galen, Ouvres Anatomiques, Physiologiques; Medicales de Galen (trans.) Daremb Paris, 1854, vol. 1, s. 627.

responsible for feeding various parts of the eye. It forms the iris, which is in front of the eye and is rather thick and different colors in different people. This part serves to screen light. In front of this section is a hole in the middle, similar to that which appears in a grape once its stem has been plucked, and this composes the pupilla.

- The Latin word "retina" (net-like layer) is derived from the translation of Ibn Sīnā's Arabic term "*tabaqa shabakiya*" for the organ.[32] Ibn Sīnā says that the innermost layer of the retina has a web-like composition. Like Galen, he says it is not a typical membrane, neither in terms of its contents nor its structure, but is rather a membrane made up of the spreading of nerve endings. For him, the retina has a spider web-like appearance.[33]
- Ibn Sīnā agreed with his contemporaries and his predecessors that there are three humors (liquids) in the eye. The first is the crystalline humor, which we refer to today as the lens. Ibn Sīnā describes this humor as being like glass. It is globular and flattened in the front and thinner in the rear. There are two humors in front of and behind it. The one in front is like an egg white, it is aquose humor. For him, it seems to be an excess of the crystalline humor, like it feeds it. The one in the back is like melted glass (called today as vitreous). Ibn Sīnā describes it as reddish and shiny. This is the humor in contact with the retina. Like Galen before him, Ibn Sīnā says the retina is sensitive.
- Ibn Sīnā mentions that the power of vision is distributed along the visual nerve. He holds that vision views return to the brain along the same path. Ibn Sīnā focused on optical sight and tried to distinguish between real and imaginary vision. He did not succeed in defining real vision and described vision as a dream. Imagining the real appearance of an object on a mirror or illuminated surface, Ibn Sīnā described the object or the observer as moving, i.e., dreams exchanging positions. For him, real dreams are constant and visions are temporary. Ibn Sīnā, like Ibn al-Haitham, says that sight is an optical vision or dream in the eye. He holds that the eye is like a mirror, and seeing an object is like it is reflected off of a mirror through air or other transparent substances. When light falls on a visible object, the vision of that object appears on the eye. Thus, Ibn Sīnā actually presents a very interesting approach to the theory of vision: Seeing rays exit an object and enter the eye, similar to what Ibn al-Haitham believed. Ibn Sīnā does not specify whether

32 Finger, Stanley (1994), *Origins of Neuroscience: A History of Explorations into Brain Function*, Oxford University Press, p. 69, p. 71, ISBN 0-19-514694-8

33 Galen, ibid.

the reflective globe is the lens of the eye or another part. The distinction he tried to draw between the two types of vision, i.e., real vision and dream vision, created a good foundation for the understanding of vision. A similar distinction was drawn in the west at a later date by Kepler.[34]

- Ibn Sīnā observed that the optic nerves are short and cross on their way to the contralateral side of the brain from their origin.
- He defined 59 eye diseases and recommended treatments.[35]
- Ibn Sīnā discussed orbitopathy. His observations determine the necessary fluidity of the lens.[36,37]
- Ibn Sīnā taught his students about strabismus and double vision.[38].
- Ibn Sīnā was the first to treat lachrymal fistula by probing and he knew the cataract was due to lens opacity.[39]
- Cautery was used by Ibn Sīnā to prevent destructive lesions, to remove putrefaction and to arrest hemorrhage. He advised the use of gold instruments for the procedure. He advised care and to use it on the tissue which is visible to the eyes and not to use it blindly.[40]

---

34 Sayili, A., A Possible Influence in the Field of Physiologycal Optics of Ibn Sina on Ibn al-Haytam. International Conference on Science in Islami Polity (19–24 Nov., Islamabad, Pakistan), c. 1, s. 328–333.

35 Kahya, Esin. İbn Sina- El-Kanun fi't-Tıbb Tercümesi. Ankara, Atatürk Kültür Merkezi Yayınları, c.3, pp 273–377.

36 Introduction to al-Umar al-Tabi'yah (Principles of Human physiology in tibb). By S. I. Ahmed, first Ed., 1980 A.D.–1401 A. H. Published by Hakim (Mrs) Nuzhat Ishtiaq, B.U.M.S (Alig.), printed by Saini Printers, Parhari Dhiraj, Delhi. pp. 80,81.

37 Ophthalmology In Medieval Islam, Compiled by World Heritage Encyclopedia™ licensed under CC BY-SA 3.0, http://www.worldheritage.org/articles/Ophthalmology_in_medieval_Islam#cite_note-4

38 Ismail M, Rafeeq MAR. *Anatomy of Eye and the Mechanism of Vision According to Ibn Sina: Bulletin of the Indian Institute of History of Medicine.* Heydarabad; 1981:146–151.

39 Shobhana Mathur and Sakait Rama Rao, G., (March-April 1402/1982). Contribution of Muslim scientists toward surgery, *Bulletin of Islamic Medicine,* Vol. III, K.F.A.S., State of Kuwait, p. 227.

40 Beg H. Surgical principles of Ibn Sina (Ibn Sina). *Bangladesh Journal of Medical Science* 2015;14(3):217–220.

### *2) Eye Diseases*

As mentioned above, Ibn Sīnā defined 59 eye related illnesses and recommended treatments for these. He was very organized in how he presented these in the Canon.

#### *a. Eyelid Diseases*

Ibn Sīnā first covered diseases having to do with the eyelids, offering information about their symptoms, causes and treatments. Among these are infections, itchiness, various lacerations, ulcers, swelling, eyelids sticking together, or to the pupil, turned eyelids, stye, small growths due to the accumulation of sebaceous substances into nodules, hypertrophic accumulations, calcifications, ticks and trachoma. Let us take some of these as examples:

**Ophthalmia (Ramad):** This is the first eyelid disease Ibn Sīnā explores. He describes the symptoms saying, "*infection* (also *inflammation*) *in the eyelids, redness, small or large nodules (papillae), sticking of the eye lids, moistness like watering, burning, pus discharging, head aches and lethargy.*"[41] For him, the larger the nodules in infected eyes, the less dangerous. The eyelids sticking is a sign that the disease has progressed. This diagnosis he makes bears similarity to various microbial diseases such as marginal blepharitis as well as to non-microbial meibomitis. We know meibomianitis today as the inflammation of the Meibomian glands, and it is characterized mainly by redness, irritation, discharge and swelling. All of these observations are in keeping with Ibn Sīnā's diagnosis of eyelid infections. However, exudation, pain and the sticking of the two eyelids brings to mind a microbial case, which means the disease could be marginal blepharitis or another microbial disease. Ibn Sīnā could also be defining a compound disease, or may not have been able to distinguish between eyelid diseases that usually occur simultaneously.[42]

In the 3rd volume of the Canon, in describing eye diseases, Ibn Sīnā refers to Ophthalmia in Arabic as *ar-Ramad*, and characterizes the inflammation of the *tunica vasculosa* (choroidea) layer of the eye (for cases of severe conjunctivitis the same name is used). In the Canon, he not only describes in detail the underlying causes of the ramed disease, climactic causes, diagnosis, prognosis and treatment, he also mentions preventative measures, dietary treatment,

41 Sayılı, A.: Mısırlılarda ve Mezopotamyalılarda Matematik, Astronomi ve Tıb, Ankara, 1982, s. 149.

42 Vaughan, D., Taylor A.: Göz Hastalıkları (Çev. Bengisu U, Sezen F), Ankara 1978, ss. 66–67.

medication options and surgery. His knowledge of ancient Greek sources is evident in his naming of the three types of ramed (ophthalmia) as 1- Tarsit (inflammation of the eyelids), 2- Chemosis (Swelling of conjunctiva), 3- Humor of *phlegm* (Balgamî).

In contrast to Al-Rāzī (Rhazes) and Ali bin Isa, he does not view discoloring and itcing as separate diseases but as symptoms of ophthalmia.

**Trachoma:** Ibn Sīnā refers to a type of Ramed (Ophthalmia) as it is called in Egypt today, as "*al-ramad al-hubaybi*" (small-grained eye inflammation). He describes the diagnosis of trachoma in the Canon. He calls eyelashes growing inward as a result of trachoma as distichiasis (*al-sha'ar al-munkalib* = inverted hairs).

**Berd(e):** Another eyelid disease is a nodule in the inner side of the eyelid. Ibn Sīnā likens this to hail and calls it *berd* or *berde* (conjunctival concretions), saying it is due to dirt or dust.

**Stye**: The information he provides resembles what we call chalazion today because Ibn Sīnā takes the stye and investigates it separately. In distinguishing between the two, he says a stye is a bloody and independent swelling. For the treatment, Ibn Sīnā recommends rose oil, an ammonia glue solution, sarcocol and narthex asafetida. He also mentions that medications used for a stye would also help with this disease.

Sarcocol, otherwise known as anzarot, has been used to treat eye diseases for many centuries. In Ottoman medicine, it was used for the same purpose and mostly as a pain reliever. Today, anzarot is no longer used in treatments. Asafetida is a malodorous plant and was used for centuries as a laxative or anti-spasmodic. Today it is used to manufacture carminative, antispasmodic and laxative medicines.[43]

Ibn Sīnā tried to treat swelling, lacerations and ulcers of the eyelids using various herbal ointments. Most of these, as seen as in other diseases, are plant-based. For example, he used rose water and rose oil in the ointments, pastes, dressings and eye baths against eye diseases. Today, rose oil is mostly used in perfumes but rose water is still used topically for eye diseases.[44]

In the same way, violet is also used to treat eyelid diseases. It is usually viewed as anti-inflammatory, so Muslim doctors and Ottoman doctors incorporated it

43 Elaus, E. V., Varro, B.: Tyler, Pharmacognosy, Philadelpihia (USA), 1968, s. 259.
44 Baytop, T.: Farmakoloji, İstanbul 1971, c. 2, s. 140.

into the contents of medicines used to treat inflammatory diseases. It contains volatile oils, so it is emollient, expectorant and diaphoretic.[45]

Ibn Sīnā often used honey, milk and the blood of various animals. Honey is also used today in various medications. We know it has laxative properties. And milk is mentioned as a diluent in various pharmacopeia.

Though rarely, Ibn Sīnā used inorganic substances in some of his ointments for treating eyelid inflammation. One of these is borax, which was previously used by the famous scientist Dioscorides. Dioscorides describes it as being white and pink, with a sponge-like texture. Ibn Sīnā's contemporary al-Biruni, in his work "Saydana", also mentions using this substance.[46]

Ibn Sīnā occasionally recommends surgical intervention rather than external medications. As mentioned before, while his predecessor Hippocrates, who was viewed as a medical authority, and other people of medicine, were vehemently opposed to surgical interventions, citing life threatening danger, he insisted that a good anatomist need not shy away from surgical intervention. Among eyelid diseases, for turned eyelids in particular, he recommends surgical intervention.

Ibn Sīnā states that this disease could occur for various reasons. Among the main causes are deformity, cutting the eyelid due to trauma or accident, and problems in the eyelid muscles. Today, turned eyelids are classified into two: turning inward (entropion) and turning outward (ectropion). Ectropion, or outward turning occurs due to paralysis and the loosening of the Orbicularis Oculi muscle. Therefore what Ibn Sīnā mentions as turned eyelid must be ectropion. Today, we also treat this disease with surgical interventions and recommend electro-cauterization on the conjunctiva side from 4–5 cm on the tars (which resembles cartilage) of the lower eyelid.[47] Ibn Sīnā said that the eyelid shortens due to the turning, precluding the meeting of the lower and upper eyelids and the closing of the eye, and recommends cutting a part of the skin of the upper lid and treating the cut with ointments.

### *b. Eyesight related Diseases*

For eyesight, Ibn Sīnā mentions these diseases: impaired eyesight, night blindness, visions, shrunken pupils, enlarged pupils, eye weakness, cataracts,

---

45 Eriş, A.: Anadolu Selçuklularında Tıp ve Eczacılık Kurumu, Ankara 1979. Ankara Ü. Basılmamış Doçentlik Tezi. s. 7.

46 Biruni S. al-Saydana. (Çev. Hakim Muhammed Said) Karachi 1973, s. 79.

47 Vaughan and Taylor, ibid, s. 68.

seeing white spots, loss of sight, farsightedness and nearsightedness. Let us choose some examples of these and compare them to what we know today.

Of all sight related diseases, Ibn Sīnā focuses most on impaired vision. The causes can be grouped as: Abnormalities or lack of normal function in various parts of the eye (cornea, iris, vitreous, aqueous humor), central nervous system related causes, (brain diseases, trauma to the brain, excess moisture or dryness in the brain, excess moisture in the optic nerve, etc.) and body related causes (due to a change in the general character of the body).

As apparent in the variety of the causes given above, Ibn Sīnā has explored the symptoms of the diseases in great detail. Among the symptoms are loss of transparency in the eye, opaque cornea, increased moisture in the eye, vision problems, increased heat in the cornea, loss of natural color, excess layers or protrusion in the eye, increased aqueous humor, and other symptoms attributed today to various eye diseases. In general, Ibn Sīnā has collected sight problems that occur due to different reasons under one umbrella, as he did with eyelid inflammations. As seen above, just as we currently distinguish among the eyelid inflammations as different diseases, citing them as microbe based, what he groups under 'impairments of the eye' is also divided into various eye disease types used today.

Ibn Sīnā takes up one disease within the group he calls eye impairment and defines it as follows: "*Sometimes the patient can see an object up close but cannot properly see an object from afar. Accurate sight means being able to see an object sharply and completely. The patient cannot make out the boundaries of the object. The reason for this disease is that the sight spirit is excessive and heavy.*"

Here Ibn Sīnā is likely referring to what we call myopia today. However, it is not known if he offers a specific treatment for it. Though the first information about lenses goes back to Pliny, Ibn Sīnā's contemporary Ibn al-Haytham, who explored lenses, is known to have more reliable and consistent information on this topic. Later, Roger Bacon in Europe (1214–1294) did some work on lenses and convex lenses became widespread in the 14$^{th}$ century. Concave lenses were used later, at the end of the 15$^{th}$ century. Though lenses were used early on, it was not until the 19$^{th}$ century that they were developed to the technical level we have today in terms of technology. Thomas Young (1773–1829) showed that the adaptation of the eye had to do with the shape of the lens and not the size of the ball nor the cornea. This meant that myopia was related with the lens.[48]

48 Singer, H.: A Short History of Medicine, Oxford, 1962, pp. 641–642.

Ibn Sīnā correctly diagnosed night blindness. He observed that some can see well in the daylight but not at night, he had to depend on the knowledge of his day, or on excess humidity. He also said that that those with darker eyelids are prone to this disease. Furthermore, a small pupil and different colors in the eye were also mentioned as causes. Ibn Sīnā also mentioned that some complaints related to the stomach and intestines could cause it.

The most interesting offering Ibn Sīnā has on this issue has to do with its treatment. He recommends eating liver or using liver to make an externally used ointment. Liver should be prepared kebab-style and eaten. Also, he holds that ointments mixing balsam oil and liver can also help.

Ibn Sīnā could not have known that liver is rich in vitamin A, the deficiency of which can cause night blindness and which was not discovered until 1913. The first person in Europe to mention and explain night blindness (nyctalopia) was William Haberden (1767),[49] but he did not offer much in the way of treatment. The first work on vitamins began in the late 19th century and continued into the 20th century. It showed that some substances except carbohydrates, fats, water and salts were necessary for the growth and health of humans. For example, Vitamin K formed in liver prothrombin was needed, but this vitamin was not among the compounds. Vitamin A, which is important for the function of the retina, was found in 1913 by McCollum and M. Davis. Vitamin A deficiency results in slowing down rhodopsin regeneration. Actually, night blindness is not an isolated disease, but an early sign of vitamin A deficiency. If a patient is given vitamin A, the disease is cured, and if not, it progresses into what we call *xerophthalmia* today, leading to impaired vision, white foamy stains on the conjunctiva, and the cornea becomes opaque, ulcerated and soft.[50]

### *c. Neuro-ophthalmology*

Among the eye diseases Ibn Sīnā mentions is loss of vision. He mostly mentions this as a malfunction of the optic nerve, citing eye pressure as the main symptom. Today, we know that optic nerve related complaints due to papilledema are usually caused by intracranial hypertension.[51] Ibn Sīnā does not offer detailed information about loss of sight, possibly because he realized it could not be treated at the time. Therefore, he does not recommend any medication or surgical intervention.

---

49 Gastiglioni, A.: A History of Medicine (Ed. E. B. Krumbhar), New York 1958.

50 Vaughan and Taylor, ibid, pp. 399 - 401.

51 Gastiglioni, A.: pp. 386–367.

Actually, it is not only nerve related cases but some diseases related to cataracts and seeing layers, which he shows in the Canon that he is knowledgeable on, that can result in loss of vision. Ibn Sīnā may not have wanted to repeat himself since here he only investigates the nerve or optic nerve aspect.

Another eye disease Ibn Sīnā mentions is impaired sight after one looks at a white or very bright light for an extended time. The person cannot see long distance and cannot tell apart the colors of even very brightly colored flowers. In other words, they have lost their normal sight. They may see spots in front of their eyes. This description by Ibn Sīnā is reminiscent of snow blindness. But he does not mention if this was transient or persistent. The first to describe this was Johan Widmark (1850–1909). Widmark especially investigated the role of ultraviolet (UV) rays, electrical ophtalmia and sun erythema in causing snow blindness.[52]

Once again, he provided useful information on the optic nerves suggesting the optic nerves cross.[53]

### Optic Chiasm

*"The origin of the first pair (means optic nerve) is the bottom of the anterior ventricles of the brain beside the excrescence mammary papilla (like breast nipples) which are responsible for olfaction. It is great and hollow. The left originated nerves turn right and the right one turn left until the two meet each other on chiasma (forming a cross). The right nerve penetrates into the right pupil. And left nerve penetrates into the left pupil. Their two holes expand to contain the humor which is called (glassy or glass-like)."*[54] He explained the Optic Nerve in detail, and the mechanism of seeing clearly to the benefits of the optic chiasma. Two eyes have one way to see an object outline where they are united to cause sight by the two eyes with one sight representing the outline in a mutual line. Therefore they see one thing as two. When one of the pupils deviates superior or inferior breaking the line to the cross and lay before the crossing point (border) for the refraction of the nerve. Each nerve will support the other and relay to it as if emerging from near the pupil.[55] The three mentioned benefits of the optic chiasma and the mechanism of seeing (reflecting current knowledge) represent the wrong scientific knowledge that prevailed in that era.[56]

---

52 Vaughan and Taylor, ibid, s. 63.

53 Stanley F (1994), *Origins of Neuroscience: A History of Explorations into Brain Function*, Oxford University Press, p. 70,

54 Ibn Sina, *al-Qanun fi't tibb*, vol. 1, p. 54.

55 Price M (2001) History of ancient medicine in Mesopotamia and Iran. http://www.iranchamber.com/history/articles/ancient_medicine_mesopotamia_iran.php.

56 Warwick R, Williams P. Gray's Anatomy, pp. 997–998, 913–914.

**Cranial Nerves**

Ibn Sīnā observed that the brain has 7 pairs of cranial nerves, which we know today there are 12. This is not surprising since the localizations of the remaining 5 pairs of cranial nerves are so tangled that they cannot be seen without detailed and meticulous dissection and taking off the bones of the cranium.

n. olfactorius, n. trochlearis, n. abducens and n. vestibulocochlearis Ibn Sīnā's explanation of the sixth pair which divides into three parts correspond currently to: the first part Glosso-pharyngeal Nerve (the 9th), the second part to the Accessory Nerve (11th), and the third part to the Vagus Nerve (the 10th).

The chapter regarding the Cranial Nerves of Al-Qanun fi't-tibb is considered to be important and forms detailed study of the cranial nerves using inductive methodical approach. Though incomplete, what he did describe is all accurate.

**Oculomotor Nerve**

In his detailed description, Ibn Sīnā says:

> *«The origin of the second pair of the brain nerves posterior to the origin of the first pair to the lateral side, goes out of the foramen of the cavity which contain the eyeballs and to separate in the ocular muscles. This pair is very thick to stand against softness and for its nearness of the origin, so as to have enough strength to move, especially that it is not supported, the third pair is deviated to move a big organ that is the mandible, and thus has no spare strength and it needs another helper as we will mention later».*[57]

## *d. Lens related issues, Cataracts*

The term "crystalline" for the lens was first mentioned by Celsus (25 BC- 50 AD). Later, influenced by the writings of both Galen and Hippocrates, Ibn Sīnā's definition of cataracts was very similar to the definition offered by Galen. The latter paid particular attention to the crystalline lens, which he described as a round lens in the middle of the eye. He concluded, "The crystalline lens was the principal instrument of vision which lay between the crystalline humor and the cornea and interfered with vision."[58]

Ibn Sīnā wrote, "*Nozul-al-maa or cataract is an obstructive disease in which external (gharibeh) moisture accumulates between the aqueous humor and the corneal membrane at the pupil and prevents images from entering the eye*". By "external moisture" Ibn Sīnā apparently meant moisture that did not originate

57 Ibn Sina, *al-Qanun fi't-tibb*, vol. 1, p.54.

58 Gordon BL. The problem of crystalline lens. Arch Ophthal 1936;15: 859–89. [doi.org/10.1001/archopht. 1936.00840170071008]

from the body and cannot be absorbed by body tissues and organs, and so accumulated as a source of infection or organ dysfunction.[59]

Ibn Sīnā mentioned the following symptoms of cataracts: seeing small floating objects of fixed size and position, blurred vision, especially in only one eye, and double vision of shiny objects. Ibn Sīnā believed that opacity could be diminished in the initial stages without surgery, and with medicines and foods only. He noted that fennel juice mixed with honey and wild marjoram is effective in treating the initial stages of cataract. Ibn Sīnā added, "The person who has cataracts should avoid fullness and drinking and sexual intercourse. He should eat just one meal (lunch) per day and must avoid eating fish and fruit and heavy meat."[60]

An important aspect of Ibn Sīnā's contribution to the medical management of cataracts was that he believed they could be cured by medication and nutrition in their early stages without the need for surgery. He also considered the patient's mental status as an important factor contributing to the postoperative prognosis.

Ibn Sīnā noted the beneficial effects of onion on the eye: "the extract of edible basl (onion) is useful for cataracts and clears vision, collyrium of powdered seeds with honey is useful in corneal opacity."[61] A century later, Nejabat et al. experimented with the antimicrobial effect of the onion juice on animal models.[62] Overall, their results indicated that onion has an inhibitory effect on the growth of normal flora on conjunctiva and eyelid surfaces. Thus, it appears that onion juice in the form of eye drops can indeed serve as a new antimicrobial therapy for ophthalmic diseases in future studies.

Another plant Ibn Sīnā prescribed was orris, which is a plant that contains flavonoids and isoflavones. It has been studied that herbal medicines containing flavonoids may slow down progression of cataracts in rats. Javadzadeh et al. found that selenite-induced cataract in rats can be prevented by an eyewash

59 Nejabat M, Maleki B, Nimrouzi M, Mahbodi A, Salehi A. Ibn Sina and Cataracts: A New Analysis of Contributions to Diagnosis and Treatment from the Canon. *Iran Red Crescent Med J* 2012;14(5):265–270.

60 Ibn Sina. *Al-Qanun fi't-Tibb*. In: Hesan Ja`far, editor. Al-Hilal, Beirut: Dar-ol-Behar; 2009.

61 Ibn Sina. *Al-Qanun fi't-Tibb*. New Delhi: Jamia Hamdard; 1998.

62 Mahmoud Nejabat; Alireza Salehi; Parisa Noorani Azad; Mohammad Javad Ashraf. Effects of Onion Juice on the Normal Flora of Eyelids and Conjunctiva in an Animal Model. *Jundishapur J Microbiol*. 2014;7(5): e9678. DOI: 10.5812/jjm.9678

prepared form onion juice which contains high content of flavonoids.[63] Another study by Goodarzi et al. showed that the consumption of some flavonoids such as quercetin reduced the accumulation of sorbitol in the lens of diabetic rats, and as a result slowed cataract progression. Tectorigenin and irigenin, two other isoflavone compounds, had similar results.[64]

Ultimately, Ibn Sīnā's decision regarding the choice of the most appropriate method of treatment was based on precise clinical observation and examination.[65] Humorism is discredited in modern medicine, but cataracts can be attributed to other health problems, such as smoking and air pollution.

His recognition of fluid build-up in the lens contributes to modern laser eye surgery, where the protein accumulation is assessed before proceeding with the operation.[66] Ibn Sīnā also considered the role of the patient's mental and psychological status in the success of surgery is an important factor contributing to the postoperative prognosis.

### *e. Corneal Edema*

It is known that outer layer of cornea (epithelium) is damaged in most of the viral effects that cause loss glassiness of the cornea.[67] Ibn Sīnā also described the sign and symptoms of this disorder as exquisite pain, elongation of eye vessels, needle irritation, and redness of the eye, headache, anorexia.[68]

Such sign and symptoms are similar to those of corneal edema. It is well accepted that these include pain in eye and headache as well as blurred vision cause due to increased pressure of the eye and inflammation.[69]

---

63 Javadzadeh A, Ghorbanihaghjo A, Bonyadi S, Rashidi MR, Mesgari M, Rashtchizadeh N, Argani H. Preventive effect of onion juice on selenite induced experimental cataract. Indian J Ophthalmol 2009;57:185–189. doi.org/10.4103/03014738.49391

64 Goodarzi MT, Zal F, Malakooti M, Safari MR, Sadeghian S. Inhibtory activity of flavenioids on the lens aldose reductase of healthy and diabetic rats. Acta Medica Iranica 2006;44:41–5.

65 The General principles of 'Ibn Sina's Canon of Medicine; Mazhar H. Shah, ibid

66 Tabei SZ, Riazi A. Medical sciences in the third millennium: An Avicennian approach. *Iran Red Crescent Med J* 2009;11(1):4–9.

67 Hamrah P, Sahin A, Dastjerdi MH, Shahatit BM, Bayhan HA, Dana R, Pavan-Langston D. Cellular changes of the corneal epithelium and stroma in Herpes Simplex Keratitis: An in vivo Confocal Microscopy Study. *Ophthalmology.* 2012;119:1791–1797.

68 Ibn Sina. The Canon of Medicine. Translated and edited by Sharafkandi A. 3rd Volume. Tehran: Soroosh; 2010, p. 224.

69 Behrens MM. Headaches Associated with Disorders of the Eye. *Med Clin North Am* 1978;62:507–521.

Also, ocular inflammation can cause redness in the eyes.[70] Others are vasospasm,[71] and sensing irritation and seeing colored haloes and also decreased visual acuity.[72]

On the other hand, ocular HSV infection causes photophobia,[73] and irritation and photophobia may lead to anorexia nervosa.[74]

### *f. Glaucoma*

The Arabic works contain unambiguous comparisons of eye color, at least in a diseased state. Tabari and Ibn Sīnā stated that the *zarqaa* (blue) hue could be associated with anterior prominence of the lens and could occur in an acquired (pathologic) manner.[75] The disease defined by the glaucous pupil in antiquity is ultimately indeterminate, as the complete syndrome of acute angle closure was not described. Nonetheless, it is intriguing that the glaucous pupil connoted a poor prognosis, and came to be associated with a large, anterior, or hard crystalline lens.[76] The Arabic authors agreed the *zarqaa* hue could occur with anterior pathology, which could be displaced by couching. Ibn Isa also noted a blue eye (*zurqa*) from forward dislocation (which did not impair the sight), or from drying, thickening, and coagulation of the humor (which did affect vision, and was difficult to cure). Then there were diseases causing the color of green plants (*akhdar*). Specifically, cataracts were described as green (*akhdar*) during that era, but Ibn Sīnā recorded that green (*akhdar*), yellow, gypsum, and black cataracts did not improve with couching.[77]

---

70 Tarff A, Behrens A. Ocular Emergencies: Red Eye. *Med Clin North Am* 2017;101:615–639.

71 Flammer, 2001: 319–349. Flammer J, Pache M, Resink T. Vasospasm, its role in the pathogenesis of diseases with particular reference to the eye. *Prog Retin Eye Res* 2001;20:319–349.

72 Aquavella JV. Chronic Corneal Edema. *Am J Ophthalmol.* 1973;76:201–207.

73 Whitley RJ. Herpes Simplex virus infection. *Semin Pediatr Infect Dis.* 2002;13:6–11.

74 Gaudiani JL, Braverman JM, Mascolo M, Mehler PS. Lagophthalmos in severe anorexia nervosa: A case series. *Arch Ophthalmol.* 2012;130:928–930.

75 Ibn Sina AA (Ibn Sina). *Die Augenheilkunde des Ibn Sina.* Hirschberg J, Lippert J, translators. Leipzig: Verlag von Veit. Available from: https://archive.org/details/dieaugenheilkund00avic. Accessed September 5, 2014.

76 Christopher T Leffler, Stephen G Schwartz, Tamer M Hadi, Ali Salman, Vivek Vasuki. The early history of glaucoma: the glaucous eye (800 BC to 1050 AD). *Clinical Ophthalmology* 2015;9:207–215. http://dx.doi.org/10.2147/OPTH.S77471

77 Ibn Sina AA (Ibn Sina). *al-Qānūn fi 'al-ṭibb.* New Delhi: Institute of History of Medicine and Medical Research; 1982:175–212.

### g. Eye Cancer

Although it is believed that eye cancer is a new concept in medicine, Ibn Sīnā propounded it with his description of *Saratan-e-Cheshm* (Saratan means cancer; *-e-* means of; and *Cheshm* means eye) in the sixth chapter of the third volume of the Canon of Medicine. Ibn Sīnā indicated that this disorder would be located on the outer layer of cornea. Corneal edema is an ophthalmic disorder which has two causes; one of them is increasing intraocular pressure that is the result of glaucoma and another reason is decompensation of endothelium that includes inflammatory and non-inflammatory types.

He also described the signs and symptoms of *Saratan-e-Cheshm* as exquisite pain, elongation of eye vessels, needle irritation, and redness of the eye, headache, anorexia, and hurt from looking at the things have humility. It can be considered as the first complete description of corneal edema as a sole ocular disorder in history.[78]

### h. Goiter and Thyroid-related Orbitopathy in Canon

The Canon described the swelling in the front of neck (goiter) in patients who had an increased appetite but could not reach satiety despite eating large amounts of food.[79] He also described the connection of swelling of the neck and protuberance of eyes in two chapters in Al-Qanoon.[80] In the chapter on exophthalmos, he discussed differential diagnosis of proptosis. He noted that exophthalmos may be produced by pressure from the back of orbit and noticed corneal edema, chemosis, orbital fat, and lassitude of extraocular muscles in the clinical presentation of exophthalmos. He described the ocular characteristics when the cause of exophthalmos is lassitude of extraocular muscles.[81] Therefore it seems likely that the idea of an association between exophthalmos and goiter had been known for centuries.

The descriptions of a clear association of goiter and exophthalmos by Ibn Sīnā around 1000 were later emphasized by Al-Jurjani around 1100. Robert Graves (1795–1853) and Carl von Basedow (1799–1854) are credited with the first modern descriptions of thyroid-related orbitopathy now referred to as

78 Levenson JE. Corneal edema: causes and treatment. *Surv Ophthalmol.* 2016; 20:190–204.

79 Al-Qanoon, Book III, part 9, chapter 6.

80 Al-Qanoon, Book III, part 3, treatise 2, chapter 15 and Book III, part 3, chapter 4.

81 Al-Qanoon, Book III, part 3, treatise 2, chapter 15.

Graves' disease.[82] The publications by Graves and Basedow in the $19^{th}$ century clearly linked the pathophysiologic association of goiter and exophthalmos and established Graves' disease as a clinical entity. However the earliest nonmedical description by the jurist Ulpianus is of great interest as well.

### *i. Lachrymal Passage*

Ibn Sīnā discusses the lachrymal pathologies giving details pertaining to acute and chronic versions, prognosis and whether they are congenital or acquired. He mentions treatment using a probe, lacrimal fistula and abscess treatment using a syringe until one reaches the sack or the bone.

### *j. Seasonal Effects and Effects of Habitat*

Ibn Sīnā discussed seasonal abnormalities leading to various affections of eyes, e.g. in summer: Pain in eyes and increased conjunctivitis.[83] He recognizes in chemosis, swelling of the conjunctiva.[83,84] Regarding prognosis of diseases, he said certain diseases are such that they cure other diseases e.g., Diarrhea cures Conjunctivitis.[83,85]

## *3) Treatment Methods Applied by Ibn Sīnā in his Canon*

Ibn Sīnā's views in his *Canon* were elucidated, as contributions to the causes, seasonal effects, diagnosis, prognosis and treatment of to various affections of eyes by prevention, diet therapy, medicines and surgery.[83,86] For example, corneal ulcers are treated by applying juice of green night-shade. For conjunctivitis, lids should be painted with barberry mixed with milk and later on the eyes are bathed with decoction of chamomile and juice of liquid basil.[87] He discussed

82 Nabipour I, Burger A, Moharreri MR, Azizi F. Ibn Sina, the First to Describe Thyroid-Related Orbitopathy. *Thyroid* 2009;19(1):7–8.

83 The General principles of Ibn Sina's Canon of Medicine; Mazhar H. Shah; Naveed Clinic; Karachi, Pakistan,1966, 2nd Ed. 1998. Printed at the Interservices Press Ltd., Karachi. pp. 166, 167, 168, 192, 295, 403, 404, 406, 407.

84 Sharafkandi. Abdolrahman. Übersetzung von Canon 3, Teheran (2009), p.200.

85 Ibn Sina's influence on the Medieval Scientific Tradition, Ibn Sina's Scientist and Philosopher, ed. A. C. Crombie, G. M. Wicken (London), p. 95.

86 Studies on Ibn Sînâ (d. 1037) and his medical works. Collected and Reprinted. Ed. F Sezgin. (Islamic Medicine. 10). 1996 Vol. I., p. 296.

87 A. C. Crombie, G. M. Wicken, ibid, p. 96.

cure for various diseases, In Section XX by Venesection; In Section XXI by Cupping; In Section XIX Effects of Baths, Sunbaths and Medicated baths.[88]

### *4) Examples of Simple Drugs Used for Treatment of the Eye Diseases*

In the book "On the Visual Organs" collected by Lale Bakhtiyar, it appears Ibn Sīnā described 192 simple drugs to be used in treating eye diseases. Some of them are below for your perusal:[89]

**Absinthe:** Absinthe is useful in treating chronic conjunctivitis when the Nabatean variety is used as a poultice below the eyes as well as for dim vision. Preparing its poultice with the addition of grape wine and water boiled down to a consistency eliminates throbbing of the eyes and their inflammation. It is also used in treating conjunctivitis. When the eyes are washed with it and warm water, it relieves conjunctivitis.

**Aloe:** Aloe is useful in treating ulcers of the eyes as well as eye pain, swelling or irritation. It dries up the corner of the eye where the upper and lower eyelids meet.

**Anemone**: The extract of anemone is useful in treating day blindness, corneal opacity and the scars of eye ulcers. It is used as a poultice in the form of the boiled down form prepared with a black grape wine for treating hard swellings around the eyes.

**Asafetida Plant:** If asafetida gum is used as a collyrium with honey, it is useful in treating early states of cataract. Asafetida resin myrrh removes and cures scars, ulcers, whiteness and pus in the eye. It softens rough eyelashes without causing irritation.

**Bamboo Ash:** Bamboo ash is useful in treating hot inflammation of the eye.

**Barberry:** Indian barberry is useful in treating conjunctivitis, cleanses the cornea, and cures trachoma.

**Basil:** A poultice of wild basil is useful in treating throbbing eyes. When wild basil is used orally, it causes blindness by thickening and evaporating the fluids in the eyes, but the extract, when used as a collyrium, strengthens eyesight

**Bitumen:** Both the white and black types of bitumen are useful in treating opacity of the cornea.

**Chamomile:** A poultice of chamomile is useful in treating eye diseases, narrow passages or ducts formed by disease or injury, blocked tear ducts,

---

88 Mazhar H. Shah, The General principles of Ibn Sina's Canon of Medicine; ibid.
89 Bakhtiyar, ibid.

conjunctivitis, cloudiness of sight, pimples, the easily spread skin disease caused by a very small species of mite or scabies, pains and itches.

## B. IBN SĪNĀ'S IMPACT ON LATER OCULISTS

In ophthalmology, Muslim physicians are due special credit as they performed almost all eye operations.[90] Within that context, Ibn Sīnā's ideas on the sight physiology of the eye and eye diseases greatly impacted Europe as well as Muslim medicine, among whom are Ammâr b. 'Ali al-Mausilî[91] and his book *Kitâb al Muntahab* (c.1040), Halifa al-Halebi and his book *Kitâb al-Kâfi al-Kuhl* (c.1275), Salâhaddin and his book *Kitâb Nur al-'Uyûn* (1290),[92] Muhammed bin Mahmud-ı Şirvanî and his *Mürshid* (1450), Mümin bin Mukbil and his *Miftah-in Nûr va Hazain üs-Sürûr* (1495).[93] Ibn Sīnā's influence is also evident in the book written by Ottoman Head doctor Gevrek Zâde Hasan Efendi in 1796 called *Risalet ül zübdet ül-kuhliye fi teşrih ül-basariye* ("Booklet on the Best Treatments of the Details of Eye Diseases").[94]

# IV. CONCLUSION

Ibn Sīnā wrote the *Canon of Medicine* approximately 1000 years ago. His treatise became the quintessential textbook of medicine throughout world and has been called the bible of medicine.[95] It was the best medical work produced in the feudal age and served as the source of knowledge for physicians of the East and West until the seventeenth century. As this rich body of literature was

---

90 Shobhana Mathur and Sakait Rama Rao, G., (March-April 1402/1982). Contribution of Muslim scientists toward surgery, *Bulletin of Islamic Medicine,* Vol. III, K.F.A.S., State of Kuwait, p. 227.

91 Wiedemann, Eilhard: Ibn Sina's Anschauung vom Sehvorgang. In: Arch. Gesch. Naturw. und Technik 4 (1913), s. 239–241.

92 'Ammâr b. Ali al Mausilî: Das Buch der Auswahl von den Augenkrankheiten; Halifa al-Halabhi: Das Buch vom Genügenden in der Augenheilkunde; Salah ad-din: Licht des Augen, Übersetzer: Julius Hirschberg, Julius Lippert, Eugen Mittwoch, Leipzig 1905.

93 Keskinbora HK, Basağaoğlu İ. Göz Nurunun Anahtarı ve Neşe Hazineleri, İstanbul, Nobel Tıp Kitabevleri, 2010.

94 Gevrek Zâde Hasan Efendi. Risalet ül zübdet ül-kuhliye fi teşrih ül-basariye. A manuscript dated 1796 is in the Topkapı Palace Treasury Library. Registered at Nr.571.

95 Ismail M, Raheem Rafeeq MA. Anatomy of Eye and the Mechanism of Vision According to Ibn Sina. *Bulletin of the Indian Institute of History of Medicine* (Hyderabad) 1981:9(1–4):146–151.

translated many times from Arabic into Latin in the eleventh through thirteenth centuries, medieval European medical practitioners had a great deal to puzzle over. On the issue of seeing and vision, generally, they were less taken with the extramission theory than their Islamic predecessors, which was partly due to the importance of Ibn Sīnā in the medieval and Renaissance medical curriculum.

It is true that the modern era in human anatomy started in the 16th century with the studies of Andreas Vesalius (1514–64). However, it should be recalled that graduates of various medical schools around Europe including this famous founder of modern anatomy and the renowned Harvey family members studied Ibn Sīnā's Canon, which features several chapters on anatomy in its first volume. The discussions of anatomy continue in the parts scattered throughout the huge encyclopedia, with the anatomy of a particular organ being discussed in the section concerned with diseases particular to that organ. In short, all of the anatomic studies of modern era include the contributions of Ibn Sīnā's anatomic studies and methods, as do all the topics of medicine.

Another contribution of Ibn Sīnā was that he trained new scientists. He was a true product of Muslim civilization at the height of its scientific growth, but he is better known today in medicine and philosophy than earth science.[96] He applied all of this background and skills as a polymath into his in-depth study into the eyes as well, to a greater extent than anyone before him had done.

There are some remarkable works such as those by Juan Cueva in 1899, Paul Uspensky, Theodor Bernikow and Elias Michailovwsky in 1900, and Julius Hirschberg and Julius Lippert in 1902 on Ibn Sīnā's contributions. A clear example is the passage below from the Doctoral Thesis of one of Julius Hirschberg students, Juan Cueva:[97] In his Preface to 'Ophthalmic Medicine of Ibn Sīnā' of Juan Cueva states:

> *"The historical influence of Islamic medicine is so important that Europeans could not comprehend Islamic medicine without consulting the Arabs. In the 16th century, the medical instructors were divided into two as Anti-Arab Medicine and its supporters because of their studies in Arabic medicine going back to ancient Greek sources. The historical and cultural importance of Arabs can be clearly understood only when the formation of Arab-Islamic Medicine is deeply analyzed.*
> *I am assigning myself to study this part of ophthalmic medicine through the help of "The Canon of Medicine" of Ibn Sina known as the Prince of Physicians. Ibn Sina has*

96 Al-Hassani STS. Ed.1001 Innovations Washington DC; National Geography, 2012, p.230.
97 J. Hirschberg und J. Lippert, Die Augenheilkunde des Ibn Sina, ibid, p. 23.

*written a huge quantity of articles not only medical but also philosophical, mathematical and astronomical works. It is rightful to regard Ibn Sina as the main representative of Islamic Medicine. He is as important for Islamic Medicine as much as Galen is for Greek Medicine.*

*Galen formed the integration and regulation of Pergamum physicians and Greek Medicine in a system, and then Greek and Arab medicine was formed on the system of Galen, especially by Razi and Ali Abbas. Not only the content of his work, but also the external form and the logical weave of Ibn Sina's crazy and nightmarish ideas deserve full praise. But the most important feature of his works is that they are independent and unique to those who preceded him, for example, in comparison with Razi.*

*Ibn Sina's Law has been an ideal Medical Work for centuries. Furthermore during this time, it causes the most famous medical works to be forgotten. Scholars of both western and eastern countries such as famous physician Ibn Rushd and authors have been inspired and influenced by works of Ibn Sina. He has also had a greater influence in Islamic schools in the west. Thanks to The Canon of Ibn Sina because of which the articles of Hippocrates and Galen had started to get lost in oblivion."*

In summary, Ibn Sīnā's Canon made immense contributions to ophthalmology. It described the physiology of eye movements, which still forms a basis of information for modern ophthalmology. Ibn Sīnā presented the anatomy, physiology and diseases of the eye in great detail. He also provided useful information on all of the parts of the eye and brought a new approach to the theory of how vision occurs, saying the optic nerve is the organ that is responsible for vision, not the lens, as it had been believed before. He also stated that the optic nerves cross. Not only did he describe sight as one of the five external senses, the Latin word "retina" is derived from the term he used in Arabic.[98] Ibn Sīnā also discussed orbitopathy and determined the necessary fluidity of the lens.[99][100] He described the dilation and contraction of the pupils and iris of the eye and their diagnostic value, and discussed the functions of the tear ducts. He described 59 eye diseases and 192 simple drugs for their treatment.

Considering all of these, one cannot help but agree with the European physician De Poure, who says:

98 Finger, Stanley (1994), *Origins of Neuroscience: A History of Explorations Into Brain Function*, Oxford University Press, p. 69, p. 71, ISBN 0-19-514694-8

99 Introduction to al-Umar al-Tabi'yah (Principles of Human physiology in tibb). By S. I. Ahmed, first Ed. 1980 A.D.–1401 A. H. Published by Hakim (Mrs) Nuzhat Ishtiaq, B.U.M.S (Alig.) printed by Saini Printers, Parhari Dhiraj, Delhi. pp.80,81.

100 Ophthalmology In Medıeval Islam, Compiled by World Heritage Encyclopedia™ licensed under CC BY-SA 3.0, http://www.worldheritage.org/articles/Ophthalmology_in_medieval_Islam#cite_note-4

*"Medicine was absent until Hippocrates created it, dead until Galen revived it, dispersed until Rhazes collected it, and deficient until Ibn Sina completed it."*[101]

## Bibliography

Al-Hassani, S. T. (2012). 1001 inventions: The enduring legacy of Muslim civilization. National Geographic Books.

Amr, S. S., & Tbakhi, A. (2007). Ibn Sina (Avicenna): the prince of physicians. Annals of Saudi medicine, 27(2), 134–135.

Avicenna (2009). El-Kanun fi't-tıbb. E. Kahya (trans.) Atatürk Kültür, Dil ve Tarih Yüksek Kurumu.

Aquavella, J. V. (1973). Chronic corneal edema. American Journal of Ophthalmology, 76(2), 201–207.

Beg, H. (2015). Surgical principles of Ibn Sina (Avicenna). Bangladesh Journal of Medical Science, 14(3), 217–220.

Behrens, M. M. (1978). Headaches associated with disorders of the eye. Medical Clinics of North America, 62(3), 507–521.

Chams, H. (2010). Iranian Ophthalmology-Past and Present. Iranian Journal of Ophthalmology, 22(4), 1.

Farhadi, M., Behzadian Nejad, G., & Bagbanzadeh, A. (1996). Papers of the international congress of the history of medicine in Islam and Iran. Iranian Institute for Science and Research Expansion, Tehran, Iran.

Finger, S. (2001). Origins of neuroscience: a history of explorations into brain function. Oxford University Press, USA.

Flammer, J., Pache, M., & Resink, T. (2001). Vasospasm, its role in the pathogenesis of diseases with particular reference to the eye. Progress in retinal and eye research, 20(3), 319–349.

Gaudiani, J. L., Braverman, J. M., Mascolo, M., & Mehler, P. S. (2012). Lagophthalmos in severe anorexia nervosa: a case series. Archives of Ophthalmology, 130(7), 928–930.

Goodarzi, M. T., Zal, F., Malakooti, M., & Sadeghian, M. S. S. (2006). Inhibitory activity of flavonoids on the lens aldose reductase of healthy and diabetic rats. Acta Medica Iranica, 41–45.

Gordon, B. L. (1935). The problem of the crystalline lens. Archives of Ophthalmology, 14(5), 774–788.

101 Al-Hassani STS, ed. 1001 Inventions: The Enduring Legacy of Muslim Civilization, 3rd ed Washington DC: National Geographic Society 2012. p. 168–169.

Hamrah, P., Sahin, A., Dastjerdi, M. H., Shahatit, B. M., Bayhan, H. A., Dana, R., & Pavan-Langston, D. (2012). Cellular changes of the corneal epithelium and stroma in herpes simplex keratitis: an in vivo confocal microscopy study. Ophthalmology, 119(9), 1791–1797.

Ishtiaq, S. A. (2009). Introduction to Al-Umur Al-Tabi'yah (Principles of Human Physiology in Tibb).

Ismail, M., & Rafeeq, M. R. (1981). Anatomy of eye and the mechanism of vision according to Avicenna. Bulletin of the Indian Institute of History of Medicine (Hyderabad), 1, 146–151.

Javadzadeh, A., Ghorbanihaghjo, A., Bonyadi, S., Rashidi, M. R., Mesgari, M., Rashtchizadeh, N., & Argani, H. (2009). Preventive effect of onion juice on selenite-induced experimental cataract. Indian journal of ophthalmology, 57(3), 185.

Keskinbora HK, & Basağaoğlu İ. (2010). Göz Nurunun Anahtarı ve Neşe Hazineleri, İstanbul, Nobel Tıp Kitabevleri.

Keskinbora, K.H., & Keskinbora, K. (2016). A systematic review of Ibn Sina's (Avicenna) studies: reflections on anatomy. European Journal of Anatomy, 20(1), 99–105.

Leffler, C. T., Schwartz, S. G., Hadi, T. M., Salman, A., & Vasuki, V. (2015). The early history of glaucoma: the glaucous eye (800 BC to 1050 AD). Clinical Ophthalmology (Auckland, NZ), 9, 207.

Levenson, J. E. (1975). Corneal edema: cause and treatment. Survey of Ophthalmology, 20(3), 190–204.

Nabipour, I., Burger, A., Moharreri, M. R., & Azizi, F. (2009). Avicenna, the first to describe thyroid-related orbitopathy. Thyroid, 19(1), 7–8.

Naderi, S., Acar, F., Mertol, T., & Arda, M. N. (2003). Functional anatomy of the spine by Avicenna in his eleventh century treatise Al-Qanun fi al-Tibb (The Canons of Medicine). Neurosurgery, 52(6), 1449–1454.

Nejabat, M., Maleki, B., Nimrouzi, M., Mahbodi, A., & Salehi, A. (2012). Avicenna and cataracts: a new analysis of contributions to diagnosis and treatment from the canon. Iranian Red Crescent Medical Journal, 14(5), 265.

Nejabat, M., Salehi, A., Azad, P. N., & Ashraf, M. J. (2014). Effects of onion juice on the normal flora of eyelids and conjunctiva in an animal model. Jundishapur journal of microbiology, 7(5).

Pollock, W. I. (1946). Arabian ophthalmology. The British Journal of Ophthalmology, 30(8), 445.

Price, M. (2001). History of ancient medicine in Mesopotamia and Iran. Iranchamber. com, October.

Sayılı, A. (1982). Mısır ve Mezotamyalılarda Matematik. Astronomi ve Tıp, Ankara.

Sina, I. (1902). Die Augenheilkunde des Ibn Sina. Aus dem Arabischen übersetzt und erläutert von J. Hisrschberg und J. Lippert, Leipzig.

Sīnā, I. (1993). Al-Qānūn fi l-tibb [English Translation], 2 vols. New Delhi: Dept. of Islamic Studies, Jamia Hamdard, 1998.

Sina, I. (2010). The canon of medicine. (Sharafkandi A, trans.), [in Persian] Tehran, 71.

Singer, C., & Underwood, E. A. (1962). A short history of medicine. Oxford University Press.

Sobotka, H. (1957). Ophthalmology during the middle ages. AMA Archives of Ophthalmology, 57(3), 366–375.

Tabeei, S., & Riazi, A. (2009). Medical sciences in the third millennium: An Avicennian approach. Iranian Red Crescent Medical Journal, 11(1), 4–9.

Tarff, A., & Behrens, A. (2017). Ocular emergencies: red eye. Medical Clinics, 101(3), 615–639.

Warwick, R., & Williams, P. L. (1980). Gray's anatomy. Churchill Livingstone.

Whitley, R. J. (2002). Herpes simplex virus infection. In Seminars in pediatric infectious diseases (Vol. 13, No. 1, pp. 6–11). WB Saunders.

## Short Biography of Kadircan H. Keskinbora

He has studied medicine at Hacettepe University, Faculty of Medicine (Ankara/Turkey). He became an Ophthalmologist in 1987, an associate professor in 1999 and a professor in 2007. He concluded his second Ph.D. in "Deontology, History of Medicine and Medical Ethics" in 2006. He still is a professor at Istanbul Bahcesehir University, School of Medicine, Head of Dept. History of Medicine and Ethics. He is a member of various national and international scientific or non-governmental organizations.

His Published Books:

**Ophthalmology:** Oftalmolojide Sorularla Eğitim (Education in Ophthalmology with Questions), Oftalmolojide Sınava Doğru (Towards Exam in Ophthalmology), Oftalmoloji İle Kesişen Bilim Dalları (Scientific Areas that Intersect with Ophthalmology)

**History of Medicine:** Göz Nurunun Anahtarı ve Sevinç Hazineleri (Key to Eye Light and Treasures of Joy), Esat Işık: Bilimde, Siyasette, Milli Mücadelede Bir Işık (Esat Isik: A Light in Science, in Politics, in National Struggle), Kanûn-u

Sagir of Ibn Sina (The Little Canon of Avicenna), The Little Qanun of Ibn Sina (Peter Lang Publish.).

**Literature:** Düşünen Beyinlerin İnsanlığa Mirası: Özdeyişler (Inheritance of Thinking Minds to Humanity: Aphorisms), Yaban Gülü (Brier Rose - poem book), Mardin Düşünceleri (Thoughts on Mardin - poem book), Ben Suyum (I am water - poem book), İddia (Claim - poem book).

Because of his studies on Avicenna (Ibn Sina), he was awarded the **"International Avicenne Prize"** in Paris/France in 2016.

e-mail: kadircan.keskinbora@gmail.com
hidirkadircan.keskinbora@med.bau.edu.tr

# Index

FSC
www.fsc.org
MIX
Papier | Fördert
gute Waldnutzung
FSC® C083411

Kolibri 360 GmbH
Ferdinand-Jühlke-Straße 7
99095 Erfurt, Deutschland
produktsicherheit@kolibri360.de

Druck:
CPI Druckdienstleistungen GmbH
im Auftrag der
Kolibri 360 GmbH
Ferdinand-Jühlke-Str. 7
99095 Erfurt